NEGOTIATING AND NAVIGATING GLOBAL HEALTH

Case Studies in Global Health Diplomacy

GLOBAL HEALTH DIPLOMACY – Vol. 2

NEGOTIATING AND NAVIGATING GLOBAL HEALTH

Case Studies in Global Health Diplomacy

Edited by

Ellen Rosskam & Ilona Kickbusch

IHEID, Switzerland
Global Health Programme

World Scientific

NEW JERSEY · LONDON · SINGAPORE · BEIJING · SHANGHAI · HONG KONG · TAIPEI · CHENNAI

Published by

World Scientific Publishing Co. Pte. Ltd.

5 Toh Tuck Link, Singapore 596224

USA office: 27 Warren Street, Suite 401-402, Hackensack, NJ 07601

UK office: 57 Shelton Street, Covent Garden, London WC2H 9HE

British Library Cataloguing-in-Publication Data

A catalogue record for this book is available from the British Library.

NEGOTIATING AND NAVIGATING GLOBAL HEALTH
Case Studies in Global Health Diplomacy

ISBN-13 978-981-4368-02-5
ISBN-10 981-4368-02-4
ISBN-13 978-981-4368-03-2 (pbk)
ISBN-10 981-4368-03-2 (pbk)

Typeset by Stallion Press
Email: enquiries@stallionpress.com

Printed by FuIsland Offset Printing (S) Pte Ltd Singapore

Acknowledgments

We are deeply grateful to the Woodrow Wilson International Center for Scholars for encouragement and assistance from the President and Director Lee H. Hamilton, Department Directors Steve McDonald, Gib Clarke, Blair Ruble, Paulo Sotero, and Lucy Jilka, Executive Assistant to the Director Nora Coulter, Information Specialist Lindsay Collins, and Senior Scholar Alexandra Vacroux, all of whom helped make this book possible.

Contents

Foreword: On Our Watch

By Jan Egeland[i]

There is one recurring question I am asked by students and young activists on each and every continent: Is the world getting better or worse in our time and age? It is indeed the big question asked again and again in each generation: are we making progress on our watch?

After having travelled or worked in more than a hundred countries the last 30 years I am convinced that the world is getting, slowly but steadily, better for a clear majority of us. There is more peace, more children in school, and more access to health care than when the Cold War ended. There is increased life expectancy in most countries and cultures.

There are also more democracies, fewer military coups, and less genocide the last decade than in each of the preceding ten decades. Child mortality has decreased markedly on all continents. The world suffered twice as many deaths due to preventable disease a generation ago — even as world population has doubled in the same period. Perhaps no sector in our global society has seen as big advances as public health care.

But there is also a darker side of our recent history: the world is also more socially unjust than a generation ago. The world's most affluent have become rich beyond anybody's wildest imaginations, while the poorest one billion live in abject misery similar to that of medieval times. We see these extremes within societies and between nations. Some 200 years

---

[i] Jan Egeland is Director of the Norwegian Institute of International Affairs.

ago the ratio between the richest and poorest nations was around one to three. Today the richest nations are a hundred times richer than the poorest. A handful of the richest individuals in our global village are richer than the total "assets" of the two billion poorest individuals combined. These contrasts are particularly stark in regard to the health care sector in particular. Much more is spent on luxurious cosmetic surgery for the affluent top million than for basic health care for the bottom billion fellow human beings. So there is, globally, reason for great optimism, but also for great anger. The new reality is that it is now generally known among the globe's many poor exactly how we live and how we consume amongst ourselves in the top worldwide billion.

Globally there are around 1.6 billion youngsters between the ages of 12 and 24 who should be either in school or in work. The bitter realities are that hundreds of millions of the young and restless know that they are and will be denied everything from a real job to education and health care. As the opinion-makers among the young and the poor can surf themselves to any kind of information from anywhere on the internet a volcanic sense of injustice builds among many because the playing field is not seen as fair; the opportunities are not equal. Access to health care, or lack thereof, is so visible, so concrete, that it plays a role of unrecognised importance as a healer or, just as often as a divider, within societies and between peoples.

Health Diplomacy

Global diplomacy, conflict prevention, and conflict resolution in the increasingly important health arena must always bear this in mind: the parties are asymmetric in how they bring resources to the table and in how they perceive the playing field. What will ultimately be "a fair, just, and durable solution" will be regarded and interpreted differently because the parties themselves are so different from the outset.

The noble aim of global health diplomacy is not only to ensure "health for all" as a citizenship right but to have this responsibility translated into action for beleaguered and threatened communities everywhere. Health diplomacy is essential because access to, or absence of health care can unite and reconcile just as much as it can divide and enrage.

I have seen how emergency medical relief can instil new hope in the most bitter and forsaken places. I have seen how the care of and eventual exchange of wounded combatants have become vital confidence builders between government armies and left-wing guerrillas, how evacuation of the sick across frontlines has been the first step on the way to a first humanitarian agreement between parties, and I have seen how a preventable death of a political activist or soldier in captivity can lead to uncontrollable strife.

In Colombia, Central America, South East Asia, Africa, and the Middle East, the International Committee of the Red Cross and its medical delegates often have been the trusted intermediaries between armed actors that shared no other contact points. The mediation of "days of tranquillity" by UNICEF and the World Health Organization to enable vaccination of children in combat areas have been notable success stories in bitter wars where the political talks among the parties have broken down. No one wants epidemics to break out in the areas they dispute or fight; everybody can see the benefit of cooperating to prevent it from happening. The fact that the armed parties to a conflict could later trust each other and cooperate on a medical campaign may help peace diplomacy on other fronts.

When negotiating humanitarian corridors and safe passage of relief convoys on the Horn of Africa, Sudan, Lebanon and elsewhere, the need to provide life-saving medical supplies often have been the most convincing arguments to hardened political and military actors. So, there is much evidence of the potential benefits of health diplomacy, but it is seldom discussed and described. This book will help fill that void.

Multilateral Action

During my years in United Nations (UN) Secretary-General Kofi Annan's senior management team I witnessed, first hand, how effective multilateral action with local and regional partners helped build health, progress, and peace. Wars ended and hope was provided in Liberia and Sierra Leone, Angola and Burundi, southern Sudan and northern Uganda, Kosovo and Nepal. We also coordinated through the UN massive, life saving international relief in the aftermath of the Indian Ocean tsunami, the south Asian earthquake, the Horn of Africa, southern Africa, the Lebanon war, and the Darfur crisis. In several of these overwhelming emergencies hundreds of thousands of lives were predicted to perish. The sombre predictions were averted because multilateral action, building on local capacities, can today be infinitely more effective than what is recognised in much of world media and national parliaments.

Too often however, we fail in acting as a collective humanity because multilateral action lacks the unity of purpose among UN member states. We fail, tragically and repeatedly, when the United Nations and regional organisations like the African Union are not provided with the political support and the minimum of economic and security resources needed from their member states. The on-going and seemingly endless suffering in Darfur, in Burma, amongst Palestinians, in Afghanistan, in the Congo, and amongst the growing numbers of climate change victims in southern nations is a product of a passive neglect or senseless bickering amongst the powerful nations that could have unlocked the situation.

Much of what is health diplomacy will, in reality, be to focus attention on the forgotten, neglected and voiceless communities in the disaster and war zones of our time and age. We prove again and again that we are great as humankind when the limelight of the news media is there. Local, national and international actors behave better and provide more resources when they know they are being watched. But we are now recording more than 400 natural disasters globally every year. There are still some 35 ongoing armed conflicts. At best one in ten of the communities that have been brought to the brink receive the minimum of attention, resources and protection that is needed.

Therefore, the health diplomat often needs to be as much the advocate as the mediator. She or he first needs to secure the attention of internal and external decision-makers and mobilize scarce resources for vulnerable people. Herein lays one of the many dilemmas that the diplomat and the advocate face. To mobilize public and political attention one needs to use the public domain and news media and speak in a plain language which describes the health situation, the brutality, the malnutrition and the mortality as it is. The *de facto* authorities that one later needs to negotiate with will, however, not like "bad publicity" on what has happened on their watch.

While we never should compromise on telling the truth we should be strategic about who will say what to whom and when. Often it is better that the field operatives and local representatives are shielded and it falls upon the headquarters of a strong institution to present the criticism and the negative, but necessary, news about what is at stake and who should be held responsible.

Vulnerable Groups

When promoting and protecting social and health rights on humanity's frontlines the special needs of women and children should be given priority. Of all the suffering I have witnessed the systematic cruelty against the most vulnerable was really the worst to stomach. The stories of the kidnapped children terrorised and brainwashed to become child soldiers for the Lords Resistance Army in northern Uganda were as heartbreaking as the stories of the raped and abused women of eastern Congo.

In 2003 and again in 2006 I visited the more the one thousand women at the Panzi hospital in Bukavu in the Democratic Republic of Congo. They had all been physically and mentally destroyed through gang rapes undertaken with total impunity by the armed militias of eastern Congo. In the Kivu provinces alone tens of thousands of women are still being sexually tortured every year. Congolese gynaecologist Dr. Denis Mukwege and his team at Panzi has slowly but surely been stitching together the rape victims, physically and mentally, trying with international medical relief to help their return to a society which often have rejected them because they had been so broken and abused. But the gang raped need security and justice more than blankets and emergency rations. Health diplomacy must therefore also foster political solutions and prevention as must as medical cure.

The bitter realities in most crisis and post-crisis situations are that pre-existing vulnerabilities are exacerbated. Women and girls suffer unbelievable human rights abuse and remain totally marginalised in all decision-making that affects their lives and their communities. It is in this context that health diplomacy must not only protect women and children, but also empower women and female leadership to make effective contributions to crisis response and to post-crisis reconstruction.

Gender programming in humanitarian response is about humanitarian effectiveness first and foremost. If deliverers of assistance continue to do "business as usual" only the strong will receive assistance. We have all seen the big trucks delivering food off the back where teaming people — all men — fight to get a bag of food. Where are the women? Who is making sure that they get services? We must have systems in place to ensure that all women, girls, boys and men have equal access to and benefit from health services and relief — if not — our job is not done and people who we are there to serve are possibly put in harms way.

Early Warnings

There was no lack of early warnings from us in the UN about the growing conflict in Darfur, but most member states were not interested. Many Asian and Arab nations wanted to protect the regime in Khartoum rather than the defenceless civilians in the western desert. There were early cease fire agreements in Darfur facilitated in part by the UN that member states did not enforce. The humanitarian workers were, as in Bosnia in the 1990s, asked to feed and shelter millions while armed men around the 140 camps planned their next massacres with impunity. It was as if Srebrenica and Rwanda were ancient history.

In the build-up to the invasion of Iraq in 2002–03 there were also countless warnings against the irresponsible inability among UN Security Council members to agree on how to deal with Saddam Hussein. There were equally clear warnings that the use of force by the US and UK-led coalition could lead to disastrous results. Those politicians chose to rely on speculative, unsubstantiated, and false intelligence rather than heed the warnings of Secretary- General Annan as well as UN staff on the ground. American and Iraqi medical experts have documented that countless Iraqi civilians died in the 40 months that followed the invasion. During the last decade, in no other place on earth have so many been killed by blunt violence as in post-invasion Iraq.

A decade with no coherent international efforts to solve the Israeli — Palestinian conflict or to end Israeli occupation and border closures of Gaza and the West Bank, caused what I called a "ticking time bomb" when I visited Gaza in 2006. Since then Gaza has seen and produced unabated strife, attacks, and horrors. Multilateral inaction resulted in precisely what the world wanted to prevent — more fertile breeding grounds for new extremism and terrorists. Locking the 1.6 million people of Gaza in a cage smaller than an average Norwegian municipality and depriving hundreds of thousands of angry youth of hope does not produce boy scouts or choir girls. It produces long lines of militants.

There would not have been a relentless increase in natural disasters produced by extreme weather if this global generation had managed to unite around curbing greenhouse gas emissions and preventing climate change as member states generally agreed in Rio de Janeiro as early as 1992. In our time seven times more livelihoods are devastated by natural disasters as by war. Humanitarian field workers cannot believe their eyes or their ears when politicians and industrialists still argue that our explosive global economic growth has not changed the climate. For many years we have seen how more and more peoples' lives are devastated by extreme droughts, hurricanes, and floods. The effects in terms of human lives lost and devastated are, as always, much greater in poor developing countries, but rich countries are not necessarily spared. In Europe the extreme heat wave of 2003 took 71,000 lives. Decades ago leading scientists agreed through the United Nations climate panels that policy and behavioural change were urgently needed. If North Americans, Europeans, Chinese, and others had started the process of change already in 1992, we would have had positive results at a lower cost.

Reason For Hope

In spite of and because of these global realities, I believe there is still reason for optimism. The coming years can and will see a revival of multilateral action because the experience of recent years has proven the costly futility of unilateral force. Since 2003 the United States has spent the incomprehensible sum of one trillion dollars on its war and still unsuccessful nation building project in Iraq. That sum is several times more than the combined cost of all United Nations health, humanitarian, developmental, environmental, peacekeeping, peacemaking, and democracy building efforts in a hundred countries during the same years.

Clearly, the age of investment in joint, collective, and coherent action through the United Nations has come for the rich and the powerful member states of the organisation. As we move from a uni-polar world of US dominance to a multi-polar world where China and India also will become superpowers, it will be as important to recognise the political importance of Beijing and New Delhi as to demand they assume their part of political and economic burden-sharing.

During the lifetime of the next generation much greater global progress can be achieved. Those of us in the growing global middle and upper classes have fewer absolute poor to lift out of abject misery, epidemic disease, and illiteracy, and fewer wars to end. Adding more promise to optimism, we have at the same time, as the incredibly fast and vast counter-recession financial stimulus-packages signal, infinitely greater resources at hand than at any time before.

We also have superior technology and information. Today experts use advanced satellite imagery and computer programmes to identify and locate displaced people and refugees and to plan humanitarian relief efforts. We use satellite data and computer projections to determine whether there is underground water or whether roads will be usable in the coming rainy seasons. Specialised agencies make use of sophisticated models projecting weather patterns, livestock availability, migration trends, and patterns in local and regional tension. We have advanced early warnings for hunger, disease, and conflict which make it impossible to claim we did not know what was brewing. Humanitarian agencies can feed, vaccinate, and provide primary schooling for children for a couple of dollars a day even in the most remote places. Such investment is, dollar by dollar, more cost effective than anything I know about in the private and public sectors in any northern or western society. These non-governmental and UN organisations will also speak up more for neglected peoples, for those whose voices are not heard.

As the UN Emergency Relief Coordinator for three and a half years I had a pulpit from which I could advocate for international action with more worldwide coverage than I had ever imagined before taking up the job in 2003. We can and must hold world leaders accountable to their obligation to defend defenceless civilians threatened in lawless places around the world. Some 190 heads of state and governments from the

United States, China, Russia, Europe, the Islamic world, Africa, Asia, and Latin America solemnly swore at the United Nations summit in September 2005 to uphold a "responsibility to protect" vulnerable communities when their national authorities cannot or will not provide such protection. This "responsibility to protect" should mean that world leaders cannot anymore be passive bystanders to carnage.

In short, more than at any time before, today we have the means to end so much of the suffering that was viewed as inevitable during previous generations. We have greater financial resources at hand, superior technology and information, advanced early warnings for hunger, epidemics, and conflict. We also have the biggest and best network of like-minded inter-governmental, governmental, and non-governmental organisations as channels of future investments in health, peace, and development. They represent great hope for us and future generations that have the responsibility and real possibility to end massive misery and to prevent conflict and disasters.

1

Introduction: The Art and Practice of Conducting Global Health Negotiations in the 21st Century

Ilona Kickbusch[i] and Ellen Rosskam[ii]

Diplomacy is the art and practice of conducting negotiations. It is a specific *method* for reaching compromise and consensus, as well as a *system of organisation* within which states — and increasingly non-state actors — pursue their interests. Diplomacy is an essentially political activity oriented towards achieving a specific outcome. States set the goals for negotiation in their foreign policies, and — as globalisation proceeds to deepen — both the private sector and civil society organisations have "foreign policies" of their own. Because of the many actors on the global stage observers increasingly comment on the need for new forms of global dialogue and decision-making that move beyond the traditional state-centred bilateral and multilateral diplomatic concepts and practices that have been the focus of 19th and 20th century diplomacy.

---

[i] Professor Dr. h.c. Ilona Kickbusch is the Director of the Global Health Programme at the Graduate Institute for International and Development Studies, Geneva.
[ii] Professor Dr. Ellen Rosskam is Senior Advisor and Consultant to the Global Health Programme, Graduate Institute for International and Development Studies, Geneva, and Professor at Webster University, Geneva.

A range of features characterise 21st century diplomacy:

- It needs to function within a multi-polar world and within a multi-level and multi-dimensional global governance structure, which increasingly includes the regional level.
- It is no longer conducted only by professional diplomats; diplomats today need to interact with many different actors, not only with other diplomats as they did in the past.
- It is characterised by *polylateral* layers of diplomatic interaction and relationships and is challenged to manage not only the relations between states (bi- and multi-lateral) but also the relations between states and other actors.
- It manages these relationships in various diplomatic venues and with a wide range of instruments.
- It is increasingly engaged in public diplomacy vis à vis an informed public and many actors at home and in the host country.
- It is involved with and contributes to a whole host of issues which are on the international agenda and which require global coordination, such as security, health, the environment, global finance, climate change, and the like.
- It needs to consider a much closer interface between domestic and international policies and cooperate with other national ministries.[1–7]

But even as one considers these features one still has not captured the full essence of the transition: the very goals of foreign policy are changing. Foreign policy is no longer only about the *"relation with external entities"*[8] *it is about achieving security, creating economic wealth, supporting development in low income countries, and protecting human dignity"* both at home and abroad.[9] As a consequence, diplomats now have a double responsibility: to represent the interests of a country as well as the interests of the global community.[10] This *"double responsibility"* implies recognition that increasingly global public goods need to be negotiated, managed, and ensured. It also means that regimes in the area of trade and economic development need to be complemented by agreements in areas of social development and on critical global trans-boundary issues, such as the environment and health. This complementarity of the national and the global interest has been expressed for example by

President Lula de Silva of Brazil in his 2003 inauguration speech: "an international order guided by values is the one which offers the broadest possibilities not just for promoting the national interests … but also for systemic stability itself."[11] This means that the dynamics between health and foreign policy have changed fundamentally in the 21st century.

As health becomes politically more relevant — in both domestic and foreign policy — it becomes a feature of the foreign policy of states and enters the realm of diplomacy. In two consecutive years, UN General Assembly Resolutions entitled "Global Health and Foreign Policy" recognize their "close relationship […] and their interdependence."[12,13] Health diplomacy as a profoundly political process is conducted at many different levels of governance; it includes various types of diplomacy ranging from the bilateral, to the multilateral, and polylateral, and it moves in different geo-political directions: North-South, South-North, South-South. The relationship can be illustrated by a continuum with two endpoints — one endpoint in which (A) foreign policy neglects or even hinders health, and the other where (D) foreign policy serves health as presented by the Oslo Declaration on health and foreign policy.[14] Along the continuum we can define a number of different relationships between health and foreign policy, two of which are of particular importance: (B) health as an instrument of foreign policy, and (C) health as an integral part of foreign policy.[15] This continuum is presented visually in Fig. 1 below.

At the multilateral level health diplomacy relates in particular to points C and D. Global Health Diplomacy — that part of health diplomacy which

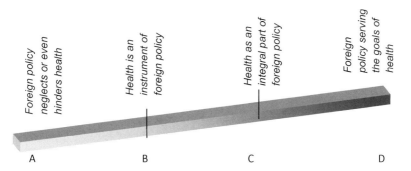

Fig. 1. The continuum of the relationship between health and foreign policy. Adapted from Kickbusch I. (2011) *21st* Century Global Health Diplomacy.

deals with the negotiation processes that shape and manage the global policy environment for health — can be considered as a *method* for reaching compromise and consensus particularly within the context of international organisations. It relates in particular to health issues that cross national boundaries, are global in nature, and require global agreements to address them both in health and non-health forums. Because of their political relevance these negotiations at the global level are conducted not only between public health experts representing health ministries of nation states but also include representatives from foreign policy, security policy, development and trade, as well philanthropists, civil society, and private players.

Global health diplomacy brings together the disciplines of public health, international affairs, management, law, and economics. New skills are needed to negotiate global regimes, international agreements and treaties, and to maintain relations with a wide range of actors. A number of factors distinguish 21st century global health diplomacy:

(1) the nature of the subject matter: health is a trans-boundary concern for all nations, it requires collective action,

(2) the role of science and scientists: the response to the spread of disease is heavily dependent on understanding the causes and as such the productive interface between diplomats and health experts is critical to successful health negotiations,

(3) the complexity of the negotiations: the interface between diplomacy and science, the multi-level, multi-factor, and multi-actor negotiations and the repercussions for trade and commerce, power relations, and values make for complicated negotiations,

(4) the unique equity issues involved: equity is a driving force of the global health agenda since its inception, but has gained force with the adoption of the Millennium Development Goals. A range of global health strategies deal with equity issues in specific ways, such as differential pricing for vaccines and other essential drugs,

(5) innovative features and approaches: throughout its history in each institutional phase health diplomacy has been highly innovative in developing methods, instruments, and organisational forms.

An additional critical feature of health diplomacy is that international health negotiations have had an institutionalised mechanism at their disposal for over 100 years ever since a permanent international agency for health was in put in place in 1907 — today this is the World Health Organization, which was founded in 1948.[16]

The intent of this book is to present a wide variety of perspectives and experiences that illustrate the defining features and characteristics of 21st century health diplomacy. They are presented in case studies contributed by a range of lead negotiators, health diplomats, Ambassadors, NGOs, technical experts, private sector, international organisations, academicians, and donors reflecting the polylateral nature of the field. The range of topics covered provides a snapshot of the diversity of levels and issues: such as negotiations in multi-lateral institutions, negotiations at national level, negotiations on specific diseases, negotiations on treaties and conventions, and multi-lateral negotiations in individual countries on issues such as health sector reform and governance.

The authors describe with as much objectivity as possible different types of enabling environments that facilitated successful negotiations, ways in which political space was captured, created, and used at a particular moment in time, types of leadership needed for successful negotiating outcomes, challenges and opportunities presented by the involvement of different actors holding differing degrees of power, creative and standard negotiating tools used, the role of and for policy, and analyses of why some negotiations were unsuccessful. Detailing different positions taken by individual countries and non state actors during multiple rounds of negotiations, the authors describe in detail various angles, perspectives, and postures adopted by the various players in the respective negotiations.

This is the first book to present case studies about *how* the different negotiations took place and it is precisely this angle that makes the book pioneering, providing learning tools for today's broad group of "new health diplomats" in the landscape of this ever-shifting, complex technical and political arena. The collection of case studies fills an important gap in both knowledge and practice by providing insight on *how* negotiations on global health issues have transpired, successes, challenges, failures, tools and frameworks for negotiation, mechanisms of policy coherence, ways to achieve global health objectives internationally, and how global health diplomacy used as a foreign policy tool can improve relations between nations.

The case studies are told as the negotiations were experienced by individuals who participated in the various debates, dialogues, negotiations, or by experts who have studied them. They highlight the art and the practice of health diplomacy. Today more than ever diplomats and negotiators need practical and technical information on global health and how to use global health as part of foreign policy to improve relations between countries. Simultaneously, non state actors need practical information to help them in negotiating and in the use of diplomacy.

In response to these needs the book is directed at representatives of ministries of health, foreign affairs, finance, and trade, staff of international organisations, and a wide range of non state actors who engage in trans-border health negotiations. It aims to increase their understanding of the dynamics as well as the art of global health diplomacy and to improve their negotiation skills. Schools of public health and international relations should also find this book highly useful for those giving more attention to this developing area. The Global Health Programme at the Graduate Institute for International and Development Studies will be using it in conducting capacity building in Global Health Diplomacy.

The editors hope that this unique collection of case studies will be useful for diplomats and other actors in this field from a wide range of countries. The diverse collection of topics, regions, and contributing authors provides a rich palette to springboard debate, which is strongly encouraged. Reader reflection about how other perspectives might present the same case study is an example of what might catalyse debate, discussion, or reaction based on the angle from which the case is told, the topic, or specific content.

References

1. Barston R. (2006) The Changing Nature of Diplomacy. In: Barston R. *Modern Diplomacy*. Pearson Longman. New York. 3rd Edition.
2. Moon S., Szlezák NA., Michaud CM., Jamison DT., Keusch GT., Clark WC., Bloom BR. The Global Health System: Lessons for a Stronger Institutional

Framework. *PLoS Med* (2010) **7**(1): e1000193 [doi:10.1371/journal.pmed. 1000193].

3. Frenk J. The Global Health System: Strengthening National Health Systems as the Next Step for Global Progress. *PLoS Med* (2010) **7**(1): e1000089 [doi:10.1371/journal.pmed.1000089].

4. Heine J. (2006) On the Manner of Practising the New Diplomacy. Centre for International Governance Innovation (CIGI) Working Paper No. 11.

5. Sucharipa E. (2002) 21st Century Diplomacy, available at: http://campus. diplomacy.edu//lms/pool/BD%20materials/Sucharipa.htm. Accessed September 2010.

6. Wiseman G. (2004) "Polylateralism" and New Modes of Global Dialogue. In Christer Jönsson and Richard Langhorne (eds), Diplomacy Vol. III, London: Sage, pages 36–57.

7. Szlezák NA., Bloom BR., Jamison DT., Keusch GT., Michaud CM., Moon S., Clark WC. The Global Health System: Actors, Norms, and Expectations in Transition. *PLoS Med* (2010) **7**(1): e1000183 [doi:10.1371/journal.pmed. 1000183].

8. Hudson V. (2008) The History and Evolution of Foreign Policy Analysis. In: Smith S., Hadfield A., Dunne T. *Foreign Policy: Theories, Actors, Cases.* New York: Oxford University Press.

9. United Nations (2009) Global Health and Foreign Policy: Strategic Opportunities and Challenges. Note by the Secretary-General (A/64/365), United Nations General Assembly, Sixty-fourth session.

10. Muldoon J. Jr., Sullivan E., Aviel JF., Reitano R. (eds.) (2005) *Multilateral Diplomacy and the United Nations Today.* Cambridge Westview Pr. 2nd ed.

11. Parola A. (2007) A Ordem Injusta; Brasília: Fundação Alexandre de Gusmão.

12. United Nations (2008) Resolution Adopted by the United Nations General Assembly on "Global Health and Foreign Policy" (A/Res/63/33), Sixty-third Session.

13. United Nations (2009) Resolution Adopted by the United Nations General Assembly on "Global Health and Foreign policy" (A/Res/64/108), Sixty-forth Session.

14. Ministers of Foreign Affairs of Brazil, France, Indonesia, Norway, Senegal, South Africa and Thailand "Oslo Ministerial Declaration — Global Health: A pressing foreign policy issue of our time", *The Lancet* (2007) 369: 1373–78.

15. Kickbusch I. (2011) 21st Century Global Health Diplomacy. In: Novotny T., Kickbusch I. (eds.) *21st Century Global Health Diplomacy*. World Scientific Press.
16. Novotny T., Kickbusch I. (eds.) (2011) *21st Century Global Health Diplomacy*. World Scientific Press.

2

Navigating the Negotiating Space Between Geneva and New York: A Case Study in Foreign Policy and Global Health

Luvuyo Ndimeni[i]

Abstract

Global health and foreign policy — as a single issue — has become a permanent agenda item of the United Nations General Assembly in New York. This case study provides first-hand insight into the multi-faceted negotiations that have brought into focus the increasingly complex relationship between these two areas, and the skillful diplomatic strategies that assembled the support of a large and growing number of countries across a North-South divide. Thorough preparation, astute understanding of the political dynamics, and good timing were critical to the process that successfully garnered high-level support in the United Nations General Assembly. The systematic engagement of an increasing number and type of stakeholders on the national and the international

[i] Luvuyo Ndimeni is the Deputy Ambassador of the South African Permanent Mission to the UN and Other International Organisations in Geneva and was the drafter of the resolution "Global Health and Foreign Policy" and its lead negotiator at the United Nations in 2008 and 2009. He has written this case study in his own personal capacity.

level has led to broadened discussions at many bilateral and multilateral meetings, and catalysed formal and informal initiatives.

The Problem

The Foreign Policy and Global Health Initiative (FPGH or Initiative) originated from the recognition by the Ministers of Foreign Affairs of seven countries (Brazil, Indonesia, France, Norway, Senegal, South Africa, and Thailand) that globalisation has provided many universal benefits, but also has increased the vulnerability of countries to communicable diseases and other health threats. The impact of cross-border movements of people, climate change, and natural disasters in terms of social and economic development and collective security[ii] highlighted the balancing act that requires sovereign states to understand that they cannot protect themselves without collaborating with other Member States of the United Nations.

In March 2007, the Ministers of Foreign Affairs of the Member States of the FPGH adopted the Oslo Ministerial Declaration[1] as the outcome of several discussions and preparation by their senior officials. The advent of the successful adoption of the Oslo Ministerial Declaration brought challenges for the founding members of the FPGH. Amongst some of the challenges were the issues of sustainability, maintaining interest, and wider involvement in the Initiative by other stakeholders such as academia, Member States of the United Nations and civil society, and the issue of adding value. The FPGH had to be seen as adding value. The Foreign Ministers' perspective on the FPGH was informed by the fact that some of them were former Ministers of Health. In addition, some senior officials involved had come from a medical background and other senior figures were working in the field of "health diplomacy."

These experiences were sufficient to convince members of the FPGH about the need to advance the idea of drawing to the attention of the global community the links identified through the three themes in the Oslo Ministerial Declaration. These themes were: "Capacity for global health

---

[ii] The notion of security though, in the context of the Initiative was understood to mean protection against public health risks and threats that by their very nature do not respect borders.

security," "Facing threats to global health security," and "Making global-isation work for all." The added value was in ensuring that United Nations organs, agencies, and funds adopted an approach that utilised a "health lens" in their programmes.

It was against this background that the idea of a resolution was conceived. One of the procedural issues to appreciate with the multilateral system is that for an issue to be on the agenda of the UN General Assembly, there needs to be a legislative mandate such as, for example, a resolution, declaration, chairman's summary, or some form of outcome indicative of an outcome of a meeting of UN Member States. For the FPGH, there was the additional dimension of convincing Member States of the linkage between "foreign policy" and "global health," which had never been introduced on the agenda of the UN, either in Geneva or New York. Furthermore, the extent to which the cross-cutting issues in the Oslo Ministerial Declaration impacted the various UN organs, agencies, pro-grammes, and funds, most of whom are located in New York, had to be clarified. The reality for the seven members of the FPGH, hereafter referred to as the "Oslo Group," was that this could be achieved through a resolution, amongst other multilateral tools.

As a result of all the above, the Oslo Group decided in 2008 to intro-duce in the 63rd Session of the UN General Assembly in New York, the highest and universal decision-making organ of the UN. The title of the resolution was entitled "Global Health and Foreign Policy."[2] The Oslo Group followed the success of the introduction and adoption of the reso-lution with a follow-up resolution in December 2009, with the same title during the 64th Session firmly entrenching the issue as a permanent agenda item that requires consideration annually by all Member States.

Needless to say, the success factor was measured by the number of the co-sponsoring delegations who were close 57 in 2008 and increased to close to 80 in 2009. The co-sponsorship was indicative of support beyond the Oslo Group.

The Local and External Players and Their Roles

A significant development in the FPGH that lead to this success by the Oslo Group was the support by the UN Secretary-General (UNSG),

Mr. Ban Ki-Moon, and the Director-General (DG) of the World Health Organization (WHO), Dr. Margaret Chan who both attended the launch of the Oslo Ministerial Declaration on the margins of the 62nd Session of the UN General Assembly (UNGA) in 2007. This development provided impetus to develop the Initiative further and the launch was attended by many Member States at the time, which was a litmus test of the extent of acceptance of the link between the two concepts "foreign policy" and "global health." Several other Member States also made statements in support of the Initiative.

This support gave impetus to the idea of introducing a resolution on foreign policy and global health. By the time the draft resolution was introduced for negotiations in October 2008, delegations were receptive to the proposal. The initial process included consultations with members of the Oslo Group in New York prior to the first presentation of the draft resolution. The purpose of the Oslo Group meetings was to ensure that the "Capitals and Geneva" were in synchronisation with developments in New York and to prevent the resolution from inadvertently landing itself in conflictual issues that would have defeated the ends and purposes of the introduction of the resolution.

The introduction of the draft resolution in New York required a lot of work, largely preparing the groundwork for the "soft landing" of the resolution. Initially, a lobbying exercise was undertaken during a visit to New York during May/June 2008. The exercise was in the form of a series of bilateral meetings with several key delegations to explain the background to the Initiative, and the forthcoming introduction of the resolution in October/November 2008. Several delegations were consulted based on their influence, positions of chairing regional and negotiating groups such as the Group of 77 and China (the group of 132 developing countries composed of Africa, Asia, Latin America, and Caribbean States), European Union, JUSCANZ (Japan, USA, Canada, Australia, New Zealand, Norway), and others.

This process of consultations required intense and repeated explanations. During the consultations, most of the questions were focused on what was the added value of this Initiative, over and above everything else happening in New York, and more pointedly, why bring a "Geneva issue" to New York where the plate was already full of political issues. The proactive situational analysis by the Oslo Group outlined above came in handy in outlining the importance of the issue of global health in the foreign policy context. In the multilateral sense, New York has always been the foreign policy domain by virtue of the annual sessions of the UN General Assembly (UNGA), which are attended by Heads of State and Governments, together with Ministers of Foreign Affairs.

Challenges Faced and the Outcome

Health as a social and economic issue was not difficult to address, however it was the process that was challenging. Many questions were asked in relation to where this issue would best be accommodated on the agenda of the UNGA. In general Member States need to trust and find logic in the rationale behind initiatives to be able to convince their Capitals. This was a process of systematically engaging with the major stakeholders. The composition of the Oslo Group of countries as a cross-regional initiative also played a significant role in convincing that this was a group of countries serious about global health.

Negotiating the first resolution 2008

The original draft of the resolution was presented to the Expert Group of the founding members of the Oslo Group in January 2008 in Chiang Mai, Thailand. This draft was conceived to be a resolution with a pre-ambular part, addressing itself to the main elements of the Oslo Ministerial Declaration and welcoming its adoption as well as the UNGA and WHO resolutions. The operative part of the resolution was omnibus in character, with the Agenda for Action which are ten specific actions, clustered under the three themes from the Oslo Ministerial Declaration:

* Capacity for global health security (Preparedness and foreign policy; Control of emerging infectious diseases and foreign policy; Human resources for health and foreign policy).
* Facing threats to global health security (Conflict; Natural disasters and other crises; Response to HIV/AIDS; Health and the environment).

- Making globalisation work for all (Health and development; Trade policies and measures to implement and monitor agreements; Governance for global health security).

The Group decided to adopt an incremental approach to the resolution, rather than introduce it in a "big bang" approach, that would have alienated potential supporters and co-sponsors. The resolution initially had headings from the ten specific actions in the Oslo Ministerial Declaration: (i) Preparedness and foreign policy; (ii) Control of emerging infectious diseases and foreign policy; (iii) Human resources for health and foreign policy; (iv) Conflict (pre, during, and post conflict, and as peace is being built); (v) Natural disasters and other crises; (vi) Response to HIV/AIDS; (vii) Health and the environment; (viii) Health and development; (ix) Trade policies and measures to implement and monitor agreements; and (x) Governance for global health security.

The initial objective and strategy was for each member of the Oslo Group to "shepherd" at least one issue during future negotiations. The Group also recognised that "diplomacy" could add value in the following areas:

- Make "impact on health" a point of departure and a defining lens to examine key elements of foreign policy and development strategies.
- Engage in developing a roadmap for what remains to be done in large-scale disasters and emergencies where foreign ministers have special responsibilities, making the use of global instruments such as the International Health Regulations and humanitarian law.
- Support national disaster planning and development of critical national capacity for emergency preparedness, including the capacity to coordinate relief efforts through the development of local relief networks.
- Strengthen the capacity of the UN Secretary General to assume a coordinating role in facilitating actions related to foreign policy in preparedness, planning, and action for global health security. Work in close cooperation with UN specialised agencies, programmes and funds.
- Identify critical gaps in capacity for effective implementation of the International Health Regulations with a specific focus on better national and transnational surveillance, outbreak investigation, and disease control.

The main element in the draft resolution was the request to the UNGA to include an agenda item on "Global Health and Foreign Policy," which was ultimately agreed during the subsequent Sixty-fourth Session of the UNGA (2009), as agenda item 123. The resolution further requested the UNSG, in consultation with the Director-General of the WHO, to prepare a report "with recommendations, on challenges, activities and initiatives related to foreign policy and global health."

During one of the preparatory meetings of the FPGH, it was observed that the three themes mentioned above together with the specific actions, were cross-cutting the work of the Main Committees of the General Assembly, in particular the First (disarmament), Second (economic) and Third (social) Committees. This led the Oslo Group to decide to introduce this issue as a plenary item. From a strategy point of view, the approach served the Group well since the allocation of issues to specific Committees would have landed global health into the polemic debates on whether it was considered as an economic or social issue. Additionally, this dimension of allocating global health to Committees had ramifications for the participants that would have shaped the nature of the resolution in the negotiations, as the slant would have been less economic than social, or vice-versa. Missions within the UN tend to allocate officials according to the Main Committees or the Principal Organs (GA Plenary, Security Council, and ECOSOC) to ensure institutional follow-up. For these reasons, the issue was firmly located in the plenary of the General Assembly.

In 2008 during the initial presentation of the resolution, negotiations began during the second week of October 2008. Participation was cross-regional from delegations such as Chile, France (representing the European Union), CANZ (Canada, Australia, New Zealand), Malaysia, United States of America, Cuba, China, Japan, Switzerland, Mexico, Egypt, Brazil, Indonesia, Norway, Senegal, South Africa, Thailand, Brunei, and Israel. Several UN agencies also attended, mainly to monitor the potential impact of the resolution on their mandates. These agencies included the International Red Cross (ICRC), the UN Population Fund (UNFPA), UNAIDS, and the WHO.

The initial concerns by participants in the negotiations centred on the potential nature of the resolution and members of the Oslo Group to prescribe to other Member States to incorporate global health issues in their foreign policies, which was the sovereign right of each member state. Other delegations highlighted their own health initiatives, which were regional in focus. The issue was that these proposals were meant to underscore that the FPGH, especially the Oslo Ministerial Declaration, was not a universally agreed document by all Member States of the UN. Ironically, no Member State raised any objection to the Initiative and this could largely be attributed to the fact that this link already had been established through another resolution that was introduced by China in 2004, entitled "Capacity-building." The Oslo Group and other co-sponsors of the resolution made the point emphasising that the Initiative was global in focus and not national or regional. The logic of the Group was based on the fact that there were so many regional initiatives that this would dilute the nature and focus of the link to include other issues outside the ten priority areas outlined in the Oslo Ministerial Declaration. The priority areas were comprehensive on their own and provide a nexus in foreign policy and global health that was logically established. In retrospect, delegations were concerned about the role of the WHO and its relationship with the General Assembly, especially possible duplication of the agendas of the GA and the WHO.

The resolution was adopted by consensus with more than fifty co-sponsors, which was a milestone for a new initiative. The resolution was entitled "Global Health and Foreign Policy" to address the concern of some delegations about putting foreign policy first and making health appear to be a secondary issue. The compromise that was reached was in the change of title, and in essence the content of the resolution address foreign policy and global health.

Negotiating the Second Resolution 2009

The second follow-up resolution, introduced by the Oslo Group during the Sixty-fourth Session in 2009, was preceded by a major decision of the General Committee taken during September. This was the decision to allocate a plenary agenda item entitled "Global Health and Foreign Policy," as requested by the UNGA resolution in 2008. This development confirmed that the link between foreign policy and global health was finally recognised by the international community and furthermore that the issue would now be a permanent agenda item of the Plenary. This marked a major shift in thinking that had taken root, and was a seminal achievement. The second resolution followed almost the same path as the initial resolution. However, the Oslo Group together with co-sponsors decided to introduce two "themes," based on the Oslo Ministerial Declaration. The themes were "Control of emerging infectious diseases and foreign policy," and "Human resources for health and foreign policy." This was part of the incremental approach agreed in Chiang Mai.

The negotiations on the follow-up resolution were fairly similar in nature and context, and required a lot of lobbying by individual members of the Oslo Group to ensure that Member States understood the introduction of themes, which were based on the ten priority areas of the Oslo Ministerial Declaration. A new and positive development in 2009 was that ECOSOC also focussed on health during its July 2009 session of the Annual Ministerial Review (AMR), with the theme "Implementing the internationally agreed goals and commitments in regard to global public health." The outcome of the AMR was a Ministerial Declaration.[3] The AMR provided an opportunity to assess the state of implementation of the United Nations Development Agenda, explore key challenges in achieving the international goals and commitments in the area of global public health, and to consider recommendations and proposals for action, including new initiatives.

The follow-up resolution for the UNGA64 was discussed and agreed during the FPGH Experts' Group meeting that was held in Paris, 8–9 October 2009. The main thrust of the resolution was to continue to raise awareness and maintain focus on the topic of global health issues in the UNGA. In 2008 the resolution successfully brought these inter-linkages to the attention of Member States in the UNGA, in its Resolution 63/33.

The approach taken during the 2009 negotiations was to incorporate the topical issues of emerging infectious diseases and human resources for health as the main focus areas for the 64th Session of the General Assembly. The resolution had two headings (infectious diseases and human resources) focussing on these areas and a section on follow-up actions. The purpose was to bring the foreign policy dimension on these issues and also link the role of political guidance of the UNGA to the entire UN system, as the only principal and universal organ of the UN mandated with the role of directing all activities within the UN system. The draft resolution also called for the policy coherence and collaboration from the UN Secretary-General with the DG of the WHO.

The second GHFP resolution in 2009 was adopted by consensus and more than sixty-five delegations co-sponsored the resolution with the same title as in 2008 "Global Health and Foreign Policy" (A/Res/64/ 108).[4] This marked a great success since the issue was also on the permanent agenda of the UN General Assembly.

Key elements of the resolution on "Global Health and Foreign Policy"

2008	2009 UNGA Resolution 64/108
1. Procedural in nature, requesting that an agenda item "Global Health and Foreign Policy" should be introduced in the UN General Assembly.	1. Linked the Annual Ministerial Outcome of ECOSOC which focussed on health with the General Assembly resolution.
2. Recognised the central role of the WHO as the primary specialised agency for health.	2. Continued to reinforce the central role of the WHO as the primary specialised agency for health.
3. Established linkages with other GA resolutions, especially the resolution on "Enhancing capacity-building in global public health," which was introduced during the SARS epidemic.	3. Underscored global health a long-term objective which is local, national, regional and international in scope and required closer international cooperation beyond emergency.
4. Recognised other initiatives in the field of global health such as the GAVI Alliance, the Global Fund to Fight AIDS, TB and Malaria, the International Finance Facility for Immunization, and the International Drug Purchase Facility, UNITAID.	4. Introduced two themes "Control of emerging infectious diseases and foreign policy" and "Human resources for health and foreign policy."
	5. Recognised the need for a fair, transparent, equitable and efficient framework for the sharing of the H5N1 and other influenza viruses with human

(Continued)

(*Continued*)

2008	2009 UNGA Resolution 64/108
5. Recognises the close relationship between foreign policy and global health and their interdependence. 6. Requested the GA to include in the provisional agenda of its sixty-fourth session an item entitled "Global health and foreign policy," taking into account the crosscutting nature of issues related to foreign policy and global health.	pandemic potential, and for the sharing of benefits. 6. Encouraged the finalization of a WHO code of practice on the international recruitment of health personnel.[5] 7. Called for the building of capacity for the training of diplomats and health officials, especially from developing in global health and foreign policy.
Adopted by consensus with more than 50 co-sponsoring Member States.	Adopted by consensus with more than 60 co-sponsoring Member States and the issue was included as an annual agenda item of the GA.

Lessons To Be Learned

Lessons learned in 2008

The major lesson that was learned during this exercise was that thorough preparations, lobbying, and consultations are critical to multilateral diplomacy. A good knowledge of the political environment and understanding its political dynamics could save a representative from unnecessary pitfalls, with the potential of undermining good intentions. Health is a "good" issue by virtue of its relevance and personal experience of individual diplomats, therefore making it undisputable. However, the introduction of the issue in an already volatile political environment demanded critical timing and judgment.

The introduction of the issue was also timely, since the outbreak of the Avian Flu virus and negotiations in Geneva on virus-sharing were also on-going. Additionally, the priority theme of ECOSOC was "Implementing the internationally agreed goals and commitments in regard to global public health," which made the resolution all the more relevant and interesting to the UN community in New York. The increasing list of countries that co-sponsored the second resolution was largely because of the ECOSOC Ministerial Declaration that brought awareness to the issues. Most delegations which attended the negotiations on the resolution on Global Health and Foreign Policy during October–November 2009 also had attended and participated in the negotiations on the ECOSOC Ministerial Declaration. This was a convergence of events that presented an excellent opportunity for the Oslo Group, and indeed, the Group strategically capitalised on it.

In a separate but related development, the participation by the UN Secretary General, Mr. Ban Ki Moon and the Director-General of the WHO, Dr. Margaret Chan as well as their staff during the launch of the FPGH Initiative in New York on the margins of the UN General Assembly, significantly increased the awareness of the FPGH issue. Their statements on September 27, 2007 in support of this Initiative brought the issue to the attention of many delegations, both in New York and Geneva.

The relevance of the priority themes had positive effects on diplomats as the inter-linkage of issues was explained. For example, the recently-established Peace building Commission could play a major role in post-conflict reconstruction and development including health infrastructure after conflicts resulting in war and destruction. Non-health issues such as trade (access to affordable medicines), crisis, and human rights were some of the issues that easily connected with practitioners.

The biggest challenge was coordination between Geneva and New York. Health is a Geneva-driven issue, however when health-related issues reach New York they compete with other important issues such as peace-keeping, peace and security issues in the Security Council, climate change and sustainable development issues, etc. In a contrasting manner, the resolution has raised the issue of global health as an important issue that needs to be considered, and it has brought a new type of awareness to the New York community.

The process of engaging many delegations during May–June 2008 in New York entailed lobbying and explaining the rationale and logic between main contributors to the UN budget, small and big delegations with influence, coordinators of the different political formations such as the Group of 77 and China, the group of 132 developing countries comprising Africa, Asia, and Latin America as well as Caribbean States. The systematic engagement at senior levels also helped in addressing issues comprehensively, to provide delegations with adequate elements for the resolution, whilst receiving feedback to ensure there was sufficient respect for all views.

After the series of consultations in both New York and Geneva during the months of May and June, the Oslo Group took into account the valuable comments of Member States and refined the language of the resolution, which was hitherto circulated to Member States where the negotiations and cross-referencing of language from other WHO resolutions occurred. The resolution requested that the UNSG, in close collaboration with the WHO DG, should compile a report in consultation with Member States. The initial report was thus compiled by the WHO Secretariat, in close coordination with the Oslo Group. The Oslo Group's main contribution was the hosting of the consultative process for the draft report on the margins of ECOSOC on July 23, 2009. These consultations were geared towards ensuring that Member States were able to provide comments before the UNSG's report was finalised before submission to the UNGA.

The importance of this report was critical to shaping the resolution that followed. The report was going to be the first test of substantive issues and it contained recommendations for future actions to be undertaken. Member States pay attention to recommended actions, more so if there is required accountability. The resolution "Global Health and Foreign Policy" (A/Res/63/33) was adopted by consensus, with more than fifty co-sponsors as Member States, which was a significant achievement for a resolution introduced for the first time where almost half of the entire membership agreed that there was a link between foreign policy and global health. The list of co-sponsors from the developed North and developing South was also indicative of the broad consensus on the link between foreign policy and global health.

Lessons learned in 2009

An overall assessment of the resolution was that it proved to be timely and relevant in the light of the current H1N1 pandemic flu crisis. The feedback from delegations during the preliminary introduction was that the draft avoided controversial issues and was focussed. The only issue that appeared difficult was the issue of the inclusion of the notion of "fair sharing" of vaccines in pandemic situations.

The tabling of the draft resolution appeared to have a positive impact on many participants of the General Assembly. The positive aspect related to the level of support received from many Member States, which provided an opportunity for outreach and networking beyond the Oslo Group. Closer consultations and coordination could have been undertaken with the relevant UN organs, funds, and programmes however, time limitations prevented this. To address this shortcoming, the facilitator for the Oslo Group on the draft resolution accepted an invitation by the Second Committee of the GA to participate in a panel discussion on "Globalisation and Health" on 24 October 2008. The panel included amongst others, Dr. Margaret Chan and Professor Jeffrey Sachs from Columbia University, New York.

One additional lesson that could be discerned from the above process was the extent to which flexibility can be exercised as a group, understanding the importance of the broader objective and the willingness to compromise. For example, when the Oslo Group was confronted by some strong views around the issue of the title for the resolution i.e. "Global Health and Foreign Policy," instead of the preferred title "Foreign Policy and Global Health," the Oslo Group realised that the entire contents of the resolution were agreed. It thus provided a small "victory" for some to remain with the title, as long as the broader picture was captured. That broader picture was to place the issue on the agenda of the UN General Assembly. This approach also minimised politicising the linkage between foreign policy and global health. This was minimised by discussing the title at the end of the negotiations on substance.

Conclusion

The processes, tools, strategies, and mechanisms outlined above constitute the experiences of diplomats in the area of global health diplomacy. However, the approach taken by the Oslo Group departed from the traditional process largely due to the cross-regional composition of its members.

The Group's ability to draw an increasing number of co-sponsors has so far been indicative of increasing interest by Member States on the subject matter. This unique cross-regionally composed Group developed strategies that allowed it to take advantage of opportunities as they presented themselves (such as the ECOSOC ministerial meeting). Of no less importance, this unique Group made use of political spaces when they appeared, and thanks to thorough preparations and the Group's "soft-landing" approach an enabling environment was created. Through that newly-created environment achievements could be realised.

The overall assessment of bilateral consultations with delegations was that the delegations were interested in procedural issues. Delegations realised and acknowledged the importance of this initiative as well as the fact that no delegation or political grouping had undertaken such an initiative before. Previous initiatives have focussed on specific epidemics and health emergencies such as Avian Flu. Another resolution focussed on the Implementation of the Declaration of Commitment on HIV/AIDS and the Political Declaration on HIV/AIDS and Roll-back Malaria.

The entire process could not have been done differently. The only other approach would have been to follow the polemic divisions of North and South which could have resulted in a resolution that was not supported, and which lacked in substance and detail.

Finally, changing the resolution's title to "Global Health and Foreign Policy" (from its original title of "Foreign Policy and Global Health") was by request of some participants during the negotiations. A compromise was reached to change the title.

The development was also timely considering the epidemics that were experienced since 2004, especially with SARS which prompted major delegations such as China to introduce a resolution in the UN General Assembly entitled "Enhancing capacity-building in global public health."[6]

In conclusion, the resolution will continue to be negotiated annually in the UN General Assembly as part of the agenda item, not excluding possibilities of complementary activities within the WHO. There is close collaboration between Member States in Geneva and New York as well the respective offices of the DG of WHO and the Secretary-General of the UN in producing the background report on "Global Health and Foreign Policy." The Oslo Group continues to meet in Geneva under an alphabetic coordination system between the seven countries and meets at least twice a year at Experts level who are representatives of the Ministers of Foreign Affairs. In 2008, Indonesia hosted followed by France in 2009. South Africa hosted in 2010 and the next meeting will be held in Brazil, with the purpose of determining "Phase II" of the Initiative.

References

1. Ministers of Foreign Affairs of Brazil, France, Indonesia, Norway, Senegal, South Africa and Thailand (2007) "Oslo Ministerial Declaration — Global Health: A pressing foreign policy issue of our time," *The Lancet* 369: 1373–1378.
2. United Nations (2008) Resolution Adopted by the United Nations General Assembly on "Global Health and Foreign Policy" (A/Res/63/33), Sixty-third Session.
3. United Nations ECOSOC (2009) Ministerial Declaration — 2009 High Level Segment. "Implementing the Internationally Agreed Goals and Commitments in Regard to Global Public Health."
4. United Nations (2009) Resolution Adopted by the United Nations General Assembly on "Global Health and Foreign policy" (A/Res/64/108), Sixty-forth Session.
5. World Health Organization (2010) WHO Global Code of Practice on the International Recruitment of Health Personnel, WHA 63.16.
6. United Nations (2004) Resolution Adopted by the United Nations General Assembly on "Enhancing Capacity-Building in Global Public Health" (A/Res/59/27), Fifty-ninth Session.

3

Public Health Diplomacy in the WTO: Experience from Developing Countries in Negotiations on Health and Related Services in GATS and Issues Related to Public Health in TRIPS

Ahmad Mukhtar[i]

Abstract

Two agreements of the World Trade Organization directly impact public health: the Trade Related Aspects of Intellectual Property Rights (TRIPS) and the General Agreement on Trade in Services (GATS). This case study describes the complex multilateral negotiations that involve a range of sensitive areas such as Health Services and the Intellectual Property Rights issues of pharmaceuticals. The tough, crowded playing field of trade negotiations involves different government arms and various other influential internal and external stakeholders. Punctuated are

[i] Ahmad Mukhtar is the lead negotiator for the government of Pakistan at the Permanent Mission of Pakistan to the WTO in Geneva, Switzerland. Mr. Mukhtar deals primarily with the negotiating areas of Trade in Services (GATS), Intellectual Property (TRIPS), and Development issues. The views expressed in this case study are entirely his own and have no association whatsoever with his employer.

the need to "do one's homework" and the types of skills indispensable for stakeholders at both the national and global levels. Along with the different interests that developed and developing countries bring to the negotiating table the discussion highlights the importance of capacity building, coordination "at home," and effective communication. The bottom line is "don't wait until the curtain rises for the final act."

The Problem

The World Trade Organization (WTO, previously the GATT) was established in 1994 (effective from 1st January 1995) as an international organization dealing specifically with trade issues. Over a period of time however, the scope and impact of WTO agreements have crossed barriers and ushered a new dimension of world trade entering into social and development issues. The WTO is, unlike most of other international organisations, a member driven organization whereby each member has equal voting rights and decisions are taking by consensus.[ii] At present 153 countries are members of the WTO and over twenty (including Russia) are in accession process. Representation, including in the dispute settlement procedures, is through Governments (mostly ministries of Trade or Foreign Affairs); however the private sector, civil society and other international organisations contribute their views through the respective government representatives.

The subject of public health is dealt with in two agreements of the WTO directly.[iii] One of these agreements covers Health and Related Services as one of the sectors of Trade in Services under the General Agreement on Trade in Services (GATS). The second agreement covers intellectual property and public health issues under the Trade Related aspects of Intellectual Property Rights (TRIPS). Both of these areas are new, incorporated during the Uruguay Round (of negotiations which took

---

[ii] The decisions are taken by consensus; however there is a provision for voting in case consensus is not possible, but this provision has never been used in practice.

[iii] There are also other agreements such as Agreement on Sanitary and Phyto-Sanitary Measures (SPS), Agreement on Technical Barriers to Trade (TBT) and GATT Article XX (exceptions) that deal with issues of health and safety.

place from 1986 to 1994) in the multilateral trading system particularly directed at developing countries. The Uruguay Round, like previous rounds of the multilateral trade negotiations, served to further liberalise trade and encapsulate it into a system which was just an agreement (General Agreement on Tariffs and Trade (GATT) between contracting parties, before the organizational set-up of the World Trade Organization (WTO) in 1995.[1] The distinctive feature of the Uruguay Round was incorporation of the Services (General Agreement on Trade in Services) and Intellectual Property (Agreement on Trade Related Aspects of Intellectual Property Rights) in addition to the Trade in Goods, which had been the main subject of various Rounds of negotiations since 1948 (when the GATT was established). Since the Uruguay Round took place, a significant amount of research and analyses reveal that developing countries did not get a fair deal out of the aforementioned two agreements. The August 2003 decision on TRIPS and Public Health did manifest however, some flexibility towards developing countries' demands. The context of this famous 2003 decision on TRIPS and Public Health[2] was a longstanding stance by the developing countries and least developed countries (LDCs) about very high benchmarks of patent protection (especially pharmaceutical patents) which serve as an obstacle to fulfill the demands of public health concerns in terms of supply and affordability of pharmaceuticals. Against this backdrop, the decision was taken, and adopted by Ministerial Meeting of the WTO (the highest level of decision-making) in 2003, that in cases of public health emergencies, the WTO member countries would be able to issue compulsory licenses[iv] for the required drug. In case of no domestic production capacity, the issuing country may request another country to produce the drugs and export them under this system. A recent example of this arrangement is Canadian production and export of HIV/AIDS drugs to Rwanda. Despite the fact that this system is in place,

---

[iv] A compulsory license for pharmaceuticals is an arrangement whereby the relevant government authority temporarily halts the "full rights" of patent holder and asks the same or other manufacturers to produce a required drug at a price which does not include "patent premium," thus making it more affordable for developing countries in particular. The patent holder is, however, given an "adequate remuneration" which is a subjective calculation.

there have not been many instances of issuances of compulsory licensing under the TRIPS and Public Health auspices.

At the time of signing onto TRIPS (along with other Uruguay Round agreements) developing and least developed country members of the WTO were granted varying transition periods (some of which are still on-going) for ensuring compliance with TRIPS obligations through national legislative and/or regulatory instruments and institutional arrangements. There was no immediate burden felt by developing country members due to this phased introduction of TRIPS obligations. However, once the developing countries and LDCs started working towards putting in place the necessary legislative and institutional mechanisms for fulfilling TRIPS obligations, they felt that the requirements of implementation and enforcement are more stringent than expected due to lack of proper anticipation at the time of signing on to the TRIPS. Moreover, the substantive areas (such as patents and trademarks duration were mostly adopted from the existing Intellectual Property conventions and protocols (such as Bern and Paris conventions) therefore no major surprises were felt in this area as compared to the implementation and enforcement obligations.

The year 2000 marked the end of the major transition/phased introduction period. Soon after, especially after the start of a new round of negotiations called the Doha Development Agenda (DDA) in 2001,[3] the developing country members felt a pressing need to re-visit what they committed to in signing these agreements. They felt a need to invoke more of the in-built special and different provisions in the TRIPS[v] as a "right" in order to balance the obligations. This need was felt the most in the area of Intellectual Property enforcement especially in the context of pharmaceutical patents which play a vital role in public health policy. The realisation was a result of the start of actual implementation, after the expiry of transition periods, and an avenue to raise these concerns in the form of beginning of a new round of negotiations, i.e. DDA.

---

[v] These provisions are in the form of transfer of technology, with fewer obligations on LDCs and transition periods for implementation, etc.

It was at this time, i.e. the launch of a new Round (DDA) in November 2001, and the start of the negotiations process, when a demand for balancing public health issues with pharmaceutical patents popped up and proved to be the lynchpin[vi] for the 5th WTO Ministerial Conference (Cancun 2003). The famous August 2003 (immediately preceding the WTO Ministerial Conference) decision on TRIPS and Public Health was the first "balancing act" of developing country members of the WTO in the TRIPS area. This historical decision in the international trade arena allowed member countries to issue "compulsory licenses" for pharmaceutical patents in case of public health emergencies.[vii] The leading WTO members in pushing the agenda for

---

[vi] The Cancun Ministerial Conference, the first after launch of the new Round, DDA, was a testing ground for relationships between the developed and developing country members of the WTO. The gap of understanding between two sides widened and the Ministerial Conference was termed as a "failure" except for the positive signs such as the decision on TRIPS and Public Health, which helped in re-gaining the trust of developing countries and LDCs in the WTO system and kept them on track for negotiations.

[vii] Compulsory licensing is one of the flexibilities on patent protection included in the WTO's agreement on intellectual property — the TRIPS (Trade-Related Aspects of Intellectual Property Rights) Agreement. Two provisions to do with least developed countries and countries that do not have production capacity directly involved changes to the rules of the TRIPS Agreement. Overall, the declaration was important for clarifying the TRIPS Agreement's flexibilities and assuring governments that they can use the flexibilities, because some governments were unsure about how the flexibilities would be interpreted.

The TRIPS Agreement does list a number of conditions for issuing compulsory licenses, in Article 31. In particular:

- normally the person or company applying for a license has to have tried to negotiate a voluntary license with the patent holder on reasonable commercial terms. Only if that fails can a compulsory license be issued, and
- even when a compulsory license has been issued, the patent owner has to receive payment; the TRIPS Agreement says "the right holder shall be paid adequate remuneration in the circumstances of each case, taking into account the economic value of the authorization," but it does not define "adequate remuneration" or "economic value."

There's more. Compulsory licensing must meet certain additional requirements: it cannot be given exclusively to licensees (e.g. the patent holder can continue to produce), and it should be subject to legal review in the country.

this decision forward were India, China, Brazil, South Africa, and the group of LDCs.

The initial proposal[4] was meant to find a way to address the concerns of developing countries due to enforcement of patents (especially in pharmaceuticals) upon implementation of the TRIPS agreement. During the course of negotiations, various proposals were tabled including another extension for enforcing TRIPS obligations. The one proposal that gained major convergence was to introduce an "exception" in the form of the issuance of compulsory licenses, which in any case was allowed in the TRIPS but did not address the situation where domestic production capacity — due to lack or absence of pharmaceutical production facilities — was not enough to utilise such compulsory license. Therefore, it was decided that in case of little or no domestic production capacity for required drugs (pharmaceuticals), the country issuing such compulsory license may import the required pharmaceuticals from another country under this regime. However, so far only one instance of imports under this decision (also known as the Para 6 system) has been reported — Rwanda imported AIDS drugs from Canada.[5] There has been a push by the developing countries in recent TRIPS Council meetings to review this system[viii] in order to determine whether there are any problems in implementation[ix] since it is perceived to be very hard to use by most of the potential beneficiary countries of the compulsory licensing system. This demand for review of the system has faced, not surprisingly, a stiff stance from the developed countries who do not find any problem with this system and who request "specific" concerns and examples of the usage or otherwise of this system. The developing countries, on the other hand, reiterate that it is not possible to come up with specific problems unless a mechanism is used a number of times. As mentioned previously, so far only one case has been reported (Canada–Rwanda) and that took more than two years between issuance of compulsory license and drugs reaching Rwanda. Developing countries insist that this one case is enough evidence to figure out the problem that the system

---

[viii] The system/mechanism under the decision on TRIPS and Public Health is also known as the Para 6 system.

[ix] Implementation issues are, for example, notification at national level, determination of public health emergency, identifying the potential source countries, time involved in production and export, and the adequate remuneration arrangement with the patent holder.

has not been used often, despite its utility and need in most of the developing countries and LDCs. The TRIPS Council, which is the WTO body dealing with issues related to TRIPS agreement, has decided, in its meeting of 14–15 June 2010, that a dedicated session would be held to review the potential flaws in this compulsory licensing system. The session is expected to be held in October 2010. This chicken and egg issue has almost frozen whatever was achieved, or perceived to be achieved, by developing countries under the TRIPS and Public Health decision of August 2003.

Put simply, the developing countries and LDCs signed on to TRIPS agreement as part of the package[x] which was an outcome of the Uruguay round, but it was evident that this agreement was and may not be attractive to the developing countries. This balancing act is proving to be tough for developing countries in recent years due to conflicts between TRIPS obligations and Public Health policies. In addition to the obligations under WTO-TRIPS, recent trends in bilateral trade agreements show a tendency to go beyond the benchmark provided by TRIPS, thus raising the bar higher and higher. One may attempt to avoid going beyond TRIPS in bilateral trade agreements, but once the benchmark (TRIPS) is there, it is not easy to resist doing something more than the starting point/benchmark set at the multilateral level (WTO). The raison-d'être of having any bilateral trade agreement is precisely that — to go beyond the benchmark set out in the multilateral commitments.

On the Trade in Services (GATS) side, the situation is even more deplorable due to the fact that under GATS, health services, which are mostly a public sector responsibility and an essential social sector instrument, are shifted to the trade paradigm and left to the unmerciful mercy of "market" interventions in, for, and of "health and related service providers."

The GATS is an agreement that deals with trade in "services." Prior to conclusion of the Uruguay Round, the GATT (predecessor of WTO) had

---

[x] The WTO negotiations work on a "single undertaking" concept which means that all members have to agree on all or nothing. The agreements in the Uruguay Round were part of this single undertaking package and the developing countries had to sign on to TRIPS even if it was not positive in balance. Since there were many other agreements, each member saw its own balance in one or another of the agreement(s).

only "goods" as the subject matter of negotiations and liberalisation. Like TRIPS, the GATS is also a recent phenomenon, agreed upon after the conclusion of the Uruguay Round. Under the GATS, the member countries are requested by other member countries to liberalise (thus commit) the market access and national treatment in various sectors, of which Health and Related Services is one (there are 12 sectors as per the existing classification[6]). "Market access" refers to commitment to allow the foreign service suppliers in the receiving country's markets through: i) cross border supply, ii) consumption abroad, iii) commercial presence or, iv) movement of natural persons.[7] "National treatment" means that the foreign services suppliers would be treated no less favourably than domestic service suppliers, in the receiving country.

Unlike the other WTO agreements, the GATS operates on a "positive list" approach, which means that a member is free to commit to the extent (and number of sectors) that it deems appropriate within the national policy framework. However, this approach is more theoretical than practical. In actual negotiations, the developing countries always receive pressure from developed countries to liberalise all sectors, particularly those of interest to the developed countries, which incidentally are the most sensitive in the developing countries.

Although not committed under GATS as much as other sectors (out of the 12 sectors as per classification used in the WTO negotiations), the Health and Related Services remains to be one of the prime targets for liberalisation by most of the demanders under the GATS negotiations. The target areas include hospital services, other human services, social services, professional services (related to medics and paramedics), and health insurance services. In this area, the developing countries are at a crossroad of choosing between the policy space/regulatory oversight and the liberalisation at the multilateral level, through bilateral and plurilateral[xi] negotiating requests and responding offers.

[xi] Plurilateral requests, introduced after the Hong Kong Ministerial Conference, is the system whereby a group of member countries make a collective request to another group of member countries. The latter group is termed as "recipients" of that request. This is a complementary approach to the bilateral request and offer approach. The results of this process, like bilateral request and offer, would be multilateral upon conclusion of the DDA.

Liberalisation in the WTO context means adhering to the obligations/ commitments of various WTO agreements. In the case of GATS, liberalisation means the granting of market access and national treatment in the sectors where that specific country has made commitments through a negotiations process, and where such commitments are scheduled in the WTO as its final binding commitment. In real terms, this becomes a choice between managing the supply of service through public sectors (which is the most predominant in most of the developing countries), giving incentives and using domestic services suppliers before using foreign ones, managing the access and cost of such services, and regulating the sector and related services from a public policy perspective rather than from market access and business motives. The latter two are the prime motivations in the case of market access and national treatment committed for foreign service suppliers.

The negotiations in GATS are done through a bilateral or plurilateral request and offer process while the resulting commitments agreed through such negotiations apply on a multilateral basis (called "MFN basis" in WTO terminology). This means that if countries X and Y negotiate bilaterally a deal on Hospital Services market access/national treatment in country X, upon agreement country X would commit that market access/national treatment for *all* WTO members and not only for country Y. This then opens the floodgates for aggressive international competition to dominate market access/national treatment in the individual sector that was negotiated by the "receiving," or newly liberalised country. The importance of maintaining a public policy perspective is self-evident.

There are certain potentially problematic issues associated with this liberalisation process. Liberalisation often is not "autonomous" but instead is done as part of a "deal." The consequences, though mostly positive as advocated by many economists, could be negative. For example, in the case of health and related services, the private supplier may fill in a gap that the government could not. Simultaneously however, there could be problems with issues of access due to affordability (in terms of price) by the general public. Affordability by the general public may not have been a problem when this service was being supplied by the government as a "duty" to the public, rather than with a profit orientation, which is the prime motive of private sector service suppliers. In the short run this might not be evident until one recognises that private service supply could actually stop the growth of public sector supply in this sector, and in certain cases even slowly replace the whole supply of such crucial services. This is one of the "fear factors" for many developing countries while going for liberalisation in the Services area.

The Local and External Players and Their Roles

The process of multilateral trade negotiations under the WTO appears relatively simple from the outside but the reality is far from simple. The negotiations process in the WTO is conducted through Rounds of multilateral negotiations, such as the on-going Doha Development Agenda, which was launched in Nov 2001.

Multilateral negotiations that involve issues related to trade, public health, health services, pharmaceuticals, health workers, intellectual property and patents, and international security are extremely complex, go very deep, and touch on extremely sensitive issues for all countries involved. It would appear to outsiders that only ministries or departments of trade and commerce would be involved in such negotiations. However, many other government arms are intricately involved, including defense and security departments, foreign ministries, finance ministries, health ministries, and labour ministries. This complex mixed playing field — even for one single country's delegation — emphasises the essential need for well concerted preparation and effort by various stakeholders at national level. At the multilateral level, i.e. the WTO, the following groups constitute the main players in the public health negotiations arena.

Developing country members

While they account for two-thirds of the total membership of the WTO, developing countries were not able to assert their proportionate weight[xii]

[xii] This is primarily due to the fact that the results of the Uruguay Round were mostly in favour of developed countries. The developing countries were not able to assess the real implications of new areas, i.e. Services and Intellectual Property (GATS and TRIPS) until the start of a new Round of negotiations which was agreed on a precondition that this would be a development oriented round of negotiations in order to balance the concerns of developing countries from the outcome of the previous (Uruguay) Round.

until the start of a new (after the Uruguay Round) Round of multilateral trade negotiations called the Doha Development Agenda (launched at the 4th WTO Ministerial conference in Doha, Qatar, November 2001). This round of negotiations kept the "development dimension" at the forefront and sought liberalisation in different areas such as Agriculture, Non-Agriculture market access, Services and Intellectual Property, amongst many other areas. The developing countries made their presence recognised in the system and since then have been trying to translate this mandate[xiii] into practical measures.

On most of the TRIPS and GATS issues, the developing countries generally act together as one block, assigning a delegate from one country in the block to speak on behalf of all countries in the block. This is advantageous for the group of developing countries since there is always a limited negotiating capital (i.e. the most important area where one country would wish to spend the most effort) with developing countries. By pooling the negotiating strategies, they can use this capital in a more efficient manner. At the same time there is also a downside to this collective action due to obvious and logical differences amongst the developing countries. These differences are certainly factors to be taken into account in terms of collective action by the developing countries. The natural differences are due to varying economic endowments and the trade policy objectives in developing countries. Some members are open in trade policy whilst others opt for conservative policies thus taking a defensive stance in most of the areas negotiated.

In broad terms, the developing country members are striving for special and differential treatment in all areas including TRIPS and GATS and upholding the development dimension in the on-going round of trade negotiations, i.e. DDA. This is being done through submitting negotiation proposals aimed at enhancing the special and differential treatment (less strict obligations on developing countries and LDCs) and achieving the macro level development objectives.

[xiii] The mandate of the Doha Development Agenda clearly instructs that negotiations in all areas would be focused on the development related outcome, and that the concerns of developing countries and LDCs would be kept prime in all areas.

Developed country members

Fewer in number but stronger in impact. That is how the developed countries act in the WTO (similar to the way they act in most of the international organizations), despite the fact that there is no proportionately weighted voting or veto system in the WTO. It is very rare to see a divide amongst developed countries in the WTO especially in the TRIPS and GATS areas. It is noteworthy that the European Union (EU) acts on behalf of its 27 members. This leaves very little political space for non-EU developed countries to form alliances. Such alliances for developed countries are very difficult to create mainly due to the fact that a vote by the EU counts as a vote from 27 countries. Yet alliances would make negotiating easier for those usually-non-existent alliances of non-EU developed countries than their negotiating directly with over 100 developing country members. In general, the developing countries act as a block but there are certain areas within the negotiations where this block is not workable and the individual members have to negotiate in their own capacity. An example of this instance is the bilateral request and offer process in the GATS negotiations for Health and related Services. It works in a way that one developed country member requests one developing country member to liberalising a certain area (although the liberalisation outcome would then be available to all members of the WTO). Thus it is the requested country that has to negotiate and in this case the block strategy is not practical.

International organisations

There are a few international organisations working on the areas of TRIPS and Trade in Services directly and indirectly, such as the World Intellectual Property Organization, the World Health Organization, and the United Nations Conference on Trade and Development (UNCTAD), amongst others. These related organisations sit as observers in the WTO and do not intervene directly in the regular and negotiating business, however the support given by these international organisations to member countries and the parallel forums that are created have made the international organisations one of the most important players in these multilateral negotiating arenas. For example, the issue of Intellectual Property is being discussed, simultaneously, in the WTO as part of the DDA negotiations in TRIPS, in the WIPO as part of the Development Agenda (a negotiations process in the WIPO to deal with Development dimensions of Intellectual Property), in the WHO as an initiative against counterfeit medicine called IMPACT, in the Universal Postal Union (UPU) as a work programme to stop piracy and counterfeiting through postal means, and in the World Customs Organization (WCO) through an initiative called SECURE which is intended to combat piracy and counterfeiting through border/custom controls.

Civil society

Civil society organisations (CSOs) have made their presence felt in recent years particularly in the area of public health and TRIPS issues. The role of civil society is most prominent in creating awareness and conducting advocacy work in national/domestic jurisdictions, which is often a difficult task for the concerned government agencies. Although the CSOs cannot speak in the WTO or make any submissions, they influence the opinion of delegations through various advocacy programmes. Most of the developing country delegates get benefit from the research and capacity building initiatives of the CSOs and often incorporate the outcome/recommendation of such work in their negotiating strategies. On the issue of Public Health, the CSOs have made a great contribution in raising awareness amongst the general public and influencing the domestic policy circles, which in turn influence the Geneva- based delegations. Some of the effective CSOs work both in Capitals and in Geneva so that the impact of their effort is strong. CSOs voice their concerns in public through various seminars, workshops, and similar events. The WTO Public Forum (which is held usually in September every year) is a good avenue for CSOs to make their points public and convey the message to concerned quarters. CSOs also actively participate in the Ministerial Conferences, though their activities are held in parallel and not as part of the formal Ministerial Conference.

Challenges Faced and the Outcomes

Capacity

The first and foremost challenge being faced by the developing countries participating in WTO negotiations is capacity at their national level, including, importantly, their capacity at the level of representation in the WTO. Oftentimes the delegates from developing countries are not well versed in the issues being negotiated and not well equipped by their respective government agencies. More often than not their actions during both official and unofficial negotiations (such as "corridor" discussions) are in a reactive mode rather than a proactive mode, even on issues and areas of importance to their own countries. A recent trend is to outsource the research and analysis burden to some inter-governmental organisations (IGOs) and to civil society organisations. This practice has both advantages and disadvantages. These externally hired groups can be effective in providing support to the government delegations, but they also can be prone to follow a set agenda and pre-determined and pre-defined thought parameters which are not known to the government hiring them, due to a lack of transparency. The most imminent disadvantage is that these external sources work on general ideas and strategies, while the one solution may not fit all. Tailor made solutions (i.e. negotiating strategies) can be achieved only when an individual effort is made by the respective delegation. This effort requires human resources, financial endowments, and well consulted (domestically with stakeholders) opinions and policies.

Stakeholder coordination at national level

In most of the developing countries essential interagency cooperation — which is crucial for a delegation to be effective in negotiations — is either absent or noticeably weak. The lack of interagency coordination and cooperation leads to a weaker stance and position for that government at the WTO negotiations. For example, on TRIPS issues the ministries or government agencies responsible for trade would have a different approach than that of the ministries or government agencies working solely on intellectual property issues, and both of the aforementioned would think and approach negotiations differently than the ministries or agencies responsible for health and related policies. This disconnect, wherever it occurs, weakens the national positions, which in turn contributes toward overall weaker collective positions by the developing countries. This phenomenon prevails mostly due to lack of understanding of the outcomes and implications of the negotiations, and absence of a collective vision and objectives by individual member countries. This is primarily due to capacity constraints, lack of institutional mechanism in the trade policy area, and tight funding positions by most of the developing countries and LDCs.

Effective communication and strategic techniques

In negotiations at the level of the WTO, experience has demonstrated that the developing countries have not been very successful in strategising their collective and individual positions in various areas. The other dimension of this dilemma is lack of effective communication techniques manifested in the form of inappropriate forum, form of communication, and timing and advocacy of various positions. Developed countries, on the contrary, strategise at least as much on process as they do on substance. The developing countries often dilute the substance due to inappropriate process and presentation.

Appropriate forum

The "appropriate" forum refers to the most relevant body in the WTO, i.e. whether an issue should be presented in General Council (the highest body in the WTO after the Ministerial Conference) or in the respective committees.

Form of communication

The negotiations in WTO or the expected results depend as much on the form that member(s) adopt to push an issue as on the substance of that issue. It is crucial to test the idea before launching it, i.e. a new proposal submitted right away in a negotiating or regular body may be shot down instantly as compared to a proposal which is shared informally in one form or another. Sometimes it is useful to launch an idea or proposal verbally before putting it in writing.

Timing and advocacy of various positions

The timing of any new proposal is also a crucial factor. One needs to choose the time of introduction of a new proposal at the time when members are relatively open to consider new ideas and not already stuck with something else. Moreover, the timing is also crucial in the context of intensity of negotiations, i.e. if it is very intensive a new idea would not find much attraction, but at the same time if it is a totally lull period the risk of not attracting attention is also high. The advocacy is a pre launch exercise that includes sharing with like-minded member countries, checking it with some not so like-minded countries (i.e. potential opponents), and with some external players such as research institutions or policy observers.

Negotiating leverage

One of the most important challenges being faced by the developing country members in the WTO is a sense of limited capacity to negotiate. They are made to believe that they have only a limited "negotiating capital" and that therefore they should exercise their wisdom in knowing when spending that capital will be the most effective for their respective countries. If a member speaks on each and every issue the reception by other members is lessened, whilst at the same time if you want too much of an ambitious outcome in an area which is more than your existing or potential trade capacity, the demand is labeled as a non-serious attitude. It is an implicit understanding that you have to use the available cards very carefully since there is no replenishment. This limited negotiating capital sometimes results in disharmony between Geneva-based delegations and respective Capitals, as the understanding of the state of affairs in both places may not be the same. In such situations, one has to exercise discretion and best judgement.

Obviously, cross-cutting or horizontal issues, such as public health, would not rank as equal to specific market access in commodities such as textiles or sugar, for example. This is due to the fact that the lobbies working for specific trade interests (in commodities or manufactured goods) are in a stronger position to influence the negotiation strategy and trade policy than the lobbies working for upholding issues such as Public Health. This situation leads to leaderless pursuit of collective objectives, such as those that are health-related, and leads to generally poor outcomes for the developing countries. Everyone wants to ride for free on some other developing country member's lead, which is often missing due to the obvious question of "why me." The "why me" syndrome causes individual member countries to wonder why they should have to use their negotiating capital in an area (such as Public Health) which is not specific to their individual concerns when instead they could use their negotiating capital for other areas where the domestic lobbies have more pressure.

Implementation issues regarding positive outcomes

As mentioned earlier, it has become all too regularly evident that developing country members lack the implementation capacity and mechanisms to achieve the positive outcomes they need in the area of public health, in WTO negotiations. There is generally a fear of "violating WTO obligations" while exercising the policy space, such as using compulsory licensing for pharmaceuticals and then the results of such positive outcomes at the multilateral level. A case in point is the very little practical application of the Para 6 system on TRIPS and Public Health to date. Moreover, the implementation issues are also linked to other instruments of national economic policy such as investment policy (to attract foreign direct investment) and other bilateral trade agreements which may have higher obligations than the WTO agreements.

Lessons to be Learned

You are always alone in the group

In WTO negotiations dealing with global health issues, the negotiators, especially from the developing countries, should bear one key thing in mind: all other members of the group of developing countries and/or LDCs — whether a formal or informal group — are focusing on their own respective trade and negotiating agendas and rarely are two negotiating agendas the same. Without all members of a delegation understanding the views and positions of the others in their delegation, there can be no coordination in the negotiations. It is this very lack of understanding and communication *within* country delegations that leads to a member government presenting fragmented and inconsistent positions during negotiations.

Effective communication and understanding of views within a delegation is fundamental to effective negotiating. Conversely, the usual scenario characterised by complete disconnect often triggers a snowball effect, the repercussions of which can be seen and felt for years, sometimes with disastrous results.

In general, the negotiating alliances in the WTO, specifically on public health-related issues, are platforms for feeling comfortable in general, and any member can and does jump out of that comfort zone if another more comfortable zone is foreseen (for example, an obvious specific gain in other areas of negotiations). These alliances are rather cults of uncomfortable members and the moment a member finds some comfort elsewhere, the obvious may happen — i.e. a negotiator or member of a delegation may leap from the position they are meant to maintain to one which is more within their comfort zone. These comfort zones are already defined at national level but not necessarily shared at the WTO level. Thus a level of uncertainty remains present in most of the cases for a potential sudden and unexpected move of any WTO member country.

This is not to say that collective actions or positions by the developing country members are essentially a bad way to proceed, but a word of caution is advised - these collective actions are extremely vulnerable and fragile, and any specific intervention by one or more members of that group can change the dynamics of that group. Moreover, the composition of such groups and thereby their actions, is always flexible and fluid. Entry of new players and exit of existing players happens as normal business since comfort and discomfort are derived from elsewhere, i.e. other areas of negotiation in the WTO.

Do your homework properly

It is absolutely crucial to be prepared for your own position in a systematic manner. This includes, firstly, having the reality check of what you have back home, secondly, what you need exactly, and thirdly, what you could expect in a given situation. If the third element is not conducive enough then the thing to do is to create the desired situation where you could expect a positive outcome of a given position.

There is positive value in working dynamically on negotiating positions and preparing for scenarios A, B, and C. The situation in WTO changes relatively quickly due to on-going negotiations and balancing acts, whereby members quickly change their positions, re-align, and leave gaps in some areas while they put up obstacles in others. It is, therefore, necessary to be adaptable, dynamic, and updated about changing positions in order to participate effectively in such negotiations.

Expect the unexpected

It is said in the WTO that things never go wrong; it is members who go wrong in following the events and outcomes. This is very true for most of the developing country members. It is hard to keep track of the happenings, of the informal and backstage processes, of members' changing positions due to external factors. And it is not easy to keep pace with the positions and changes in positions in the respective WTO body. All of these factors together or any one of them alone could certainly lead to unexpected outcomes. But such unexpected outcomes do not occur by chance; these are very well orchestrated outcomes. In fact, they are so well orchestrated that the "outsiders" (those who are out of the informal and small group processes) have no other option but to face these "unexpected" outcomes, ill-prepared as they are. There is little room left in the end game scenario to stand up and say "no" in a last-resort attempt to resist the adoption of such "unexpected" outcomes. The best way to avoid this situation is to keep on repeating your points/positions of interest in whatever form of meetings or groups you represent so that one cannot ignore these once you raise them when faced with the ushering in of "unexpected outcomes." In this way, you could be in a position to expect some way of balancing your concerns.

The bottom line is to not be quiet and wait until the curtain is raised for the final act.

Conclusion

Supposedly negotiations in the WTO are on trade transactions and appear from the outside to be very simple, clear, and logical at the outset, unless of course one gets in over one's head and hits the bottom. The issue of public health is a social sector instrument which is given to trade policy professionals who have only one prism through which they can see and that is "how to multiply trade and transactions." That is far from the prism through which public health specialists see. There is a clear divide between trade policy and liberalisation objectives, and the policy space or social considerations that should be fundamental to any negotiation dealing with public health issues that are also trade-related. The divide is primarily due to stakeholders of trade policy as compared with stakeholders of public health policy, for example. The stakeholders of trade policy (the private sector and big business corporations) usually have more influence in government and policy circles than those who advocate for the public health concerns.

Even though there have been attempts to narrow this gap through various instruments at the multilateral level (such as the decision on TRIPS and Public Health), a lack of trust prevails amongst developing country members. This lack of trust is deep-rooted due to the fact that trade amongst developing countries is not comparable to developed-developing country trade. This leads to a natural tendency that a developing country would look more towards its existing or potential developed country trade partner, both at the multilateral (WTO) and bilateral levels. Thus, the reality is that South-South economic cooperation is more of an interesting theory than practice, at least at this point in time. The area of public health, being no exception, also carries a natural flow from developed to developing in terms of supply of pharmaceuticals, investment in the health sector, related technology transfer, and similar initiatives which are not yet there between the developing countries. This in turn affects the negotiating strategy in the WTO when it comes to an issue that is divisive between developed and developing countries.

There has been some visible movement in a few instances, as mentioned above, where the developing countries showed a collective negotiating strategy, but the optimum level is still far away. It would come with time and take its natural course, which is largely dependent upon an increase in South-South trade and economic cooperation. Moreover, the developing countries would have to graduate from the pursuit of "market seeking" to a level where they think more about "economic growth and development," in which trade is just one component.

References

1. Marrakesh Agreement establishing the World Trade Organization and the Marrakesh Declaration 15th April 1994.
2. The WTO General Council Decision on Implementation of Paragraph 6 of the Doha Declaration on the TRIPS Agreement and Public Health. WT/L/540 and Corr.1 adopted on 1st September 2003.
3. WTO Ministerial meeting Doha, November 2001, Document No. WT/MIN(01)/DEC/1.
4. Paragraph 17 of the Doha Declaration, Document No. WT/MIN(01)/DEC/1.
5. WTO Document No. IP/N/9/RWA/1 dated 19th July 2007.
6. WTO Document No. MTN.GNS/WTO/120 dated 10th July 1991 (based on UN-CPC system).
7. Article 1.2 of the WTO General Agreement on Trade in Services (GATS).

4

Negotiating the Framework Convention on Tobacco Control: Public Health Joins the Arcane World of Multilateral Diplomacy[i]

Kenneth W. Bernard[ii]

Abstract

Responding to the tremendous global health and economic burden of tobacco — the leading preventable cause of death worldwide, the World Health Organization's (WHO) Framework Convention on Tobacco Control represents the first multilateral treaty covering a significant public health issue. Sharing experience from the front line, this chapter describes the complexity and the intrigue of the multidisciplinary

---

[i] This case study is written from the point of view of a single head-of-delegation experience negotiating the Framework Convention on Tobacco Control (FCTC). Others have drawn different conclusions from the same set of facts.[1,2] The intent, however, is not to necessarily write a consensus history of international tobacco control efforts, but rather point out issues, some not so obvious, that may affect future treaty negotiations when public health and diplomacy inevitably intersect.

[ii] RADM Kenneth W. Bernard, MD, USPHS (Ret.). Consultant on Security and Health. Joy Epstein, public health consultant, tobacco expert, and US delegation coordinator for the Framework Convention negotiations, provided numerous substantive suggestions for this case study.

negotiations. For 191 governments to reach consensus is a tremendous challenge. The negotiating process, involving the WHO Secretariat and government delegations, is revealed as one intricate in dynamics, skills, and personalities. Good intentions, trial and error, politics, and economic interests all played out during the difficult deliberations which covered a broad range of issues from the structure of the convention and the health consequences of passive smoking, to cross-border advertising, taxation, and trade.

The Problem

A new public health convention

Tobacco is a killer. As summarised by a World Health Organization (WHO) Report in 2009, tobacco use continues to be the leading preventable cause of death, killing more than 5 million people per year. The annual death toll could rise to 8 million by 2030. More than 80% of those premature deaths would occur in low- and middle-income countries.[3] WHO, the United Nation's specialised agency for international health, had for years publicised the dangers of tobacco use to global public health. The WHO Programme for Tobacco or Health, while well meaning, was relatively powerless in the 1980s and 1990s to bring about major reduction in the use of tobacco worldwide. Their reports and frequent World Health Assembly (WHA) resolutions recited apocalyptic statistics and exhorted countries to enact legislation to reduce production, trade and consumption of tobacco — to little avail.

In 1993–94, however, a number of public health activists, including American law professors Ruth Roemer and Allyn Taylor; Judith MacKay, a British anti-tobacco advocate working in Hong Kong; and Neil Collishaw, a Canadian who ran the tobacco programme at WHO, proposed that WHO become more proactive and prepare an International Convention on Tobacco Control. In 1996, the World Health Assembly adopted resolution WHA49.17, calling on the WHO Director-General "to initiate the development of a framework convention in accordance with Article 19 of the WHO Constitution."[4]

The majority of WHO's normative constitutional authorities do not carry the weight of enforceable international law. Because of that, most resolutions of its governing bodies, the WHA and its Executive Board, use non-committal words like "calls upon" or "urges" when recommending action to member governments. Moreover, almost all of the public health resolutions from the World Health Assembly are adopted by consensus of all member governments in order to avoid "yes or no" voting. Controversial decisions are thereby eliminated, avoiding potential contentious, difficult, or costly obligations for any one country or political or regional group.

Yet, Article 19 of the 1948 WHO Constitution gave the organisation additional, and as yet unused, power: "The Health Assembly shall have authority to adopt conventions or agreements with respect to any matter within the competence of the Organization…which shall come into force for each Member when accepted by it in accordance with its constitutional processes."[5]

Meetings and discussions were held over several years to look at the structure and content of a future Framework Convention on Tobacco Control (FCTC) as requested by the WHA, and authorised by the Constitution. But WHO leadership in the mid-1990s under Director-General Hiroshi Nakajima was viewed as weak by many governments, including the US and the European Union (EU). The initiative floundered in the absence of commitment, support, and promotion from the organisation's highest level leader.

In May 1998, Dr. Gro Harlem Brundtland, former Prime Minister of Norway, was elected the new Director-General of WHO. In her acceptance speech she said: "What is our Key mission? I see WHO's role as being the moral voice and the technical leader in improving health of the people of the world. Ready and able to give advice on the key issues that can unleash development and alleviate suffering. I see our purpose to be combating disease and ill-health — promoting sustainable and equitable health systems in all countries." The FCTC had found a champion — a necessary step to move the international bureaucracy.

New leadership

Dr. Brundtland quickly established a special project called the "Tobacco Free Initiative (TFI)" under Dr. Derek Yach, a well-spoken and self-confident public health expert from South Africa. She also convinced the UN Secretary General, Kofi Annan, to move the "UN Focal Point for Tobacco" from the United Nations Conference on Trade and Development (UNCTAD) to WHO. Brundtland had embarked on a personal mission to get the FCTC completed, and her experience as a Prime Minister as well as a physician and development specialist made her the perfect person to help create this new treaty.

In May 1999, one year after Brundtland's election, the WHA passed resolution WHA52.18, "Towards a WHO framework convention on tobacco control," that established a technical working group to prepare draft elements for the treaty and created an Intergovernmental Negotiating Body (INB) to actually negotiate the Convention and possible related protocols.[iii,6] The technical working group met twice — once in October 1999 and a second time in March 2000. Dr. Kimmo Leppo from Finland was elected chair. It was open to all member nations, but since many of the poorest countries could not afford to attend the meetings, WHO announced it had set aside $125,000 to assist with travel for the poorest participants, and over $1,000,000 initially to support the process in 2000–2001.

The two technical working group sessions created a series of draft papers laying out the various topics in a very complex document. Elements included not only issues concerning the clear public health impact of tobacco, but also tobacco trade, farming subsidies, smuggling, taxes, advertising, promotion and sponsorship, surveillance, package labeling, second-hand smoke, access to tobacco products by youth, media and communications, liability and compensation for damages, aid resources, and research.

[iii] The terms "treaty" and "convention" are different names for the same legal instrument, so long as the content follows the rules and obligations of international law. It is the content — not the label — that determines the scope, impact, and validity of the agreement. A Protocol, while having the same legal obligations, is usually written as an amendment that complements or adds to a treaty or convention. In the case of the FCTC, Protocols are only binding on an individual party to the convention if they are also ratified separately, thereby leaving the possibility that some protocols will be binding on a lesser subset of countries than those which signed the entire Framework Convention.

It became clear that creating a useful international legal document would require input from a much broader group of experts than those with a public health background. As shall be seen later, this was the biggest impediment to progress during the subsequent INB negotiations, and one of the primary reasons the Convention today is not more muscular.

In May 2000, at the 53rd WHA, member governments felt that sufficient preparatory work and drafting had been done, and called on the INB to begin formal negotiations of the Convention.[7]

Local and External Players and Their Roles

World Health Organization Secretariat

By May 2000, WHO had everything it needed to move forward with the formal FCTC negotiation: subject matter experts, either on staff or under contract; adequate resources; direction from the governing bodies; and strong support from the Director-General and WHO Secretariat. The personalities involved and their individual attributes, biases and sensitivities, are underestimated in the eventual success or failure of a negotiation. This was true for the FCTC as well.

The support and process functions for the negotiation were headed by senior international civil servants working for WHO: Dr. Derek Yach (South Africa), Executive Director for Non-Communicable Diseases and Dr. Douglas Bettcher (Canada), Coordinator of the new WHO Framework Convention on Tobacco Control Office in the TFI. Tom Topping (USA) and Gian Luca Burci (Italy) from the WHO legal counsel's office provided much needed legal expertise (unfortunately, neither was an expert in treaty law), and Denis Aitken (United Kingdom) and Bill Kean (Australia), long-time senior policy and administrative advisers to WHO, worked the political backrooms and ensured that the negotiations ran as smoothly as possible.

WHO hired Allyn Taylor, a US law professor with long experience in tobacco issues, as an adviser, and legions of administrative, documents, and translation staff were assigned as needed to assist in the process. It was decided that it would be most cost effective to conduct all of the formal INB negotiations in Geneva, where WHO headquarters could support the administrative functions, including translation and interpretation services. However, between formal sessions, WHO's six geographic regions were encouraged to hold additional regional consultations (which totaled nearly 40 separate meetings over 3 years) to discuss Convention draft language of joint concern.

Nongovernmental organisations

In October of 2000, WHO held public hearings on the Convention at which interested parties gave written or verbal statements. Over 160 members of the public health community, tobacco industry, farmer groups and Non-Governmental Organisations (NGOs) participated. During and after these meetings, it became clear that there was going to be some hostile rhetoric during the negotiations. The NGO community joined together behind two umbrella organisations presenting a unified voice for many smaller consumer-based, public health oriented NGOs: *Infact* and the *Framework Convention Alliance* (*FCA*).

Infact (now Corporate Accountability International) and its Executive Director, Kathy Mulvey, represented civil society on many issues but had one primary focus: the tobacco industry's fundamental conflict of interest with public health. It took the firm position to encourage governments to reject partnerships with the industry for any reason whatsoever, including such things as financial contributions to antismoking educational programmes. The tobacco industry, to no great surprise, objected. Countries quickly lined up in support of *Infact*'s position, and the tobacco industry was removed from any participation in the negotiations.

Unfortunately, *Infact* also intensely distrusted the motives of the United States, Japan, China and other major tobacco producing or exporting States, accusing them of being "fronts" for the big tobacco companies. For the US this was simply not true. Japan and China, as opposed to the US, have significant national financial investments in their tobacco industries, and the influence of those industries on country negotiating positions has been open to speculation from others.[8] Interestingly, both Japan and China have ratified the FCTC.

Contrary to some personal opinions and dubious press reports appearing at various points during the 2½ years of negotiations, at no time did "big tobacco" have any direct or indirect input into any of the US positions or try to influence the delegation so far as we could discern.[iv]

United states delegation

The first INB negotiation took place in Geneva from October 16–21, 2000, and from the beginning the US took the negotiations very seriously. The first US head of delegation was Dr. Thomas Novotny, Assistant Surgeon General, Deputy Assistant Secretary, and Director of the Office of International and Refugee Health at the Department of Health and Human Services (HHS) and a career US Public Health Service officer. He had a long history of work in the Office of Smoking and Health at the Centers for Disease Control and Prevention (CDC).

He was aided by a large multidisciplinary group that included a critical staffer on contract to HHS, Joy Epstein, a longstanding tobacco control expert. Joy was the intellectual and administrative glue who ensured the US delegation (USdel) had the historical background it needed and who developed useful delegation documents and appropriate cross-agency position clearances. This was no small task given the different organisational cultures at the White House Office of Domestic Policy, the Departments of State, HHS, Commerce, Agriculture, Justice, Treasury (Bureau of Alcohol, Tobacco and Firearms [ATF] Customs and Tax Policy), as well as the Environmental Protection Agency (EPA), US Trade Representative (USTR) and the Federal Trade Commission (FTC). All of these agencies participated in the planning and drafting of the US negotiating positions on various parts of the Convention. In addition, agencies within HHS, including the Office of Smoking and Health at the Centers for Disease Control and Prevention (CDC), the Food and Drug Administration (FDA), and the National Institutes of Health (NIH) had significant input.

Because the Framework was so broad in concept and scope, a large group of agency stakeholders was either consulted or actually participated on the USdel. One of the difficult "treaty negotiation" skills that the US public health experts learned in the process was how to ensure all

---

[iv] The author was the Head of the US delegation at each of the last four INB sessions beginning in November 2001 through FCTC completion in March 2003.

agencies of the US Government (USG) with equities in the outcome of the treaty had the opportunity to have input. As was previously noted, some issues, such as tobacco smuggling, advertising on television, farm subsidies, taxes, etc, were mostly trade, communications, agricultural or fiscal in substance, and did not require primary public health expertise (even if they resulted in public health impact). Dr. Novotny and the other members of the public health leadership learned, sometimes the hard way, that broad public health issues were not always first on a list of agency priorities for those agencies such as the Department of Commerce or Justice.

Among the most influential of the USdel members was John Sandage, a brilliant career civil servant lawyer from the State Department's Office of the Legal Adviser. Tall, thin, dark-haired, with a regal manner, unflappable demeanor and dry wit, he provided superb advice and legal interpretations of treaty and international law for the sometimes "legally challenged" public health experts on the delegation. He also was the target of many of the NGOs verbal and written criticisms — often aimed at him as a visible proxy for the US negotiating positions. Perhaps it was his competence or appearance, but more likely it was his habit of taking the most venomous attacks with a polished combination of serious consideration and good humour. He was just fun to spar with, and as a result, far more effective than his remit on the delegation would have indicated. This was a lesson lost on some of the NGO representatives, who frequently took themselves a bit too seriously. Moreover, there were so few other treaty lawyers in the room most of the time that his ability to achieve US negotiation objectives was often successful.

Chair of the intergovernmental negotiating body: First of two brazilian diplomats

When the INB first met from October 16–21, 2000, its initial task was selecting a Chair for the negotiations. Based on previous discussions among the country Missions, WHO Secretariat and others, the first Chair was selected: Ambassador Celso Amorim, Brazil's Permanent Representative to the UN Agencies in Geneva. It was generally held among the diplomatic community that Brazil's diplomats were among the most professional, well trained and talented in the world, and Ambassador Amorim was considered their best.[v] This was extraordinarily good luck for the FCTC. An experienced Chair in a complex negotiation can have an immense impact on the outcome — and he did.

Ambassador Amorim's approach was influenced by long experience with the multilateral UN system, especially in New York. He knew that there is a pattern and tempo to negotiations related to the time frame allocated for completing the document. Little real progress is made in resolving the differences at the beginning while deliberations near the end pick up pace and resolve issues much more quickly under the pressure of time and delivery schedules.

A six-member Bureau, or Executive Committee was established to advise the Chair on the flow of work for the negotiations. The Region of the Americas chose the US as its representative. During the first of the six INB sessions, Ambassador Amorim ensured that any country that had a political point to make — especially those who brought speeches from capitals — could speak during the session, even when that produced little progress in the actual construction of the Convention. The Chair, with considerable support from Dr. Yach and his team, had prepared a draft FCTC text, a document consisting mostly of the papers prepared by the previous two technical working group sessions. After the end of the first INB, a draft working paper was distributed, but little had been agreed.

In fact, the only way Ambassador Amorim could make any progress at all was to repeat many times the statement, "Nothing is agreed until everything is agreed." Wisely, he understood that attempting to lock down text in the first of many negotiating sessions would be a waste of effort. At the beginning of long negotiations, participants tend to give rather long speeches, thanking others and outlining their most fervently held positions.

The second session of the INB met from April 30-May 5, 2001 (INB2). By now, the Chair realised that to make any progress on a document with so many issues to resolve, he had to divide the drafting into three working groups. These met in parallel and would then submit their text to him for merging into a single document. Countries with large delegations could

---

[v] Celso Amorim had been Brazil's Ambassador to the UN in New York, went on to be Brazil's Ambassador to the United Kingdom and its Foreign Minister, a post he has held since 2003.

simultaneously attend all three working groups. Those with only one or two members had to choose — and provide proxy input to the others through regional or political groups.

The three working groups covered such a breadth of issues that the task initially seemed unapproachably daunting:

Working Group I

Passive Smoking
Regulation of Contents of Tobacco Products
Packaging and Labeling
Education, Training and Public Awareness
Advertising, Promotion and Sponsorship
Tobacco Dependence and Cessation
Elimination of Sales to and by Young Persons
Research

Working Group II
Price and Tax Measures
Illicit Trade in Tobacco Products
Protocol on Smuggling
Licensing
Tobacco Manufacturing and Agriculture
Surveillance
Exchange of information

Working Group III
Scientific, Technical and Legal Cooperation
Conference of the Parties
Secretariat
Reporting and Implementation
Financial Resources
Settlement of Disputes
Liability and Compensation

In addition, each working group was assigned parts of the FCTC Guiding Principles and General Obligations Articles to draft that were most relevant to the other topics.

By the end of INB2, Ambassador Amorim had cobbled together a new working draft Convention consisting of a merging of the original paper with the literally hundreds of suggested changes, deletions and additions suggested by the working groups (indicated in brackets to signify that they have not necessarily been agreed to). At this point, no one was willing to move to the "horse-trading" on contentious issues or to agree on language necessary to make real progress.

A new administration and a change in the US delegation

In November 2000 the US held its presidential election to replace President Bill Clinton, who was completing his second and last term. It was perhaps the most contentious election in recent US history. After much political wrangling and an eventual Supreme Court decision, Democratic candidate Al Gore conceded defeat in December and Republican George W. Bush was sworn in as President in January 2001.

The new US President took office three months before INB2. Bill Steiger, a political appointee and senior adviser on global health issues to new Secretary of Health Tommy Thompson, asked that the negotiating positions for INB2 immediately be reviewed for consistency with the new Administration's approach to international agreements. He cited concerns for Constitutional federalism, states' rights, fair trade issues, and the role of the federal government in regulatory affairs regarding tobacco. The review was not completed prior to the start of INB2 Negotiations in Geneva in April, 2001, and the USdel was still relying on previously established positions developed in an administrationwide working group under the Clinton White House Domestic Policy Council.

Dr. Thomas Novotny, the Head of the USdel for the first two INB sessions, anticipated that there would be political differences between the set of positions put forth by the USdel in INB1, and what he perceived as the new Administration's lack of support for pro-public health and anti-tobacco policies approved in the previous US negotiating positions during the Clinton Administration.

As a result of the review by Bill Steiger and the White House, a number of US positions were changed to reflect the new political landscape after the election. Dr. Novotny was notified of these changes only after the start of INB2, and was ordered by phone to bracket (i.e., not agree to) all previously agreed positions and to remain silent regarding any new ones. He was outraged. Most of the changes concerned the new Administration's approach to federalism issues related to separation of powers and states' rights issues rather than directly aimed at public health. But he and some other members of the USdel felt their impact would damage the US leadership position on the FCTC hoped for by tobacco control activists and public health professionals involved in the negotiations. Because of Novotny's public antipathy toward Bill Steiger and the new Administration, Steiger began directly phoning John Sandage, the delegation's State Department lawyer, late at night with instructions on issues likely to be debated in INB2 the following day.

After INB2, devastated by what he considered inappropriate interference in the delegation's prerogatives to sustain previously developed public health positions on the FCTC, Dr. Novotny gave an interview to a reporter very late one night. Although it was "not for attribution" and did not cite him by name, the published news report was critical of the new Administration, implying that its new positions on the FCTC were being influenced by the tobacco industry whose views it claimed were contained in a position paper from the tobacco giant Philip Morris. The Administration was furious at this criticism, insisting that the changes in the US positions were not related to industry influence or lack of support for public health issues, but rather to constitutional and legal differences of opinion regarding treaty negotiations and their attendant obligations.

What happened next is unclear, but Dr. Novotny soon resigned his position as Delegation Head as a matter of principle and retired early from his career in the US Public Health Service, moving from government into academia. The official reason he gave was to "pursue personal interests," but from his academic position, he continued to critique the US approach to tobacco control (and later criticised the failure of the Administration to ratify the FCTC).

Bill Steiger took over the Office of International and Refugee Health (later renamed the Office of Global Health Affairs), and began searching for a new Delegation Head for the next INB — the third — scheduled for November 22–27, 2001.

The author [K.B] had recently returned to HHS from a 2-year detail to the Clinton White House as the first ever Senior Adviser on Health and Security on the National Security Council Staff. A medical doctor, Assistant Surgeon General and career member of the US Public Health Service, he formerly had served as the Associate Director of the Office of International and Refugee Health and as the Health Attaché at the US Mission to the UN in Geneva. Previously, he had had no specific involvement in tobacco control programmes.

Tommy Thompson, Secretary of HHS, asked Dr. Bernard to serve as Delegation Head based primarily on his Geneva-based experience with multilateral negotiations and his White House experience with interagency consensus building. At about the same time, David Hohman, long a senior staff member in the Office of International and Refugee Health, was named Health Attaché at the US Mission in Geneva, and simultaneously became the representative for the Americas Region on the FCTC Executive Committee (referred to as "the Bureau"). While there were minor adjustments in the other delegation members, mostly because of scheduling issues, the rest of the USdel remained relatively stable.

Dr. Bernard chaired the ensuing interagency preparations for INB3 throughout the summer and autumn of 2001. Diana Schacht, a Special Assistant to the President at the White House Domestic Policy Council, conferred final USG approval for positions. Before coming to the White House, she had been Chief Counsel on the House Judiciary Committee staff. She was assisted by Garry Malphrus, a White House lawyer who had been a former Counsel on the Senate Judiciary Committee. It also should be noted that the White House interagency approval process was not an original Bush Administration creation, but had been put in place during the Clinton Administration because the State Department required the interagency process as a condition for HHS to take the lead (rather than State) for the treaty negotiations.

The delegation guidance documents were painstakingly prepared by Joy Epstein, with input from each relevant department and office and then cross-cleared before submitting them for White House final approval. Particularly important, the White House, while supportive of the public health-specific issues, had little to say about their content. They only seemed to have input on the issues that overlapped with a strict "federalism" and states' rights political agenda.

A delegation guidance document was prepared for each INB session. For each section of the Convention, it would include the working Chair's text, any changes recommended by the U.S., discussion, draft talking points, "redline" (cannot cross) positions, and fallback positions when possible. Literally hundreds of pages of carefully reviewed documents were included in the US negotiation guidance for each INB. Few who were not intimately involved realise the amount of staff work required to negotiate a legally binding international Convention. Importantly, public health professionals from CDC and elsewhere came to realise that legally binding international treaties are actually written in the end, by lawyers, not people with public health degrees.

The Second Brazilian Chair

At the end of 2001, after INB3, Ambassador Amorim left his position in Geneva to become Brazil's Ambassador to London. His Geneva replacement for the last three INB sessions, Ambassador Luiz Felipe de Seixas Corrêa, had similar expertise and provided a common and well-oiled approach to chairing what was becoming a very contentious meeting.

Of interest, his selection as the Chair was contested by the Minister of Health of South Africa, Dr. Manto Tshabalala-Msimang. Public health officials from many countries were aghast. Dr. Tshabalala-Msimang was the Minister who had sided with South African President Mbeki in voicing doubt that HIV caused AIDS, and who took actions that slowed the use of anti-retrovirals in government clinics in South Africa. She was also known as being very difficult, the antithesis of the two Brazilian diplomats. Luckily, the diplomatic community saw the logic of continuing with a Brazilian Chair who had excellent political and negotiating credentials. A potential leadership crisis, one that could have completely undermined the FCTC negotiation, was averted.

The new Chair was also very gracious, in and out of the conference rooms. At one point during INB4, Ambassador Seixas Corrêa invited me along with his staff up to his Geneva residence to discuss the US positions and his desire to move the negotiations forward. After sharing more than a few jokes, single malt Scotch whiskies, and discussion of treaty sticking points, we ended with a much better understanding of our common interests regarding the negotiations, as well as the legal constraints leading to some difficult "red lines" for the US. Social graciousness is yet another unappreciated skill in a Chairperson that can help move negotiations forward. However, late that evening, given the convivial discussions, and perhaps a bit too much very good scotch, I decided to take a taxi home, coming back the next day to pick up my car.

Challenges Faced and the Outcomes

At this point, I will deviate from the roughly chronological description of the negotiations and its stakeholders. Rather than consider the last three INB sessions separately, I will deal with them together as a rolling series of issue negotiations, and select a few of the challenges that shed light on the negotiation process itself. In fact, these examples point out the difficulties in reaching consensus when the topics of the Convention are broad, and the number of participating parties is large and diverse.

Delegation membership

A primary difference among the many delegations throughout the negotiations was the breadth of subject matter experts that countries brought to the meetings. The US was lucky because the government supported a delegation consisting of experts ranging from international law to trade to public health to law enforcement, and others as needed. Many large countries, like Japan, China, UK, Russia, France, Canada, Australia, and others — especially the European Union (EU) — did similarly. But many smaller countries would send only one or two people from their capitals or sometimes only a representative from their diplomatic mission in Geneva. This gave them a major disadvantage when the topic turned arcane or highly technical (such as advertising or trade law). Often they would join an ad hoc regional or political group joint position, associating with others (like the G-77 or Africa Group) that had similar geographic or political background. As a result, single positions would be put forth with dozens of "co-sponsors," i.e., all the countries in the group or region. These would be powerful levers, because changing a group position requires an agreement among the members of the group, not an individual speaking as head of a country delegation.

Of particular note was the case of the European Union. The 15 nations in the EU plus another 10 candidate members would vote as a block on some issues and separately on others. It all depended whether the EU had been ceded authority for all the members of the Union on the specific issue. For example, individual countries had competency on most public health issues, while the EU/European Commission was responsible for trade.

The structure of the convention — the case of tobacco advertising

Surprisingly, one of the most contentious battles fought intermittently throughout the INB process was over the basic form of the Convention itself. Originally, when discussing the structure of the Convention, the member governments had the option to create a "Framework Convention" of overarching principles, such as exist in a number of environmental conventions. These would include what in the FCTC are encompassed by the Guiding Principles and General Obligations (Articles 3, 4 and 5), as well as the mostly non-contentious areas of education and public awareness, illicit trade, surveillance, scientific cooperation, research and exchange of information.[9]

Under this proposal a variety of "Protocols," or complementary and optional sub-agreements, would then be negotiated (either simultaneously or subsequently) by interested parties to the Framework. Each protocol could be joined by either all of the Framework signatories or by a subset. The image of a Christmas tree (Framework) with ornaments hanging on the tree (protocols) was used as a descriptive representation. The advantage to this approach, as argued repeatedly by the USdel, was that the most difficult areas for global consensus, including tobacco advertising, taxes, and other major politically charged issues could be stronger in a Protocol if the few countries who did not or could not participate for constitutional or political reasons opted out of that section, leaving the majority to agree to a strong set of actions.

For example, many countries wanted a total ban on advertising for all tobacco products. They initially included Ireland, Norway, Belarus, and Zambia speaking for the entire African region, New Zealand and Indonesia, among many others. The EU, Canada, Argentina speaking for 19 Latin countries, and Japan could only agree to "progressively eliminating" tobacco advertising over time. The United States clearly stated that because of First Amendment Constitutional concerns about free speech, it would be unable to agree to language that totally banned advertising, but could accept "prohibited tobacco advertising promotion and sponsorship targeted at persons under 18," or other more circumscribed prohibitions.

An intervention given by Kenneth Bernard at INB3 in November 2001 summarised the US position on these issues at the time:

We want to thank Australia for their comments on issues related to the relationship between the Convention and the development of protocols.

We share their concern that development of protocols not interfere with the negotiation of the strongest possible consensus language in the Convention itself.

There are clearly two roles for protocols that have been outlined by Australia:

1) They can produce details that elaborate on the general treaty obligations in the framework.
2) They can set out new obligations and agreements on areas in which all parties cannot reach agreement.

We would like to highlight the issue of smuggling as a good example of the first role — an elaboration of details in the convention. We appreciate the support of the African region, just expressed, for moving forward on a smuggling protocol....

I would also like to briefly comment on the second role for protocols — that of setting out new obligations in areas on which we cannot reach consensus.

Advertising has been mentioned by some as one in which some countries may want an agreement that is stricter than what others may be able to accept under their Constitutions.

While we think it is premature to begin a protocol on advertising until the Convention language is closer to consensus, we continue to believe that some like-minded countries may want to have preliminary and informal discussions on this issue sooner rather than later.

We believe that this may be the best way to make rapid progress towards our objective of a final agreement on the framework in 2003.

However, the concurrent "Convention with Protocols" approach survived in name only. The US was shouted down — literally — by almost everyone, from the NGOs, to the African group to the EU to the Chair. Virtually everyone else wanted a strong Framework (including an advertising ban or at least progressive restrictions imposed directly in the Framework Convention). Many argued this would force recalcitrant countries to do what they would not do if they were given an easy "out" to not participate in a protocol.

The US, under instructions from the Department of Justice, simply could not go along. The reasons had virtually nothing to do with tobacco, despite *Infact's* and *FCA*'s insistence that "Big Tobacco" was controlling the US position. It was entirely based on legal opinions promulgated by the Justice Department based on Supreme Court decisions, that the banning of advertising would violate the protection of commercial free speech in the US that was granted by the First Amendment to the Constitution. While others (especially US Representative Henry Waxman) argued that this was not the case, the Bush Administration went with its ideological preference and left the USdel no room for movement.

The US continued to push for the use of parallel protocols to find a practical solution to issues, like advertising, in which consensus could not be reached. The US argued that a protocol banning advertising could be written and signed by those who could, concurrently with the Framework, thereby taking a big step to the reduction of tobacco advertising worldwide. The assumption is that others would join over time, as domestic political conditions permitted. At one point, an informal tally showed that approximately 80 of the 191 negotiating countries could agree on a complete ban. The US failed miserably in convincing virtually any country or WHO staffer that this approach would be beneficial overall. Derek Yach and the NGOs were apoplectic — saying it was an attempt by the US to undermine the strength of the treaty.

In fact, the consensus wording on advertising in the final FCTC was necessarily weak to reach consensus: "Each Party shall, in accordance with its constitution or constitutional principles, undertake a comprehensive ban of all tobacco advertising, promotion and sponsorship. This shall include, subject to the legal environment and technical means available to that Party, a comprehensive ban on cross-border advertising, promotion and sponsorship originating from its territory."[10] As it is written, there are loopholes in the Convention allowing countries to proceed with advertising bans at their own pace. As a result, without the strong advertising protocol, as of 2010 only 26 countries have a complete ban on advertising. Under the protocol proposal, one could hope that up to 80 would have initially signed up, with others potentially being added.

Second-hand smoke

At another point, the US tried to take a strong role on restricting passive smoking and made the following statement:

> In recognition that involuntary exposure to environmental tobacco smoke is a common and completely preventable public health hazard, the U. S. Delegation seeks to expand upon and strengthen the Chairman's text in several important ways:

> First, we propose that the convention prohibit smoking rather than providing systemic protection in several environments, including: 1) Places providing services to children, and 2) Enclosed public places, public transport, and indoor premises of government agencies.

> We also support the promotion of systemic protection from exposure to tobacco smoke in restaurants and/or private workplaces.

Second, recognizing the importance of an informed general public for the successful implementation of policies related to passive smoking, the USdel proposes a strong position for effective educational campaigns to inform the general public of the health risks associated with exposure to second hand smoke.

Third, the USdel proposes that the definition of vulnerable groups be expanded to include persons with chronic lung diseases, such as asthma, and persons with heart disease.

Interestingly, many countries, including the EU, spoke out against these measures, calling them too strict. The final wording in the Convention, Article 8, says: "Each Party shall adopt and implement in areas of existing national jurisdiction as determined by national law and actively promote at other jurisdictional levels the adoption and implementation of effective legislative, executive, administrative, and/or other measures, providing for protection from exposure to tobacco smoke..."[11] Again, this was the weaker consensus language. But that was the typical outcome of any negotiation when the Chair had to get all 191 WHO governments in 2003 to agree. Many other delegations faced the same frustrations on areas they felt strongly about when muscular language lost out to consensus agreement. Consensus, after all, is what nobody likes but everyone will agree to.

Federalism and criticism of the US

Much of the criticism of the US negotiating positions resulted from fallout from the strict political/legal federalism arguments that guided the US positions. There was never any specific anti-health or pro-tobacco sentiment from the Administration injected into the language at any point in discussions of negotiating positions. The two lawyers representing the "political" wing of the government, Garry Malphrus and Gregory Jacob (from the Office of Legal Counsel in the Justice Department), were involved primarily to ensure the US positions were compatible with these legal interpretations — and, as a result, there was some effect on the final language of the FCTC.

Few other delegations could understand why federalism issues were so important. In the Bush Administration's strict interpretation of the United States Constitution, the federal government's authority to agree to treaty commitments is limited to the extent that it could not enter a treaty that imposed duties on a state or any of a state's political subdivisions to take certain actions inconsistent with the powers reserved to the states by the Constitution. The Administration accordingly insisted that it was necessary to add language qualifying the obligations of the national government to those that would not infringe upon governmental powers reserved to the states by the Constitution. In the final discussions, this argument was most relevant in the sections on sale of tobacco to and by youth, and national licensing of tobacco retailers.

Another interesting discussion with Constitutional implications revolved around the mandated size of the warning label on cigarette packets. The US Administration argued it was a prerogative of the US Congress, representing the States, to determine the size and specific language to be placed on tobacco packages, not the federal government. Other delegations were perplexed. "Why can't the federal government just intercede when it is in the clear best public health interest of the population?" they would ask. In fact, the US Congress had no real problem with the size of warning labels, and was already considering mandating a larger label. However, the White House and Justice Department made it clear that the Constitutional separation of powers was the overriding consideration and the decision was not the Executive Branch's to make — much to the annoyance of many who said the US Constitution should not restrain good international public health.

Then there was the acrimonious debate over the use of terms like "low tar," "light," and "mild" on cigarette packages and in advertising, which most negotiators wanted banned. While the US supported a ban of any language that was deemed false, misleading, deceptive or unsubstantiated, it claimed the Constitution's First Amendment right to commercial free speech prevented a broader application of a ban unless the ban met those conditions.

The US, particularly the State Department, took as its starting point that the US takes its treaty obligations seriously and will not agree to something in a negotiation that it knows it cannot or will not honour. It also views many other countries as posturing when they insist on provisions in the negotiation that they are unlikely to either implement or enforce. On the other side, many countries took as their starting point that the US would never ratify the treaty under negotiation and that it just throws its weight around to influence provisions it will not be a party to in the end. These opposing viewpoints resulted in a certain amount of ill will in the negotiations.

Final sticking points

By the final negotiation, INB6 from February 17–28, 2003, there were a number of non-agreed issues — most hinged on simple but critical word changes, such as changing "shall" to "should" or adding a preambulatory line such as, "In accordance with national law," or "in accordance with its Constitutional principles." The push to agreement was influenced in part by the Director-General's desire to complete the document during her tenure at WHO, and the real problem of insufficient funds to continue the expensive negotiation process for much longer. Final issues included:

1) Advertising, promotion and sponsorship, especially cross-border advertising
2) Liability and Compensation of those harmed by tobacco
3) Funding of poorer countries to implement tobacco control programmes
4) Size of the health warning labels on tobacco packages
5) Banning duty free sales of tobacco
6) Taxation of tobacco
7) Whether to include a "reservations" clause in the final treaty
8) Federalism language to accommodate the situation in federal states.
9) Definitions of critical terms

A non-starter for the US (and a number of other countries) was detailed proposed language on increasing domestic taxes on tobacco products. While it had been shown that increased taxes on tobacco leads to decreased smoking (because of increased cost), it was also clear from both Democrats and Republicans in the US Senate that the Senate would not ratify an international agreement that attempted to set tax requirements for Americans — taxes were strictly domestic decisions to be voted on in Congress, not at a meeting of WHO member governments in Geneva. Had the final language in the FCTC overstepped that line, and in the absence of a "reservations" clause, the US would never be able to sign or ratify the FCTC. However, with the help of the experienced Chair, Ambassador Seixas Corrêa, the final text included the language, "Without prejudice to the sovereign right of the Parties to determine and establish their own taxation policies…" This obviated the problem.

Another interesting outcome concerned the provisions for Liability and Compensation of those harmed by tobacco (Article 19), support for implementation of the Convention in poorer countries (Article 26) and support for viable alternatives to tobacco production for farmers (Article 17). In none of these sections was the language strong enough to "force" the richer countries to finance or pursue these issues based on the Convention language alone. Despite much discussion of the financial obligation pursuant to those Articles, they remained general and anodyne.

As the Negotiations came to a close in February 2003, virtually all of the problems were eventually worked out with the exception of whether or not to include Article 30, "No reservations may be made to this Convention."[12] The US argued that having the option of filing formal reservations was necessary for ratification because of the US Senate's longstanding antipathy towards treaties that prohibit them. Such treaties have been regarded by the Senate, not unfairly, as infringing on their constitutional "advice and consent" prerogatives by precluding the opportunity for the Senate (or for that matter any other national parliament) to modify or comment on a treaty's obligations through legal reservations.[vi]

The remainder of the delegations and all of the NGOs, knowing that the Convention would be accepted by virtually everyone else at this point

---

[vi] The pre-eminent 1969 Vienna Convention on the Law of Treaties permits reservations under rules in Article 19: "A State may, when signing, ratifying, accepting, approving or acceding to a treaty, formulate a reservation unless: (a) the reservation is prohibited by the treaty; (b) the treaty provides that only specified reservations, which do not include the reservation in question, may be made; or (c) in cases not failing under subparagraphs (a) and (b), the reservation is incompatible with the object and purpose of the treaty."[13]

(i.e., that it could be adopted by a vote, if necessary), turned a deaf ear to the US arguments. The US gave up. Article 30 forbidding reservations remained in the final Convention. The NGOs cheered. The EU cheered. Even our political allies cheered. The US knew it had lost and would not be able to add reservations — which effectively made eventual US ratification very difficult.[vii]

The almost universal objection to the US desire to allow reservations to the Convention appeared to be a proxy for significant anti-US sentiment especially late in the negotiations. INB6, and to some extent INB5, were taking place during the run up to invasion of Iraq. The hostility to the US and the USdel engendered by the impending invasion was almost palpable in the halls.

Lessons to be Learned

Civil society and the convention

The NGO community at the negotiations was a very serious group of advocates. One or another of them followed the USdel around, hoping to catch a US delegate talking (by mobile phone) to a tobacco company representative, presumably to get "secret" instructions. They seemed quite disappointed when none of those secret meetings ever happened.

The group of NGOs at the INBs published a daily newsletter about the negotiations, called the "Alliance Bulletin" — identifying who was supportive of their positions and which delegations were not. As would be expected, the USdel was frequently criticised for its position. The Bulletin awarded a "Dirty Ashtray Award" for what its editors considered the countries that were trying to undermine the public health agenda of the negotiations. On October 17, 2002, during INB5, the US and Germany got the Dirty Ashtray Award for, "using their constitutions to inflict tobacco advertising on the rest of the world."

After winning the award many times, the editors decided it was time to move on to other egregious violators, so they gave the USA the "Dirty

---

[vii] The US unsuccessfully attempted to have the "no reservations" clause removed later when the FCTC was presented for approval at the May 2003 World Health Assembly.

Ashtray Lifetime Achievement Award." John Sandage, the State Department lawyer, decided to cut out the award from the Bulletin and pin it to his lapel, partly to make a point, and partly to lighten the atmosphere. The *FCA* and *Infact* were not amused, accusing the US of diminishing the importance of the negotiations by not seriously considering criticisms that were deserved. With a perfectly straight face John responded that he had never received a lifetime achievement award for anything, so he would take what he could get.

What the NGOs forgot along the way is that a Convention or Treaty is inherently an international legal instrument between sovereign states or groups of states. For whatever their intrinsic worth or use, the opinions of the NGOs are not positions of governments. They may be influential constituencies, but often they have single points of view that do not, by their nature, require much compromise. As the public health community discovered, international diplomacy is the art of compromise. If done properly, the few things in a negotiation your government must get, you fight for. For those things you may have an opinion about but do not really need, you can bargain away. And, most importantly, you do not confuse the two because no government in a multinational negotiation ever gets everything it wants.

An important lesson has been lost in the self-congratulatory post-Convention rhetoric. The FCTC negotiators (mostly public health professionals) had a conflicting requirement both for consensus on anti-tobacco mandates to be adopted by all 191 WHO Member Countries, while simultaneously adopting strong international legal obligations to implement those mandates. In the end, this political *naivité* undermined the strength of the final text.

Throughout most of the approximately eight weeks of formal INB negotiations, and hundreds of hours of informal issue and regional discussions, consensus was hammered out on the majority of issues. By the end, the US, Germany, and Japan had the most problems with the text and the NGOs and some governments were wild in their accusations against the US as a country determined to "undermine" a strong Convention. Toward the end of the negotiations, especially in INB5, many NGOs called for much more directive language with a strong advertising ban and other mandates that made it clear that "health trumped trade" in all jurisdictions and sectors. They wanted the US and other countries considered to be non-cooperative to withdraw from the negotiations because they saw such countries as moving the group toward a banal consensus draft rather than a strong proactive treaty. The Chair, wise as always, refused to move in that direction, perhaps knowing that he would then not gain the consensus necessary to complete the negotiations.

It is interesting, however, to remember that early on the US proposed a Convention structure that consisted of a general Framework with specific, strong protocols that would have allowed as many countries as could agree to strong legal mandates (banning advertising, for example) to lock down those obligations without excluding anyone from the Convention. Because the most ardent anti-tobacco advocates pushed for a single overarching treaty with the strongest consensus language, political realities ensured that the result was weaker than what could have been achieved had they not reflexively rejected the US proposal.

As a result, the US and others insisted that to reach consensus, qualifiers such as "in accordance with its constitution or constitutional principles," must be added to difficult sections to reach political consensus. This provided the flexibility necessary to allow rapid ratification and implementation of the FCTC by many countries, some of which would have had problems with a variety of specific obligations. It also would allow potential room for ratification by the US — even in the absence of reservations.

Money

In addition to the breadth of legal and other non-health expertise necessary to negotiate a legally binding international health instrument such as the FCTC, there is another major ingredient in the recipe that is often overlooked — money. It is phenomenally expensive to negotiate a treaty with 191 governments. WHO estimated that each week of INB negotiation cost approximately $1.5 million. That included payment for the increased staffing, rental of meeting halls, and especially the continuous translation and interpretation services (both written and simultaneous) in the six official languages of WHO (Arabic, Chinese, Spanish, Russian, French, and English). But perhaps the largest expense was the decision to pay for the travel of one plane ticket and per diem in Geneva for all developing countries to encourage participation, even by the smallest. That was well over 100 countries being supported by WHO Headquarters. And this does not account for the approximately $100–300 thousand average for each of the nearly 40 intercessional and regional meetings interspersed between the formal INBs. For one intercessional meeting on Illicit Tobacco trade hosted (and funded) by the US Bureau of Alcohol, Tobacco and Firearms in New York, the cost approached $1 million.

All in all, WHO spent somewhere over $15 million to negotiate and conclude the FCTC — not including the funds spent over three years by developed countries such as the US, Japan and the EU.

Definitions

One of the lessons learned by the public health representatives during this negotiation involved "definitions," something that on the surface seemed innocuous. Words in treaties are very important because they imply obligations and duties, and the definitions of those terms must be clearly agreed upon.

The public health experts had little previous experience with the importance of terms. For example, defining the commonly used phrase "health for all" in the legal sense is much more difficult than it would appear. In the Convention, what is meant by "tobacco advertising, and promotion?" Does it include only commercial advertising, or can it include personal promotion? How about the European Commission? Is it considered a state or a regional economic integration organisation? Or neither? More importantly, does it matter? What exactly is the "tobacco industry?" Does it include tobacco importers as well as manufacturers? Are small family tobacco farmers considered part of the industry?

When negotiating a treaty in six official languages, the issue of definitions is even more acute. The sensitivities of translation must also be taken into account.

The INB faced two options for dealing with the definitions issues. 1) Define terms before starting the negotiations, which could lead to hundreds of definitions done in advance to be used if needed, or 2) Wait until the Convention is nearly done, and then define just those terms necessary to reach agreement. The INB chose the latter. In the end, after discussing literally hundreds of terms, it was decided to restrict formal definitions in the FCTC to only seven terms (one included giving the European Commission status equivalent to a state in areas for which it has been ceded competence by its Member States).

Other lessons for the public health community

A "savings clause" originally was proposed for the Convention to be included in its guiding principles (Articles 2–4): "Priority should be given to measures taken to protect public health when tobacco control measures contained in this convention and its protocols are examined for compatibility with other international agreements." This was the contentious "health trumps trade" issue. It did not survive the final negotiation, not because there was not a good argument for giving health issues precedence, but because trade and political interests were, and continue to be, more powerful in most countries. Trade and Foreign Affairs Ministries were not about to allow a WHO-negotiated Convention to trump their own treaties. Plainly stated, nations have more interest in empowering the World Trade Organization than the World Health Organization.

As has been alluded to throughout this case study, public health experts stand on strong moral ground for their anti-tobacco and other pro-health positions. That does not cause any problems when health people talk to other health experts. However, in the world of international diplomacy, trade, constitutional law, and global political hegemony, international health is almost never first on a government's list of priorities. It receives rhetorical support, but real action waits in line after other pressing issues.

Perhaps the biggest take-home lesson from this negotiation is the extent to which international lawyers write treaties, not public health experts. The ability to move those who write international legal agreements to a position of understanding of the health issues is critical to moving the agenda forward in these fora.

Conclusion

Negotiation of the Framework Convention on Tobacco Control was instructive and resulted in a reasonably good final product — an excellent "first" health treaty for WHO. Unfortunately, much of the language is hortatory and most of the real work for implementing tobacco control and health promotion measures will require national action and laws to enforce the ideas promulgated by the treaty. In part, this is secondary to the inexperience of the public health community in the ways of international diplomatic negotiation, and the insistence that all of the 191 WHO Member Countries agreed by consensus on even the most contentious political issues.

However, many governments subsequently have used the Convention to justify new laws within their own national governing process, and that is a great secondary benefit. Perhaps just as important, the lessons in diplomatic negotiation helped make WHO's second global health treaty, the 2005 "International Health Regulations," a better document than it would have been without the basic preparatory work and lessons learned in successfully negotiating the Tobacco Convention.

Importantly, the public health community must persuade foreign policy, diplomatic, trade, justice, and defense officials that international health is an integral part of what they do. At the beginning of the 21st century we have many important concerns vying for our leaders' attention, such as a worsening economic picture, global warming, ethnic hatred and regional conflicts, radical fundamentalism, terrorism, and inequitable economic development and trade. WHO Member States must convince powerful foreign affairs officials in their countries to embrace relevant health issues in the first tier of policy and budget concerns. We can start by learning to speak their language and eliminating the sanctimonious lecturing for which global health advocates are known.

Tommy Thompson, US Secretary of Health and Human Services, signed the Convention for the United States in May 2004. It has not yet been submitted to the Senate for ratification, although neither the Bush nor the Obama Administrations have voiced objection to Senate ratification. As of June 2010, 169 countries are party to the FCTC. The Conference of Parties has met three times and will convene again in November 2010 (absent ratification, and therefore membership and financial support of the US). Hopefully, the Secretary of State and the President will submit the Convention to the Senate for ratification as a high priority.

References

1. da Costa e Silva VL, David A (eds.) (2009) History of the WHO framework convention on tobacco control. WHO Press, World Health Organization: Geneva.
2. Alcazar S. (2008) The WHO framework convention on tobacco control: A case study in foreign policy and health — A view from Brazil. Global Health Programme Working Paper No. 2, The Graduate Institute: Geneva.
3. World Health Organization (2009) WHO report on the global tobacco epidemic, 2009: implementing smoke-free environments, p.8. Available at http://www.who.int/tobacco/resources/publications/en/World Health Organization: Geneva.
4. World Health Organization (1996) International framework convention for tobacco control. (WHA Resolution Number: WHA49.17) World Health Organization: Geneva.
5. Constitution of the World Health Organization (2009) In: *Basic Documents.* pp 1–18. World Health Organization: Geneva.
6. World Health Organization (1999) Towards a WHO framework convention on tobacco control. (WHA Resolution Number: WHA52.18) World Health Organization: Geneva.
7. World Health Organization (2000) Framework convention on tobacco control. (WHA Resolution Number: WHA53.16) World Health Organization: Geneva.
8. Assunta M, Chapman S. (2006) Health treaty dilution: A case study of Japan's influence on the language of the WHO Framework Convention on Tobacco Control. *J Epidemiol Community Health* 60: 751–756.
9. World Health Organization. (2003) WHO Framework convention on tobacco control. Available at http://www.who.int/fctc/text_download/en/index.html World Health Organization: Geneva.
10. *Ibid.*, Article 13, pp. 11–12.
11. *Ibid.*, Article 8, p. 8.
12. *Ibid.*, Article 30, p. 26.
13. United Nations, *Vienna Convention on the Law of Treaties*, 23 May 1969, United Nations, Treaty Series, vol. 1155, p. 331, available at: http://www.unhcr.org/refworld/docid/3ae6b3a10.html

5

Negotiating the Revised International Health Regulations (IHR)*

Rebecca Katz[i] and Anna Muldoon[ii]

Abstract

The Revised International Health Regulations adopted in 2005 by the World Health Assembly of the World Health Organization marked an important shift in global cooperation and coordination in the fight against infectious diseases and other acute public health emergencies. With the urgency of Severe Acute Respiratory Syndrome in the background, there was little debate that the existing health regulations had to be amended. This case study describes the interplay between health concerns, security, and sovereignty which created a dynamic framework in which divergent national interests had to be defended. The complicated but speedy process of the drafting, revising, and agreeing upon flexible and universally accepted provisions highlighted the importance of balancing health expertise and professional diplomatic skills in complex international negotiations.

* We are grateful to the many people who graciously spoke with us about the IHR negotiating process. Any errors in this paper, however, are the authors' responsibility.
[i] Rebecca Katz is an Assistant Professor at the George Washington University School of Public Health and Health Services, in the Department of Health Policy.
[ii] Anna Muldoon is a Research Assistant in the same department. Any matters regarding this paper should be addressed to Rebecca Katz.

Introduction

In May of 2005, the World Health Assembly of the World Health Organization adopted the Revised International Health Regulations, following almost a decade of discussion and negotiations. These regulations, known as IHR (2005), marked a shift in global cooperation and collaboration in the fight against infectious diseases and other acute public health emergencies, particularly public health events that have the potential to cross national borders. Not only did the regulations establish networks for better transparency, cooperation, and governance, but they also called for the development of core capacities by all Member States. IHR (2005) entered into force in the summer of 2007. This case study describes the impetus for revising the regulations, the process by which the revisions took place, challenges and obstacles to the negotiation process, and lessons for future negotiation efforts. This case study also highlights the importance of having the appropriate people at the negotiating table, and the need for high level diplomats, health professionals with technological expertise, and experienced negotiators to best argue for national interests.

The Problem in Context

History of the international health regulations

The international community has long recognized the fact that infectious diseases know no borders, and that nations must set regulations and standards for cooperation in order to control the spread of disease. Such international agreements, though, reflected the threats of the time and the state of knowledge regarding specific pathogens. Early agreements focused almost entirely on cholera, as Europe had experienced repeated waves of cholera epidemics throughout the 19th century, each one spreading further than the last.[1] The first International Sanitary Conference (ISC) was called in 1851 in response to these repeated cholera outbreaks in Europe, generally thought to be imported by ships bearing trade goods and workers from Asia.[2] While cholera brought nations together at first, disagreement on the cause of the disease would lead to intense disagreement among the delegates and end the first several ISCs. The lack of scientific agreement fueled diplomatic debate on appropriate containment and quarantine measures, and even as an increasing number of nations joined the ISCs, theories on the cause and spread of cholera abounded and scientists continued to argue vehemently at each conference.[3] This intense debate prevented an acceptable agreement from being reached at the first six conferences. It was not until 1892 — at the seventh ISC — when a narrowly focused agreement finally was signed.[4]

Cholera was the nearly exclusive focus of the ISCs until the 10th conference in 1897, when on-going plague epidemics and the fear of plague spreading throughout Europe by way of pilgrims returning from Mecca broadened the discussion.[3] At the end of 1897, there were four International Sanitary Conventions in force: Maritime Quarantine (1892), Land Quarantine and Disease Reporting (1893), Pilgrims to Mecca (1894), and Plague (1897). These four agreements were complied into the new International Sanitary Convention of 1903, which also codified the practice of de-ratting certificates (certificates stating when a ship has been inspected for rats or fumigated) and established an international health office in Paris.[5] Despite the increasing focus on international cooperation, it was not until the 1907 conference in Rome that the "Office international d'hygiène publique" in Paris was formed, funded, and agreed upon by the European nations, the United States (US), and Brazil to oversee international health agreements.[3] The inclusion of the US and Brazil in the founders of the Office would cause difficulties after the founding of the League of Nations Health Office in 1919. The US blocked the combination of the two offices (the US was not a member of the League of Nations), so the offices worked side-by-side until the founding of the World Health Organization.

When the World Health Organization (WHO) was founded in 1946, the duties of the Office international d'hygiène publique were transferred by a protocol to the WHO Constitution, and the International Sanitary Conventions were re-named and re-negotiated to become the International Sanitary Regulations of 1951.[6] These regulations remained focused on control of disease at borders, and addressed a list of six diseases, primarily, though, cholera, plague, and yellow fever.[7] Despite major social changes, these regulations did not change significantly between 1951 and 1969, when they were slightly amended (including dropping two louse-borne diseases — relapsing fever and typhus — from the list of notifiable diseases) and re-named the International Health Regulations (1969)

[IHR(1969)]. They were again amended in 1973 to alter cholera practices[8] and in 1981 to remove smallpox from the list of notifiable diseases.[9] By the Constitution of the World Health Organization, all Member States who did not submit significant reservations were party to the regulations.[10]

Push to revise the international health regulations

Despite the existence of the 1969 International Health Regulations, there was neither specific discussion of the appropriateness of the IHR requirements nor universal compliance among the WHO Member States.[11] By the late twentieth century, the IHR (1969) was an outdated agreement, with a focus on nineteenth century diseases and control measures. Although the agreement had been updated repeatedly since its first iteration in 1892, the body of the agreement had changed little in response to emerging concerns.

The emergence and global spread of HIV/AIDS throughout the 1980s and 1990s, the re-emergence of diseases such as cholera, and the largest outbreak of Ebola since 1976 in the Democratic Republic of Congo (then Zaire) in 1995 made it clear to the WHO that the stagnant IHR (1969) was not flexible enough to respond to the threat of emerging infectious diseases and needed to be updated.[12,13] In 1995, the World Health Assembly (WHA) passed Resolution WHA 48.7, calling for the revision of IHR (1969) to include response to emerging infectious diseases and a framework that better reflected the emergence of global networks and rapid travel. Specifically, the resolution noted "that there is a continuous evolution in the public health threat posed by infectious diseases related to the agents themselves, to their easier transmission in changing physical and social environments, and to diagnostic treatment capabilities."[14]

Although the resolution passed and there was some interest in revising the IHR, little was done.[iii] In May 2001, the WHA adopted another resolution (WHA 54.14) on Global health security: epidemic alert and response,[15] addressing the importance of detection and response to public health emergencies of international concern, and in 2002, the Assembly

---

[iii] The WHO held a series of expert consultations and working groups between 1995 and 1997 in order to gain support and consensus on the direction of the revision process, and a report was produced and reported to the 54th WHA.[18]

adopted WHA 55.16 regarding public health responses to natural, accidental or deliberate uses of biological, chemical or radiological material.[16] Both of these resolutions highlighted the importance of revising the IHR. Still, nothing of any consequence happened.[iv]

In 2003, the outbreak of SARS dramatically demonstrated the potential international danger of emerging infectious diseases and specifically highlighted the importance of transparency and global cooperation as essential elements to contain public health emergencies at the source.[17] The detection and response to SARS also showed where the WHO needed more regulatory power if the organization was to be effective in responding to emergencies. The threat of SARS brought significant political and technical will to negotiate a new agreement — one that would address the realities of the twenty-first century.

Procedures for the negotiations

In the midst of the SARS outbreak, the World Health Assembly adopted Resolution WHA 56.28, reiterating calls to revise the IHR and establishing an Intergovernmental Working Group (IGWG) to begin the revision process.[18] Work began almost immediately. The first draft of the new IHR was created in 2003 by technical experts at the WHO Secretariat, intended to be a starting point for negotiations. By January 2004, the first Secretariat draft was sent to Member States for comment.[19] The following spring, written comments were collected and two rounds of regional consultations took place. New sub-working groups formed within the IGWG to look at information sources, scope, intentional use, armed forces, and the decision algorithm for determining a public health emergency of international concern.[20] Three subsequent meetings of the IGWG were held in November 2004, February 2005, and in May 2005. Following the last round of negotiations, the WHA adopted the Revised International Health Regulations (2005) on 23 May 2005, with entry into force in June 2007.[21] The Chair of those negotiations, a diplomat by training, has described her own experiences in that process.[22]

[iv] Again, workshops and meetings were held in 2001 and 2002, particularly around notification instruments and core capacities, but there was no further movement towards a revised text.[18]

Table 1.   Major Components of the International Health Regulations — 1969 and 2005

Area of focus	IHR (1969)	IHR (2005)
Type of threats	Infectious diseases	Any public health emergency
Focus of activities	Control disease outbreaks at ports and borders without hampering trade and travel	Detect, report, and contain any public health threats at ports, borders, and anywhere they might occur within borders to prevent international spread
Risk assessment	Specific diseases of historical significance (cholera, plague, yellow fever)	Decision instrument to evaluate the risks and potential impact of the public health event (Annex 2)
Response	Pre-determined public health controls at points of entryt	Flexible, evidence-based responses adapted to nature of threa
Communications	Nations identify appropriate authorities on an ad hoc basis	Notifications to and from WHO via designated IHR National Focal Points
Capacity requirements	Public health and infection control measures at ports of entry	Capacity to detect, assess, report, and respond to public health threats in near-real time at national and community levels

Source: Fischer J, Katz R. International Health Regulations 101. Stimson Center IHR (2005): from the global to the local. March 2010. Available at: http://www.stimson.org/globalhealth/GHS_IHR_ website/Policy%20Brief_1-%20IHR%20101.pdf

The Players and their Roles in the IHR (2005) Negotiations

The intergovernmental working group

An Intergovernmental Working Group (IGWG) was formed, comprised of representatives from 151 member countries of the WHO and 25 organisations representing United Nations agencies, European and African Unions, and various non-governmental entities.[23] Members of the IGWG were solicited from all WHO countries, with a limit of three official delegates per State Party. Most nations sent technical and health experts for the IGWG, although some nations sent more political representation, which had a clear impact on tone and content of the negotiations.

Key delegates

While IHR (2005) is more or less a consensus document, and all nations were given equal weight in their opinions for or against the regulations, several nations and blocks of countries stood out as major contributors to the negotiation process, be it because of particular concerns or delegates' ability to broker agreements. The concerns raised during the negotiations were primarily defined by national country interests, based on political concerns, previous experiences, or governments' positions on other international negotiations.

China

China was a significant player in the negotiation of IHR (2005), particularly around issues of national sovereignty. Concerns about sovereignty were manifested in discussions over verification processes, the ability for WHO to rely upon non-state reporting (discussed in more detail below), cross-border access of WHO investigative teams, and implementation of health measures. China entered the negotiations particularly sensitive to international condemnation over the country's failure to report in a timely fashion to WHO authorities the 2003 SARS outbreak, further complicating the discussions over non-state reporting mechanisms. In addition to staunchly defending national sovereignty, China's position regarding Taiwan had the potential to derail negotiations early in the process.

Iran

The negotiator from Iran played a key role on the issue of including chemical, biological, and radio-nuclear events in the revised IHR, as well as any language pertaining to intentional and deliberate release of the aforementioned. The Iranian position was to remove any of these words from the text of the regulations, which led to intense debate on several articles. Iran's position was based on their concern that the IHR could be used as a security agreement if intentional events were directly included.

The United States

The US came into the negotiations with several national interests it wished to pursue. First, the US delegation believed it was essential, from a public health perspective, for the IHRs to address both intentional and accidental release of agents that would cause a public health emergency. Second, the US, having just pulled out of the negotiation of a verification protocol under the Biological and Toxins Weapons Convention (BWC), was strongly opposed to the inclusion of specific references to or ad referendum language on a verification mechanism under the Revised IHR. In defending its national infrastructure, the US tried to get other federalist nations to push for inclusion of language regarding public health authorities in a federalist form of government. Lastly, the US took a strong stance on operational security and other concerns regarding how the IHR would apply to armed forces. The US was not able to gain support for such provisions in the text and instead submitted a formal reservation on federalism and understandings regarding intentional and accidental releases of agents and application of the regulations to the armed forces.

The United Kingdom

The United Kingdom played a significant role in the negotiations on two issues: health measures and border restrictions. The discussion of health measures focused on whether or not a nation could impose health measures which were not supported by scientific evidence. Although there was a large debate about limiting health measures and national sovereignty, Britain's interest was specific to the question of scientific evidence. Their concerns likely focused on several common health measures, such as the use of masks, self-isolation, and quarantine, which are presumed to be effective even where little scientific evidence exists.[24]

The second issue, border restrictions, focused on developing countries' fear that restrictions on entry under the IHR would be used to prevent immigration. In particular, countries with higher rates of endemic diseases were concerned the disease burden could be used as an excuse to prevent immigration. Britain, along with other developed countries, spoke out strongly against this argument.

Cuba

Cuba had multiple concerns throughout the course of the IGWG process, and close to the end of the negotiation process the government planned to re-open debate on several already agreed upon articles. There was, however, virtually no support for this action. At the close of the negotiations, Cuba made a final statement regarding the process of the IGWG, how the text was not adopted by consensus, and that the process was undemocratic. The chair of the IGWG heard these concerns and promised to note them in her report to the WHA. Cuba did not enter any formal reservations, declarations, or understandings to IHR (2005).

Switzerland

While Switzerland had few strong national interests aside from the scientific content of the text, delegates from this country served an essential role in brokering discussions and building consensus around contested issues.

Regional groups

As in many international negotiations, groups of nations with similar interests and regional issues banded together to support or oppose parts of the text. These blocks included a group of African nations particularly concerned about how health measures might be applied unfairly to discriminate against travelers from selected areas. These nations and another group of Latin American countries also worked to ensure that health measures could not serve to modify immigration policies.

Challenges Faced and the Outcomes

While the negotiations were successful in the end, the process encountered several complex issues, both within and outside the traditional domains of public health. The original drafts of the IHR (2005) produced primarily by technical experts included many scientific and public health principles that the international community supported. The language of the initial text, however, did not reflect political needs and requirements. Additionally, several major issues need to be addressed in negotiation. Here we discuss some of the primary issues that were problematic during the negotiations and describe how various obstacles were eventually resolved. We discuss these by the relevant section in the actual IHR.

Non-state reporting

The WHO established the Global Outbreak Alert and Response Network in 1997 and by 2005 it was receiving 77% of its information from non-state sources.[25] A major issue during the IHR (2005) negotiations, however, was whether the WHO Secretariat would be able to use information obtained from unofficial sources, including media and private sector organisations, to identify potential public health emergencies of international concern. China and Iran, in particular, opposed WHO accepting reports from non-state sources, insisting that verification of outbreaks needed to come exclusively from official governmental reports of affected countries. Other nations, such as Argentina, suggested that the WHO be allowed to receive information from unofficial sources, but that the source must be named and shared with the affected nation.

The first working drafts of IHR (2005) included the reporting of "rumours" of events, which caused a significant amount of tension in the negotiations. The IGWG changed the language to be more politically astute and re-worded the provisions so that China, Iran, and the other nations expressing concern were willing to accept the revised article.

WHO Secretariat Draft	Final Language
Article 8 Verification	**Article 10 Verification**
1. WHO, in consultation with the health administration of the State concerned, shall verify **rumours of public health risks** which may involve or result in international spread of disease and/or possible interference with international traffic, subject to these Regulations.	1. WHO shall request, in accordance with Article 9, verification from a State Party of reports from **sources other than notifications or consultations of events** which may constitute a public health emergency of international concern allegedly occurring in the State's territory. In such cases, WHO shall inform the State Party concerned regarding the reports it is seeking to verify.

Sovereignty

National concerns on sovereignty issues can be linked to several of the key roadblocks in the negotiations of the IHR. The concern over national sovereignty is not unique to the IHR. There are persistent concerns by nations with regard to international organisations, the power they are given for governance, and the ability of those organisations to take actions that affect the economic and political situation of a given nation. Specific to the IHR debate, nations were concerned about the power WHO would be given regarding accepting unofficial sources of information, verification of such information, enacting health measures, conducting investigations, and the granting of power to a health organisation to coordinate the response to chemical, biological, radiological, and nuclear incidents- all very much linked to national security concerns.

Several states were specifically concerned about issues of sovereignty and the potential for the new IHR to become an invasive document. This led to careful and touchy negotiations around any issue that had implications for

countries' notions of sovereignty and the removal or alteration of several articles from the draft IHR. The debate on sovereignty played out strongly
through original articles on intentional use reporting and samples, application
of health measures, information-sharing, and WHO verification teams. In the
final draft, the Articles referring to intentional use reporting and samples were
entirely removed, while the Articles on health measures and verification were
significantly altered to address concerns about sovereignty.

The issue of Taiwan

China was very concerned with if and how Taiwan would be recognised
as a partner in the IHR. Taiwan's quest for independence and China's
insistence on "One China" had caused problems in multiple international
agreements in the United Nations, World Trade Organization, and the
WHO.[26] Several nations were able to work with representatives from
Taiwan and China to secure language in the 'Principles' section of the IHR
to ensure that Taiwan was covered under the regulations without including it as an individual party in the negotiations. Article 3.3 refers to the
protection of "all peoples of the world from the international spread of
disease" and sets a goal of universal application of the IHR.[27]

Concern by the Chinese over Taiwan also surfaced in discussions
regarding the reference to other international organisations since some of
the other organisations recognised Taiwan, while others did not. This was
partially resolved by the drafting of issue #4 in the Preamble of the IHR,
which states that the WHO is expected to cooperate and coordinate activities with other international organisations.[27] The World Trade
Organization was removed from the list because Taiwan is an active member of the organization. The Office International des Epizootics, which
includes Taiwan as a member, was agreed to be listed last.

Finally, China submitted a declaration that the IHR (2005) applies to
the entire territory of the People's Republic of China, including the
Taiwan Province.[27]

Health measures

Several states objected to articles disallowing national implementation of
health measures that were more restrictive than recommended by the WHO.

The states viewed this as an infringement on their sovereignty because it would prevent them from exercising public health authority within their own borders. The British also advocated for the right to impose measures not supported by scientific studies — most likely measures such as hand washing and social distancing, for which there is significant historical basis but little scientific evidence. In the final meeting of the IGWG, nations agreed on provisions that would allow Member States to adopt protective health measures beyond those recommended by WHO, but that those measures must be based on scientific principles, reported to the WHO and other States Parties, and not be more restrictive of travel and trade. In addition, States Parties affected by health measures, such as border controls, also have the ability to request the scientific evidence for and/or challenge those measures through the dispute process of the WHO as defined in Article 56.[27]

Verification

Early drafts of IHR 2005 included the ability for the WHO to send a team into a country to verify an incident. In the original working paper on the IHR, States Parties would have had to "collaborate…in conducting on-the-spot studies by a team sent by WHO, with the purpose of ensuring that appropriate control measures are being employed"[19] under an article titled "Verification." The US was strongly opposed to this language and thought it echoed the failed verification protocol negotiations under the Biological Weapons Convention (BWC). China and Iran in particular also were strongly opposed to what was seen as an article allowing the WHO to violate state sovereignty at will. One of the strongest fears was that a verification mechanism would create an intrusive WHO regime with inspection measures that would violate states individual political sovereignty. Several nations pushed for language specifically referencing verification, but in the end, concerns regarding sovereignty and fears of creating an alternate BWC verification protocol combined to remove any kind of explicit language on verification from the IHR.

Other international agreements

The US was concerned that some articles of the draft IHR would force the government to violate WTO agreements or were not aligned with the

Sanitary and Phytosanitary Agreement (SPS) or the Technical Barriers to Trade (TBT). Conflicts with the International Atomic Energy Agency (IAEA) reporting requirements concerned many nations party to IAEA agreements. In addition, nuclear safety professionals in the US appeared concerned that the IHRs might conflict with IAEA requirements or, at the very least, require double reporting that would be onerous for the industry.[28] There was significant discussion about the BWC and Chemical Weapons Convention regarding the need to ensure there was no overlap and that the agreements would not come into conflict at any point. The final language reads:

1. WHO shall cooperate and coordinate its activities, as appropriate, with other competent intergovernmental organisations or international bodies in the implementation of these Regulations, including through the conclusion of agreements and other similar arrangements.
2. In cases in which notification or verification of, or response to, an event is primarily within the competence of other intergovernmental organisations or international bodies, WHO shall coordinate its activities with such organisations or bodies in order to ensure the application of adequate measures for the protection of public health.[27]

Although this language does not preclude WHO action to protect health, it limits the organisation's measures to those specifically related to health impacts and places the rest of the authority with the appropriate organisation.

Definition of "disease" and inclusion of Chemical, Biological, Radiological and Nuclear Events

During the negotiations, a long and contentious discussion ensued about including Chemical, Biological, Radiological or Nuclear (CBRN) events in the definition of disease, particularly in the early drafts, when the definition included both accidental and intentional release. The US, European Union, New Zealand, Canada, Nicaragua, and Australia wanted to make the range of events covered by the IHRs explicit in the text, with inclusion of language on all kinds of CBRN events, and intentional or accidental release of specific agents, in the definition of disease and of Public Health Emergency of International Concern (PHEIC). However, other nations were vehemently opposed to that position. Iran, the Eastern Mediterranean Region, and African countries were very concerned that by including intentional release, the IHR 2005 would become a security, rather than health, focused agreement and fervently opposed language including the topic. China and Cuba criticised nations that wanted CBRN mentioned in the IHR but which had opposed the BWC Verification Protocol. Although the governments of developed countries insisted that the inclusion of intentional release would not change the character of the treaty, the inclusion of intentional release made it very difficult to convince the objectors that there was no security motive behind the inclusion. To break the impasse, Switzerland convened a small group and led informal discussions to reach a compromise. The final text does not specifically name chemical, biological or radiological materials. The language focusing on "events of any origin" was the compromise that allowed the negotiations to move forward. The final language reads:

> If a State Party has evidence of an unexpected or unusual public health event within its territory, irrespective of origin or source, which may constitute a public health emergency of international concern, it shall provide to WHO all relevant public health information.[27]

The US however, submitted a formal understanding that the US sees the IHR as referring to public health emergencies of international concern, including those events caused by the natural, accidental or deliberate release of CBRN materials.[27]

Inclusion of a reference to WHA 55.16, "Global public health response to natural occurrence, accidental release or deliberate use of biological and chemical agents or radio-nuclear material that affect health," was also a contentious point in the negotiations.[16] After the long debate with Iran about the inclusion of deliberate or intentional release, the inclusion of a reference to WHA 55.16, which deals specifically with that topic, was a victory for the nations that had pushed for inclusion of language explicitly covering deliberate events.

Decision instrument for assessing potential public health emergencies of international concern (PHEICS)

The final text of IHR (2005) contains Annex 2, known as the decision instrument for the assessment and notification of events that may constitute a public health emergency of international concern. The purpose of this instrument is to help nations evaluate public health events and determine if they are required to report the event to the WHO. The Annex 2 decision instrument became a point of contention in the negotiations and the final version differs significantly from the original. Both the final and draft versions are shown below side by side.

The debate over the decision instrument emphasized the disagreement on whether to include a list of specifically reportable diseases. With the focus on emerging infections in the 2005 IHR, several delegates did not want to specify any list of diseases. In contrast, many developing countries argued that they would be unable to get grant or government funding for surveillance without a specific list to show their focus. Discussion about the inclusion of intentional and deliberate events also played out in the debate over the decision instrument, particularly once a list of diseases and events was included. In the end "Any event...including those of unknown causes or sources and those involving other events or diseases...shall lead to utilization of the algorithm"[27] was the compromise language that allowed the decision instrument to move past this roadblock.

The decision instrument was drafted by a separate ad hoc committee of experts, focusing on creating the simplest possible instrument. After the debate about a specific list emerged, the committee added a top tier allowing multiple ways to enter the matrix. While the original instrument only assessed the severity, novelty, and likelihood of international spread, the final instrument allows an immediate decision for a short list of diseases and an assessment path for unknown events or a longer list of potentially serious infections. This compromise satisfied both sides and retained the ability to assess novel pathogens through the IHR.

Cost of implementation and financing the IHR

A financing mechanism was another highly contentious issue in the final negotiations of the IHR, particularly given concerns about the cost of

Comparison of Draft Annex 2 (right) and Final Annex 2 (left)

The top layer of the right version was added in negotiations to address concerns over having no specific list of notifiable diseases in the original.

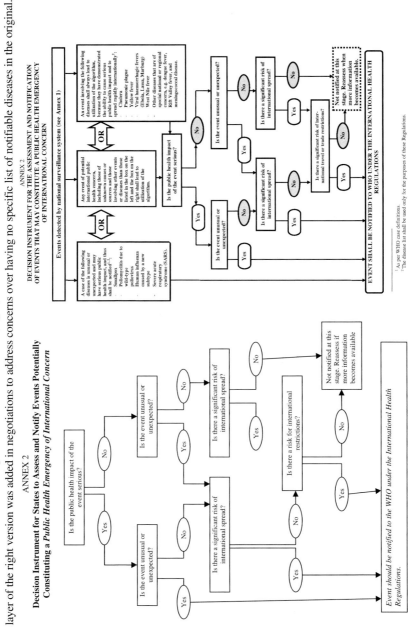

reaching compliance with IHR and how compliance would be defined. It was noted several times during negotiations that developing countries would have a difficult time reaching the surveillance and response goals laid out in the new IHR. There was also discussion of creating a financing mechanism to fund implementation in poorer countries, but this fell by the wayside over the course of negotiations.

From the US perspective, putting a financial commitment into the IHR was never an option. The US Congress would never have authorised an agreement that committed the US government to give money to another government. The general language in the final agreement left open the possibility to aid other nations without committing any group of nations to a specific mechanism or amount of money.[27]

Travel restrictions and immigration

Restrictions on borders and travel caused concern among many nations during the negotiations. African countries in particular were concerned that restrictions created through the IHR would be used to prevent immigration from any country with endemic disease. Developed nations and particularly the European Union attempted to reassure the developing world that this was not the case, but the wording in the final text had to be carefully crafted so that the IHR would not become a tool to deny immigration.[27]

Emergency committee

The emergency committee is a body of experts that can be assembled by the Director- General of the WHO to evaluate potential PHEICs and create recommendations to slow the spread of disease. The developed countries were concerned that any decision to declare a PHEIC could significantly damage the economy of the affected country. The fear was that the emergency committee could declare a country dangerous based solely on scientific opinion and might do so too quickly. Developed countries in particular were insistent that their country representatives be involved in the determination process to ensure their positions would be heard. Another fear was that the WHO would gain too much power through the Emergency Committee. This was resolved through two additions to the agreement. First, it was agreed that the WHO Director-General would appoint one member to the roster of experts at the request of each State Party.[27] Second, it was agreed that the Emergency Committee would include at least one member who is an expert nominated by "the State Party within whose territory the event arises."[27] Third, the affected State Party has the opportunity to present to the Emergency Committee before any decision is made.[27] Combined, these provisions ensure that the view of the affected State Party is taken into account and reassured concerned nations.

Points of entry

Ideally, every State Party would have the ability to control the entry and exit of disease along all borders, but in the negotiation of the IHR it rapidly became clear that this was not the case. As a result the phrase "as far as practicable" appears repeatedly in Part IV of the IHR 2005, which focuses on "Points of Entry." This section allows nations to designate Points of Entry, rather than attempting to assess disease risk along the entire border, limiting the resources necessary to comply with the IHR.[27] In addition, each section of Part IV calling for specific measures to prevent disease, for example vector control, sanitary measures, or control of ship behaviour at ports, includes the phrase "as far as practicable." While the phrase may appear rather insignificant, the extent to which it relieves State Parties of unachievable expectations for compliance is very significant, particularly for developing countries.

Lessons Learned

Negotiating the IHR 2005 was unusual compared to many international agreements in that there was universal agreement by all Member States from the outset that a new agreement was needed and that the new agreement had to address a specific set of issues, including emerging infectious diseases. The universal agreement that the IHR had to be changed affected the content of the negotiations. All delegations went into discussions knowing agreement had to be reached. Although there were many difficult and political points to be debated, the universal investment enabled the negotiations to focus on technical issues and not on the validity of or need for the IHR, or on the importance of the primary issues.

While this background made negotiations easier in some respects, it also affected the type of negotiators governments sent to the IHR meetings. Those countries that viewed the IHR as an exclusively health-focused agreement sent technical experts — scientists, doctors, public health professionals. It is clear in the first working paper for the negotiations that the political complexity around some issues was not fully understood by the technical expert groups and this caused significant difficulties initially. In contrast, countries that viewed the IHR as a potential security agreement sent highly experienced negotiators, particularly arms control experts, who were powerful figures in the debates and more knowledgeable about the political ramifications of certain lines of argument. In particular, because there were few high ranking diplomats from the health-focused nations decisions could not be made quickly and bottom line positions could not be updated rapidly during negotiations. This imbalance had a clear effect on the final outcome of the negotiations and is something to examine when choosing health delegations for future negotiations.

Conclusion

Overall, the negotiation of the IHR 2005 was a success, both in its speed and in the creation of a flexible agreement that is universally accepted. Although the negotiations experienced some road-blocks, none were contentious enough to sink the agreement as a whole. Many of the issues that arose in the course of IHR negotiations are consistent issues on the international stage. Taiwan's status has caused incidents in both the UN and the WTO and tension will continue to be an issue in negotiations over future international agreements. Sovereignty is a concern for nations whenever they are negotiating international agreements; it has been an issue in every version of the IHR, from the first ISC to the 2005 discussions, and will likely come up again in the next discussion of IHR revisions.

The inclusion of an all-hazards approach to health in the IHR 2005 is a victory for international health security and sets the stage for future agreements to address a broad range of issues affecting human health. Although chemical, biological, and radio-nuclear events are not specifically mentioned in the IHR 2005, inclusion of these hazards is clear in the final language and the international community clearly understands that these issues are included on a de facto basis. While the issue presented a significant point of contention during the negotiations, the discussions nonetheless concluded with a solution that both advances international public health efforts and accommodates the security concerns of nations opposed to the inclusion of the full range of health hazards.

There was little debate that the IHR needed to be revised, but there was significant disaccord over what the final agreement would look like. Overall, the end result is more open to future updates and evolution than previous iterations. The speed with which the new IHR were drafted, revised, and agreed upon is a clear success of the negotiations. In addition, the legally binding nature of the new IHR and the inclusion of all WHO Member States in an opt-out treaty was a significant achievement for participants. With the 2007 entry into force of the IHR (2005) the WHO took a major step forward in protecting the world from public health emergencies.

References

1. Huber, V. The Unification of the Globe by Disease? The International Sanitary Conferences on Cholera, 1851–1894. *Hist J* (2006) 49: 453–476.
2. International Sanitary Conferences. (2010) Contagion: Historical Views of Diseases and Epidemics. *Harvard Open Collections Program*. Available at: http://ocp.hul.harvard.edu/contagion/sanitaryconferences.html
3. Howard-Jones, N. (1975) *The Scientific Background of the Internaitonal Sanitary Conferences 1851–1938*, World Health Organization: Geneva.
4. *"Protocoles de la Conférence Sanitaire Internationale: Ouverte à Paris le 9 avril 1859"*. (1892) Impr. Nationale de J. Bertero: Rome.
5. *"Conférence Sanitaire Internationale de Paris, 10 octobre–3 décembre 1903: Procès–Verbaux"*. (1897) Forzani et Cie, Imprimeurs du Sénat: Rome.
6. Proceedings and Final Acts of the International Health Conference Held in New York From 19 June to July 1946. *Official Records of the World Health Organization, No. 2*.

7. The New International Sanitary Regulations. *Am J Public Health* (1952) 42: 194–196. Available at: http://ajph.aphapublications.org/cgi/reprint/42/2/194.pdf

8. World Health Assembly. (1973) Additional Regulations amending the International health Regulations (1969). (WHO Document Number: WHA26.55) World Health Organization: Geneva.

9. World Health Assembly. (1981) Amendment of the International Health Regulations (1969). (WHO Document Number: WHA34.13). World Health Organization: Geneva.

10. Constitution of the World Health Organization. (2006) In: *Basic Documents:Supplement.* pp1–18. World Health Organization: Geneva.

11. Fidler D. (1999) *International law and infectious diseases.* Clarendon Press: Oxford.

12. Know Cases and Outbreaks of Ebola Hemorrhagic Fever, in Chronological Order. (2006) Centers for Disease Control and Prevention. Available at: http://www.cdc.gov/ncidod/dvrd/spb/mnpages/dispages/ebola/ebolatable.htm

13. Centers for Disease Control and Prevention. (1995) Update: Outbreak of Ebola Viral Hemorrhagic Fever — Zaire, 1995. *Morbidity and Mortality Reports Weekly* 44: 468–469. Available at: http://www.cdc.gov/mmwr/preview/mmwrhtml/00038026.htm

14. World Health Assembly. (1995) Revision and Updating of the International Health Regulations. (WHO Document Number: WHA48.7) World Health Organization: Geneva.

15. World Health Organization. (2001) Global health security: epidemic alert and response. (WHO Document Number: WHA54.14) World Health Organization: Geneva.

16. World Health Assembly. (2002) Global public health response to natural occurrence, accidental release or deliberate use of biological and chemical agents or radionuclear material that affect health. (WHO Document Number: WHA55.16) World Health Organization: Geneva.

17. World Health Assembly. (2003) Revision of the International Health Regulations. (WHO Document Number: WHA56.25 addendum 1) World Health Organization: Geneva.

18. World Health Assembly. (2003) Revision of the International Health Regulations. (WHO Document Number: WHA56.28) World Health Organization: Geneva.

19. World Health Organization. (2004) Intergovernmental Working Group on the International Health Regulations: Working Paper for Regional Consultations. (WHO Document Number: IGWG/IHR/Working Paper/12.2003) World Health Organization: Geneva.

20. Silberschmidt, G. (2009) "Negotiating IHR: International Health Regulations." Presented in Nairobi.

21. World Health Assembly. (2005) Revision of the International Health Regulations. (WHO Document Number: WHA58.3) World Health Organization: Geneva.

22. Whelan M. (2008) Negotiating the International Health Regulations, Global Health Programme Working Paper No. 1, The Graduate Institute of International and Development Studies, Geneva.

23. World Health Organization. (2004) Groupe de Travail Intergouvernemental sur la Révision du Règlement Sanitaire International: List of Participants. (WHO Document Number: A/IHR/IGWG/DIV/3 Rev.1). Geneva, Switzerland.

24. European Center for Disease Control and Prevention. (2009) Guide to public health measures to reduce the impact of influenza pandemics in Europe: 'The ECDC Menu'. Available at: http://www.ecdc.europa.eu/en/publications/Publications/0906_TER_Public_Health_Measures_for_Influenza_Pandemics.pdf.

25. Tucker JB. Updating the International Health Regulations. *Biosecur Bioter* (2005) 3: 338–347.

26. Roberge M, Lee, Y. (2009) China-Taiwan Relations. Council of Foreign Relations. Available at: http://www.cfr.org/publication/9223/chinataiwan_relations.html

27. World Health Organization. (2008) *International Health Regulations* (2005): 2nd Ed. World Health Organization: Geneva.

28. International Atomic Energy Agency Secretariat. (2007) Report of the Fourth Meeting of the Representatives of Competent Authorities Identified Under the Convention on Early Notification of a Nuclear Accident and the Convention on Assistance in the Case of a Nuclear Accident. International Atomic Energy Agency: Vienna.

6

Transformative Diplomacy: Negotiation of the WHO Global Code of Practice on the International Recruitment of Health Personnel[*]

Allyn L. Taylor[i] and Ibadat S. Dhillon[ii]

Abstract

The May 2010 adoption of the World Health Organization Global Code of Practice on the International Recruitment of Health Personnel created a global architecture, including ethical norms and institutional and legal arrangements, to guide international cooperation and serve as a platform for continuing dialogue on the critical problem of health worker migration. Highlighting the contribution of non-binding instruments to global health governance, this case study describes the preparation process for the Code from early stages to adoption. Detailed are the dynamic negotiations

[*] The opinions expressed herein are those of the authors alone and do not necessarily reflect the views of the World Health Organization or Realizing Rights.
[i] Allyn L. Taylor is a Visiting Professor of Law at Georgetown University Law Center. She has also been a legal consultant to the WHO Human Resources for Health Division in the development of the WHO Global Code.
[ii] Ibadat S. Dhillon is the Associate Director of Health Workforce at Realizing Rights: The Ethical Globalization Initiative.

amongst key stakeholders, including the active role of civil society. The analysis emphasises the importance of political leadership, appropriate sequencing, and support for capacity building of developing countries' negotiating skills to successful global health negotiations.

Introduction

The loss of highly skilled personnel, colloquially referred to as 'brain drain,' has been a central concern of developing countries for the last half century. Despite a call by developing countries, limited international structure has emerged to equitably manage the gains and losses from the largely asymmetric movement of skilled workers.

Over this last decade, in the context of a global health workforce crisis, the international migration of health personnel and associated negative impacts on health systems in source countries has been identified as a particular concern by many developing and some developed nations. The escalating demand for health workers in middle- and high-income nations is increasingly being met through reliance on foreign health workers, very often from low-income countries. The Organization for Economic Co-operation and Development (OECD) recently identified that 18% of physicians and 11% of nurses working in OECD nations were foreign born and that the international migration of health workers to OECD nations was increasing.[1]

The migration of health workers to middle- and high-income countries is exacerbating existing inequities in the health workforce. For example, over half of the physicians from Angola, Antigua and Barbuda, Grenada, Guyana, Haiti, Liberia, Mozambique, Saint Vincent and the Grenadines, Sierra Leone, Tanzania, and Trinidad and Tobago — many already facing critical health workforce shortages — practice as expatriates in OECD countries.

The challenges associated with health worker migration at its core points to a lack of coherence between the global health-related development agenda and the domestic health workforce policies of many donor nations. Ameliorating the negative effects of health worker migration demands an international structure to further dialogue and guide cooperation amongst states on issues related to the international recruitment and migration of health workers.[2]

The May 2010 adoption by the World Health Assembly (WHA) of the World Health Organization (WHO) Global Code of Practice on the International Recruitment of Health Personnel (hereafter "the Code") puts in place a global architecture, including the identification of ethical norms as well as institutional and legal arrangements, to guide international cooperation on the issue of health worker migration and serves as a platform for continuing dialogue.[3] Only the second code of its kind promulgated by the WHO, the process towards development of the Code evidences a growing maturity of global health diplomacy. Multilateral agreement amongst all 193 WHO Member States has been achieved on an issue of long-standing concern to developing countries, one that until recently was viewed as irreconcilable with the interests of high-income nations. The choice of a non-binding approach to address an issue that is dynamic, complex, and highly sensitive also reflects more nuanced understanding by Member States of the nature and utility of binding and non-binding international legal instruments to further global health.

Key Points

- Despite being a priority concern for developing countries over the last half century, limited international structure has evolved to address the challenges associated with the international migration of high skilled workers.
- The international migration of health workers is exacerbating critical health worker shortages in many developing countries.
- Adoption of the WHO Global Code of Practice provides important global architecture towards furthering dialogue and coordination between relevant stakeholders on the challenges associated with the international recruitment and migration of health workers.

The Development of the WHO Global Code of Practice

Initiation of the WHO Global Code process

In order to advance a global framework for dialogue and cooperation amongst states on international health worker recruitment issues, in May 2004 the World Health Assembly, the legislative body of WHO, adopted Resolution 57.19 mandating that the Director-General develop a non-binding code of practice on the international recruitment of health workers in consultation with Member States and all relevant partners. The resolution marked the first time that the Health Assembly had invoked the constitutional authority of WHO to develop a non-binding Code since the 1981 International Code of Marketing of Breast Milk Substitutes.

The WHO Global Code process was preceded by a number of initiatives to address international health worker recruitment concerns on a country-by-country, multilateral, or transnational basis. Over the last decade countries have adopted a number of non-binding instruments aimed at tackling the challenges associated with international health worker recruitment, including the Commonwealth Code of Practice on the International Recruitment of Health Workers, the Pacific Code of Practice for the International Recruitment of Health Workers in the Pacific Region, and the United Kingdom National Health Service Code of Practice for the International Recruitment of Healthcare Professionals. During this period there has also been a proliferation of non-binding instruments adopted under the auspices of professional associations and unions, such as the World Medical Association, the International Council of Nurses, and the European Federation of Public Service Unions. Bilateral agreements between source and destination countries that formalise ongoing dialogue and address rights and responsibilities in ethical international recruitment also multiplied over the ten years prior to the adoption of the Code.[4]

Existing voluntary codes of practice and other similar non-binding instruments have been widely criticised as weak and ineffective in addressing the core challenges of health worker migration and its impact on health systems. Critics have argued, for example, that such non-binding instruments have been largely ineffective in limiting health worker migration from poor countries or protecting the human rights of health workers because they lacked meaningful mechanisms to collect data and to monitor national compliance.[5] In addition, unlike the WHO Code, none of the earlier instruments set forth a global approach necessary to addressing a global problem or mobilised the funding required for implementation.

Despite early support for the development of a WHO Global Code, the initiative lacked political support, resources, and policy direction. However, in early 2008, the Code effort re-emerged as the issues surrounding health systems and health worker recruitment rose in stature in the global health policy agenda of states. Development and drafting of the Code were led by the World Health Organization's Human Resources for Health Division (WHO/HRH) and a framework for the proposed Code was first presented by WHO/HRH at the Global Forum on Human Resources for Health in Kampala in March 2008.

The efforts of the Health Worker Migration Initiative ('HWMI'), a partnership between Realizing Rights, the Global Health Workforce Alliance ('GHWA'), and WHO were also critical to the renewed focus on developing the WHO Global Code. The Health Worker Migration Initiative is composed of two closely linked entities, the Global Policy Advisory Council ('the Council'), whose secretariat is Realizing Rights, and the Technical Working Group ('TWG') whose secretariat was WHO/HRH. The idea of the partnership, linking rigorous research and evidence with high level political leadership and engagement, emerged in 2006 on the occasion of the UN General Assembly Special Session on Migration and Development. The HWMI was officially launched during the World Health Assembly in May of 2007 as a formal initiative of Realizing Rights, GHWA, and WHO.

The Council, co-chaired by Hon. Mary Robinson, former President of Ireland and UN High Commissioner for Human Rights, and Dr. Francis Omaswa, former Executive Director of GHWA, played a significant role in supporting the development of the WHO Global Code. The Council was comprised of forty high-level sitting and former policy makers from sending and receiving nations, as well as high-level representatives from international organisations. The Council included current and former ministers of labor, development, and health, as well as high level representatives from WHO, the International Labour Organisation, and the International Organization for Migration. The Council aimed to further mutually acceptable solutions to the issue of health worker migration in a manner that honours both the right to health and freedom of movement. Through its members and meetings, the Council provided both political and technical support to the work of the WHO Human Resources for Health Division in the development of the Code.

Despite growing support for the international cooperation many observers continued to dismiss the potential contribution that a non-binding code of practice could make to issues surrounding international health worker recruitment. It was argued that the proposed Code was not 'legal' or could have no impact in state practice because it would be technically non-binding as a matter of international law. To gather and respond to such concerns, as well as galvanize stakeholder interest, at its May 2008 meeting in Geneva, the Global Policy Advisory Council commissioned a paper to facilitate critical discussion on the potential strengths of non-binding instruments in international legal practice and how the proposed code could best be structured and negotiated to advance global consensus and action on international health worker migration issues.[6] In addition, WHO, GHWA, and Realizing Rights in March and April 2008 hosted a two-week Online Global Dialogue to further disseminate this information and to engage discussion on the potential value and content of the Code. The Online Dialogue included 749 participants from 102 countries.

Preparation of first draft text and early stages in the negotiation process

Technical legal work and the preparation of the first draft of the Code commenced in earnest in July 2008 at WHO headquarters in Geneva and the draft of the Code prepared under the auspices of the WHO/HRH, headed by Dr. Manuel Dayrit, was ready for consideration by Member States by the end of the summer in 2008.

The first draft of the Global Code endeavoured to establish global architecture for national and international dialogue and action on international health worker recruitment and migration. The brief first draft, consisting of eleven articles, did not aim to address and resolve all of the substantive issues raised by the international recruitment of health personnel or the substantial challenges to the health systems of low-income states raised by health worker migration. Rather, the goal of the first draft was to set forth a brief, straightforward framework and platform for substantive negotiations. It was expected that WHO Member States would negotiate more detailed commitments in the final text of the Code or in later instruments.

Notably, the first draft of the Code did aim to respond to criticisms of other non-binding instruments in this realm by recommending voluntary measures to promote national compliance. Consistent with contemporary international practice in other realms of international law, the first and all of the following drafts of the Code recommended a robust and transparent framework for global governance, including voluntary mechanisms for effective and periodic information sharing, reporting, and supervision of implementation.[7]

In September of 2008, the WHO Secretariat launched a web-based global public hearing on the first draft of the proposed Code. In addition, the draft text was presented by the WHO Human Resources for Health Division and considered at WHO Regional Committees in September and October 2008 in the European Region, South-East Asian Region, and Western Pacific Region. The Council also met for two days in September 2008, with members including the then-Chair of the WHO Executive Board reviewing the text line-by-line and providing specific input through the online process. Based on the input provided by the regional committee meeting, the global public hearing, and the comments provided by the Council, the WHO Secretariat prepared a second draft of the proposed Code in November 2008.

The second draft of the Code was considered by the Executive Board in January 2009 at one regular session and in one closed informal session. Whilst there was wide agreement on many parts of the text, there was also a divergence on some key aspects of the draft that reflected the underlying complexity of the issues and differences amongst states surrounding health worker recruitment and migration. For example, a number of industrialised countries, including the United States and Hungary on behalf of the European Union, expressed concern that the Code was overly prescriptive for a non-binding instrument. Japan, the United States and other delegations intervened that provisions on monitoring and implementation were inappropriate for a non-binding instrument. In contrast however, a number of countries, including Mauritania on behalf of the WHO Afro

Region, as well as Malawi and South Africa, emphasised that the Code needed to be "enforced."

As a further example, Member States of the WHO AFRO region, Sri Lanka, and others expressed the view that the Code must also include mechanisms to compensate developing countries for the migration of health workers to high-income states. Other participants, in particular some destination states, indicated that bilateral support was a preferred alternative and that a compensatory mechanism should not be included in the Code.

Notably, many Member States, including Mauritania on behalf of the WHO AFRO region, Hungary on behalf of the European Union, Brazil, Djibouti, Bahamas, and China expressed the view that the second draft paid insufficient attention to the impact of migration on the health systems of developing countries. Some delegations also argued that the draft overemphasised the rights of health workers at the expense of the health systems of source states and could be interpreted as encouraging migration.

In recognition of the important differences amongst countries on issues surrounding health worker recruitment, there was widespread agreement that the draft Code required further consultation amongst Member States and subsequent revision before it could be forwarded to the Health Assembly for negotiation and adoption. At the same time, some state delegates privately expressed the view that delaying negotiation and adoption of the Code for one year could create a more fertile negotiating environment by allowing time for a new United States presidential administration to take office and establish policy that might be more supportive of the Code effort. Consequently, it was agreed that the Secretariat should initiate a consultative process on the draft Code, including consideration of the draft Code at the WHO regional committee meetings in the fall of 2009 before the issue of the Code would be revisited by the Executive Board in January 2010.

Following the January 2009 Executive Board session, issues related to the Code were considered in national, regional, and international meetings in preparation for fall 2009 regional committee sessions. Some Member States held national consultations, and some regional offices convened regional and sub-regional meetings. In addition, a draft WHO Code was highlighted in international settings. In July 2009, the G8 countries at their Summit (L'Aquila, Italy, 8–10 July 2009) encouraged WHO to develop a Code of practice on the international recruitment of health personnel by 2010, and the ministerial declaration of the 2009 High-level Segment of the United Nations Economic and Social Council called for the finalisation of a WHO Code. In September and October 2009, all six regional committees discussed the key issues relating to a Code.

The Secretariat revised the text and prepared a third draft of the Code in order to take into account the views and comments expressed by members of the Board in January 2009 and the outcome of the subsequent sessions of the Regional Committees.[8] In particular, the Code was deftly revised to considerably strengthen the emphasis of the text on the interests and concerns of source states in the health worker migration process, but, at the same time, reflected the views of destination states by, amongst other things, softening the perceived 'prescriptive' language of the draft text.

In January 2010 the draft Code was once again before the Executive Board. Whilst some states expressed disagreement with some aspects of the draft text, or proposed mechanisms for improvement, it was unanimously agreed that the draft Code was a good basis for negotiation and should be forwarded to the May 2010 Health Assembly for negotiation and possible adoption. Mauritania on behalf of the AFRO states, Hungary on behalf of the European Union, Canada, Samoa, Moldova, Russia, New Zealand, India, Bangladesh, Paraguay, France, Switzerland, Bahamas, Japan, Oman, South Africa, Zimbabwe, and Iran all spoke in favour of forwarding the draft Code to the Health Assembly for negotiations.

Alongside the formal WHO process, Council members and others supported a political process to both inform and engage Member States around support for a substantive WHO Code. Norway's leadership, both in its capacity as a Member State and as an active member of the Council, in this process was invaluable.

The Council, through its meetings and partnerships, additionally worked to highlight the content and import of a substantive WHO Code to both source and destination Member States. Particular emphasis was placed on engaging constructively with President Obama's incoming administration. Hon. Mary Robinson and others reached out to the highest level of US government, including to President Obama through his advisors, on numerous occasions to encourage support for the WHO Code.

Whilst it was African countries that championed the call for development of the Code, their engagement with the initial drafts of the proposed WHO Code was relatively limited. The Council endeavoured over the course of the Code development process to inform and engage source countries, particularly sub-Saharan African countries, with the Code text. A week before formal Code negotiations at the World Health Assembly in May 2010, Norway and the WHO EURO region supported the Council to host a two-day Inter-Regional Dialogue around the text and contentious issues of the Code. Norway in particular supported the Council in ensuring strong representation of African nations at the meeting. The meeting included 55 participants from 32 countries, fifteen from Africa. Some of the national governments represented at the meeting included South Africa, Norway, the United States, Botswana, Ghana, Uganda, Kenya, Brazil, Zimbabwe, the United Kingdom, France, Hungary, and Spain (which held the European Union presidency) — many of whom were to play a leading role in Code negotiations. The two-day meeting was perhaps most important in familiarizing some participants with the text and underlying points of contention associated with the draft Code before formal negotiations took place, as not all of the Member States had participated in the Executive Board deliberations over the past two years. The participants were united in recognising that the areas of contention could not be allowed to jeopardize adoption of the Code.

Negotiation of the WHO Global Code at the May 2010 World Health Assembly

The Sixty-Third World Health Assembly, on its opening day, May 17, 2010, established a "drafting committee" open to all Member States to negotiate the text of the Code of Practice that had been forwarded by the January 2010 Executive Board. Under the chairmanship of an experienced negotiating chair, Dr. Viroj Tangcharoensathien of Thailand, and the support of the WHO Secretariat, led by Dr. Manuel Dayrit, the Director of the WHO Human Resources for Health Division, the final text of the WHO Global Code was negotiated in this closed drafting group that met over three days during the May 2010 World Health Assembly, including a final negotiating session that lasted until 4:30 AM on Thursday, May 20, 2010.

Over 30 countries, including many of the key players in the global health recruitment debate, such as the South Africa, Norway, the United States, Botswana, Switzerland, Uganda, Kenya, Brazil, Thailand, Zimbabwe, New Zealand, Australia, Canada, and the European Union, represented by Spain (as well as some of its Member States such as the United Kingdom, France, Belgium, and Germany) participated in the global negotiations. Whilst many of the major players participated throughout the negotiations, notably missing from the drafting group were countries such as India and Japan that had been vocal participants in debates at the Executive Board and the regional committees.

Whilst there remained important differences between countries, under the keen stewardship of Dr. Viroj, the negotiating group forged a consensus document that contains voluntary recommendations on many of the issues surrounding international recruitment of health personnel. The draft was negotiated by first identifying the key issues in dispute and then proceeding through the text provision by provision until consensus was achieved.

Global health workforce recruitment and migration is a complex and multidimensional global health challenge and a number of the critical issues that had challenged the development of the text throughout the negotiation process were central to the debates of the drafting group. However, as the draft text had been revised several times prior to the Health Assembly by the Secretariat, the differences amongst countries had been considerably narrowed. Consequently, the final text of the Code can be fairly described as only subtly different from the last draft prepared by the Secretariat: reflecting fine differences in tone and precision, but only limited substantive changes.

A recurring issue in the discussions leading up to the Health Assembly and the drafting group itself was the perceived "prescriptive" nature of the voluntary Code. As described during the Executive Board debates a number of high-income countries argued that the tone of the draft Code was too prescriptive or mandatory for a non-binding instrument. Most of the high-income countries present in the drafting sessions joined in support for modification of the draft Code during the Health Assembly, including

Canada, New Zealand, Spain on behalf of the European Union, the United States, Monaco, and others. Without any objection from low-income states, the draft Code was revised to eliminate terms such as "standards" and "comply." At the same time, Member State commitments under the Code were modified throughout the text from the word "should" to terms such as "should consider" or "should encourage." It can well be argued that since the Code is non-binding and only makes recommendations to governments that these subtle changes have no impact on the substance of the Code and are likely to make no meaningful difference in state practice. However, the case can also be made that such changes, by undermining the precision of the commitments in the text, could potentially impact or even soften the sense of duty amongst Member States to comply with the underlying norms in the Code.

Another key issue that arose during the consultations surrounding the draft Code was whether the instrument should narrowly focus on estab-lishing voluntary principles and practices related to international recruitment or whether the scope of the instrument should be broadened to address the impact of health worker migration on health systems gen-erally. Revisions to the text during the drafting committee did not fully clarify this issue. Early in the drafting group, high-income states tailored the text of the Code, particularly the Objectives in Section 1, to focus exclusively on recruitment and to leave out the larger issues of migration. However, a careful reading of the final text of the Code reveals that broad issues of health workforce migration, the 'brain drain' from developing countries, comprises a substantial part of the substance of the text. For example, Article 5 focuses on general issues surrounding health system sustainability and Articles 6 and 7 are centred upon collection and exchange of information on health personnel migration.

An important area of concurrence amongst high and low-income states during the drafting group revolved around human rights issues under Article 4 of the Code. As described above, issues surrounding how to honour the right of developing countries to strengthen their health sys-tems and the rights of health workers to migrate to countries that wish to admit and employ them was a long-standing concern in the drafting of the Code. During the Health Assembly deliberations, the right to health of source countries became the dominant concern in this balance as interests amongst high-income and low-income participating states aligned. Consistent with international human rights law and pre-existing codes, such as the Commonwealth and the Pacific Codes of Practice, the draft WHO Code had emphasised the human rights of health workers in Article 4 to fairness and equality of treatment in several articles. High-income countries modified the language in this Article by, amongst other things, subjecting rights to "applicable law." The effort of high-income countries to limit the broad recognition of rights aligned with the interests of developing countries who had long argued that the draft Code had overemphasised the rights of workers at the expense of the health systems of developing countries.

Another key area on which there was significant discussion during the negotiations was the way in which the Code should reflect and encourage an appropriate balance between the interests of source states and destination states. The United States led a wide consensus to modify the draft text of the Code in Article 5 to address issues of "health workforce development and sustainability" rather than "mutuality of benefit," reflecting more of a change in tone and not substance. Other modifications proposed by destination states to the text, however, highlighted the interests of high-income countries. One important area of divergence amongst states was whether the Code should promote bilateral and other arrangements amongst source and destination states. Whilst low-income states had emphasised the importance of such agreements in discussions leading up to the Health Assembly, the draft language calling upon states to abstain from active international recruitment unless there exist equitable agreements to support recruitment activities was deleted from the final text of the Code.

Throughout most of the negotiation process at the Health Assembly, high-income states, particularly the participating states from the European Union, Canada, the United States, and New Zealand, dominated the interventions and advanced recommendations for change in the draft text. Developing countries, particularly the delegates from African States, remained frequently silent during discussions of the substantive provisions of the draft Code with Norway and Brazil often voicing the position of source countries. However, an important change occurred after midnight on May 20 as the delegates moved from negotiations of the substantive aspects of the Code to discussions of the detailed procedural mechanisms involving data collection, information exchange, monitoring, and implementation, and the ranks of negotiators thinned from a high of over thirty participating states to a core group of delegates from just over twenty Member States. As described above, a number of high-income states had strongly opposed the Secretariat's detailed inclusion of these critical procedural and institutional mechanisms in the voluntary instrument. An information document prepared by the Secretariat, consisting of Member State proposals to the draft text, evidenced that countries such as Canada, the European Union, and the United States preferred that such provisions be strictly circumscribed or deleted.[9] However, starting with the deliberations on data collection the delegations from African States, including South Africa, Zimbabwe, Kenya, and Botswana established a united front in favour of maintaining the strong legal and institutional provisions in the draft text against all efforts to modify and limit such provisions In the end, the detailed legal, institutional and data sharing provisions established in the final text remained substantively unchanged from the draft prepared by the Secretariat.

In addition, whilst developing countries had long pushed for strengthening the financial mechanisms to promote "compensation" from destination states to source states during the early stages of the Code process, there was no effort to negotiate more detailed commitments on financial provisions in the final negotiations. Indeed, there was a keen recognition amongst developing country delegates at the Health Assembly that high-income states would simply not agree to deeper provisions on financial support to developing countries. As the delegate of Brazil essentially noted, the Code effort should not be held back by lack of agreement on compensation and that maybe, in the future, there could be meaningful discourse on compensation.

The three-day negotiation of the WHO Global Code of Practice occurred during what was a well-attended and highly charged World Health Assembly. The agenda of the Health Assembly included negotiation of contentious issues in other substantive and procedural areas. It also saw the launch of President Obama's new Global Health Initiative. Whilst negotiations on the WHO Global Code were occurring at Committee A, there were negotiations around WHO governance structures, in particular the process to appoint the Director General, occurring in Committee B.

Delegates to the negotiations were highly sensitive to shifts in alliances due to negotiation positions taken on other topics.

The linkages between the various different sessions at the Health Assembly and their impact on the Code negotiations was made especially evident during discussions hosted by the United States on President Obama's Global Health Initiative on the second day of the Health Assembly. During this session, which was open to all Member States and civil society, the United States found its efforts to highlight the good works of the Obama Global Health Initiative hampered as delegates from other Member States as well as other participants specifically and repeatedly brought up the challenges of health worker migration and the US negotiating position in the closed "room next door."

Key Points

- Strong technical work from the WHO Secretariat and effective partnership between WHO and civil society from the very inception of the Code development process was critical to the development and successful negotiation of the WHO Global Code of Practice.
- The WHO Human Resources for Health Secretariat was able to address concerns related to the non-binding voluntary nature of the instrument by including strong procedural mechanisms in the various iterations of the draft WHO Global Code of Practice.
- The three-year efforts towards development of the WHO Global Code of Practice, supported through formal WHO and informal civil society mechanisms, enabled informed engagement during negotiations from both high-and low-resource nations.

The WHO Global Code of practice

The drafting committee's final text of the Code was brought forward on May 21, 2010 to Committee A for further discussion before the text was to be accepted by Committee A as final. Many of the negotiators from both source and destination countries privately expressed the view that they remained apprehensive that that the process towards adoption achieved by the drafting group could still be derailed by ongoing discussion and negotiation at Committee A. However, the WHO Global Code of Practice elicited no discussion at Committee A. Once accepted for adoption, there was spontaneous applause by all present in the room. According to observers, the applause in the room reflected both the magnitude and urgency of the challenge of health worker migration, as well as the ability to achieve multilateral agreement on such a complex and sensitive subject.

The WHO Global Code of Practice on the International Recruitment of Health Personnel was officially adopted in the evening, on Friday, May 21, 2010 at the closing session of the Sixty-Third World Health Assembly. Director-General Margaret Chan identified the adoption of the WHO Global Code as one of the major achievements of the Assembly, referring to adoption of the Code as a "real gift to public health everywhere."

The final text of the WHO Global Code includes a preamble and ten articles, including: Objectives; Nature and scope; Guiding principles; Responsibilities, rights, and recruitment practices; Health workforce development and health systems sustainability; Data gathering and research; Information exchange; Implementation of the Code; Monitoring and institutional arrangements; and Partnerships, technical collaboration and financial support.

The WHO Global Code of Practice is a voluntary instrument that identifies global ethical norms, "principles and practices." around the international recruitment and migration of health workers. The instrument's norms link to an array of critical challenges associated with the migration of health workers — encouraging health personnel development in countries with critical shortages, the development of sustainable health workforce in all countries, greater cooperation on issues of recruitment and migration, equitable treatment of migrant health personnel, coordination and collection of relevant data, and discouraging active recruitment of health personnel from countries with critical health workforce shortages. The WHO Code is explicitly a dynamic text to be updated based on the changing nature and impact of health worker migration.

Most importantly, the WHO Code incorporates strong procedural mechanism for data collection, information sharing reporting, monitoring, and systematic review by the Health Assembly. WHO, through the Director-General, in particular, is called to report to the Health Assembly on implementation of the Code every three years, after initial data reporting in 2012.

The WHO Global Code is neither a perfect text nor a solution to the challenges associated with health worker migration. The substantive norms advanced by the Code remain relatively general and are advanced in a soft manner to Member States. It should be recognised however, that the WHO Global Code was never intended to be the final answer or encompass the whole solution to the challenges associated with health worker migration. Rather, the goal of the drafters was to establish a global platform that could provide a framework for continuing dialogue and cooperation amongst states. The WHO Global Code, in particular the key legal and institutional arrangements, does provide a robust instrument for ongoing global cooperation that may lead to a deepening of commitment over time.

Key Points

- The WHO Global Code of Practice on the International Recruitment of Health Personnel was officially adopted on May 21, 2010. Adoption of the WHO Global Code was a major achievement of the Sixty-Third World Health Assembly and identified as a "real gift to public health."
- The WHO Global Code is a non-binding instrument that articulates global ethical norms surrounding the international recruitment of health personnel, as well as containing strong procedural and institutional mechanisms to support Member States in data collection, information sharing, and implementation.
- The WHO Global Code is not the solution to the challenges associated with health worker migration. It is however, a significant step forward towards international cooperation and dialogue on a topic of significant complexity and sensitivity.

Lessons Learned for Future Negotiations

In any political context, the organisation of negotiations is a question of political mapping that must respond to political realities and resource constraints. Issues, interests, and strategies need to be organised to reduce complexity and promote coalition building and consensus. With that said, there were certain aspects of the legislative process that contributed to the success of the WHO Global Code endeavour.

The lessons to be learned from the WHO Global Code negotiations go beyond the mere spectrum of the nuts and bolts of international negotiation processes, and provide some deeper insight into the evolution in global health diplomacy over the past decade. The senior author of this case study initiated the idea of the Framework Convention on Tobacco Control (FCTC), the first treaty negotiated under the auspices of WHO, with the late Professor Ruth Roemer and was a legal adviser to WHO during the negotiations of the FCTC and during the negotiations of the WHO Global Code.[10] A comparison of the negotiating processes of the Code and the FCTC clearly is not a scientific endeavour that can fully reveal transformations in global health diplomacy over the past decade. Amongst other things, there are important differences between the two processes, including the fact that the analysis involves a comparison of the negotiations of binding and non-binding instruments. As described further below however, the experience of the Code negotiations does appear to evidence some growing maturity and, perhaps, an evolution, in global health diplomacy at WHO amongst the different actors in the process: the Secretariat, civil society and, most importantly, Member States.

The potential contribution of non-binding instruments to global health governance

Recent developments in global health diplomacy have led to increasing calls for international standard setting. However, consistent with other international realms the pattern that is beginning to emerge is a marked preference for binding global health law instruments. This preference for expanding treaty law appears amongst state actors, civil society, and academia and is reflected in the proliferation of proposals for new global health treaties over the last decade.

The experience of the WHO Global Code evidences the important and largely overlooked contribution that non-binding instruments can make to global health diplomacy and may serve as a model for future global health law negotiations.[11] Undoubtedly, there is no alternative to treaties when states want to make credible commitments. However, treaties are not the only source of norms in the international system. It is increasingly recognised that the challenges of global governance demand faster and more flexible approaches to international cooperation than can be provided by traditional and heavily legalised strategies. Consequently, in other realms of international concern ranging from the environment to arms control the world community is increasingly turning to the creation of non-binding international norms.

Like binding international instruments, non-binding instruments have important strengths and limitations as international legal tools. Chief amongst the limitations of non-binding instruments is that such voluntary agreements are not subject to international law and, in particular, its fundamental principle of *pacta sunt servanda*. There are no rules of international law that regulate or supplement non-binding instruments like the Vienna Convention on the Law of Treaties. Many non-binding instruments are purposefully designed as way stations or even detours from hard, binding legal commitments. Consequently, many if not most non-binding instruments are purely rhetorical and have no impact on state practice.

However, non-binding instrument have some important advantages as a mechanism for international cooperation and can, at times, make an important contribution to shaping state behaviour. A key advantage of non-binding instruments is their flexibility. Flexibility is an essential component of international negotiations. Non-binding agreements can facilitate compromise and agreement may be easier to achieve than binding instruments, especially when states jealously guard their sovereignty since non-binding standards do not involve formal legal commitments. Notably, the FCTC was negotiated in six separate rounds of two-week negotiation sessions open to all WHO Member States over five years whilst the WHO Global Code was negotiated in just a fraction of that time. In addition, by removing concerns about legal non-compliance, non-binding instruments may, at times, promote deeper commitments with stricter compliance mechanisms than comparable binding instruments. Notably, the WHO Global Code incorporates procedural mechanisms to advance implementation that are more potent than those incorporated in the FCTC. Whilst both the FCTC and the Global Code set forth a shallow substantive framework, the Global Code sets forth a deep legal and institutional framework.

The WHO process: Development of a simple draft text early in the negotiations

An important factor contributing to the success of the Code negotiation process is that the Secretariat introduced a simple negotiating text early in the process and maintained control of the drafting of the text until formal negotiations at the World Health Assembly in 2010. At first instance, a key strategy was to establish concise and carefully drafted commitments for states to bargain over and flush out. In addition, Secretariat control over the drafting process helped prevent the document from spiraling out of control.

The first draft of the Code and process of developing subsequent drafts can be contrasted sharply with the negotiating experience during the FCTC. During the FCTC negotiations, the first draft text prepared by the Secretariat for the negotiating chair contained an entire catalogue of potential substantive obligations.[12] In addition, during the process of negotiating the FCTC in six formal rounds of negotiations open to all Member States, each and every recommendation by Member States, sometimes amounting to nothing other than mere wording and stylistic differences, were incorporated into the draft leading to remarkably complex texts and unnecessarily prolonged negotiating sessions. In the case of the Code, the Secretariat contributed to advancing negotiations by maintaining control of the drafting process and incorporating the key themes proposed by Member States and not verbatim text during the early stages of the negotiation process.

The WHO process: Staging and sequencing

Negotiations tend to be marked by a series of stages that narrow the agenda and differences amongst countries. There is not one formula for successful negotiations and different structures can be used. In some respects, the Code negotiations reflect a good example of sequencing in that Secretariat draft text went through several political scrubs by a small group of states representatives at the WHO regional committees and the WHO Executive Board before it was opened up for broader negotiation for all WHO Member States at the WHA. Consequently, the text was largely acceptable before it was opened up to broad negotiations. However, a critical last stage of the negotiation process involved the Member States taking control and ownership of the document in the final negotiations at the WHA.

Cementing broad stakeholder participation is critical in a negotiation process and a cautionary tale is provided by some international negotiations that fail to incorporate effective participation by relevant stakeholders, particularly states. For example, in the case of the United Nations Guidelines on Internal Displacement, the draft text of the Guidelines were developed by an expert group and never negotiated by governments. When brought for adoption to the United Nations General Assembly, certain countries complained that since states were not involved in the drafting, the Guidelines lacked legitimacy. Such objections were overcome only by the arguments that the Guidelines merely reflected existing international law and did not set forth new standards.

With that said, it should be recognised that the Code negotiation process was also hampered by the absence of a truly global negotiation prior to the WHA in May 2010. Issues surrounding health worker recruitment and migration reveal important political divides amongst high-income and low-income states. Although the Code was considered at various international fora and regional committees prior to the Health Assembly negotiations, there was no formal global consultation necessary to advance consensus, and to move the text and the consensus forward.

Political leadership

Political leadership is a critical factor in international negotiations to broker deals and bring innovative thinking. Leadership can come from many sources, including the executive head of an international organisation, as was the case of Dr. Mostafa Tolba for many years at the United Nations

Environment Programme. It can also be brought by states. Notably, it is often mid-sized countries such as Australia, Canada, Switzerland, New Zealand, and Norway that have provided leadership in areas ranging from the environment to health.

In context of the WHO Global Code negotiations, Norway led the way amongst the states. Recognising the challenges associated with health worker migration, Norway had previously engaged across its ministries to make coherent its domestic need for foreign health workers with its international development efforts. In February 2009, Norway released its internal policy coherence strategy. However, Norway also recognised that singular action alone could not meaningfully address the global nature of the challenge. As such, Norway was a strong advocate for development of a WHO Global Code of Practice. Moreover, Norway was cognizant throughout the process of its own unique economic position and the need to engage other, particularly source country, champions.

In addition to country leadership, a strong chair is an essential ingredient of effective negotiations and the Code negotiations were expertly steered throughout the WHA process by Dr. Viroj Tangcharoensathien.

The role of civil society

The unique partnership between WHO/HRH, GHWA, and Realizing Rights was integral to development of the Code. Realizing Rights' formation of the Global Policy Advisory Council, an independent body and authority, in particular, allowed for a channel that could run parallel to the formal WHO process in shaping and advancing negotiations. The Council, through its secretariat, members, and meetings, was able to complement WHO Secretariat's efforts by reaching out to specific Member States and hosting an inter-regional discussion in order to clarify and further consensus around contentious issues. The Code effort reflects a new type of civil society participation in global health negotiations at WHO. Through the Health Worker Migration Initiative partnership, Realizing Rights, an organisation with experience in global governance, was involved with the Code development from the very inception of the process. Realizing Rights' method of work focused on supporting its partners and Member State capacity to move forward mutually acceptable solutions. Moreover,

Realizing Rights staff — led by Hon. Mary Robinson — had knowledge and experience in international law and global negotiations and were able to bring this depth to Council meetings and its contacts with Member States. Mary Robinson's ability to convene and engage stakeholders and key decision makers was undoubtedly an important additional asset.

Notably, neither the Council nor or its Secretariat were ever directly involved in drafting the text of the Code, but rather worked with Member States to provide detailed commentary on draft text and raised awareness and support for a substantive Code. Moreover, enabled by the technical legal work of the WHO Secretariat on the WHO Global Code, the Council was able to point to a tangible vision and action that political leadership, from both source and destination nations, could further.

The role of civil society in the negotiation of the Code stands in contrast with that of the negotiation of the FCTC from 1998 to 2003. Civil society played a much more limited role in participating and guiding the FCTC negotiations primarily because of its lack of expertise and experience in international lawmaking and the limited opportunities to work with Member States and WHO in closed negotiation sessions that dominated the negotiation process. It should be recognised, of course, that FCTC was the first binding treaty negotiated at the WHO. Civil society organisations participating in the treaty negotiations were largely domestic tobacco control organisations, with no experience in international law and negotiations. In recent years however, through the Framework Convention Alliance, civil society acquired depth and experience in the international lawmaking process and has played an increasingly important role in guiding the implementation of the FCTC.

Member States and the evolution of diplomatic capacity

Similar to the apparent growth in legal capacity amongst members of civil society, the Code negotiations evidence a deepening or maturing of diplomatic capacity to engage in global health negotiations amongst low-income country delegations. Indeed, there was a striking difference between delegations engaged in the FCTC negotiations and the Code negotiations. During the FCTC negotiations, the vast majority of low-income Member States delegations was new to international law negotiation process and was comprised of representatives from health ministries accompanied by junior mission lawyers or no lawyers at all. During the FCTC negotiation process, such inexperienced delegates were simply and frequently out-lawyered by the experienced negotiators, including highly skilled international lawyers, from high-income states.

The difference in negotiating capacity, including legal expertise, largely, though not exclusively, explains the textual outcome of the FCTC that consists of soft substantive obligations and shallow institutional and procedural mechanisms. A lack of realistic assessment about the scope of the treaty and the depth of commitments haunted the negotiations of the FCTC. Health ministers from low-income countries clearly thought it possible to have deep and wide substantive commitments on tobacco control without losing any participants. During the final days of the negotiations, high-income states were able to negotiate substantially softer substantive commitments in the seventeen articles of the text that set forth tobacco control commitments. But, at the same time that low-income delegations were focused on the substantive obligations, they neglected attention to the key procedural and institutional mechanisms necessary in a framework convention to strengthen and deepen the regime over time. Although a robust procedural framework had been set forth by the Secretariat in the drafts of the FCTC, many of the key legal and institutional mechanisms of global governance were deleted in a side meeting open to all Member States in the final negotiations round in March 2003 in which no developing countries participated. Although the FCTC has, in practice, been remarkably successful in a number of respects,[13] an important consequence of a lack of negotiation experience amongst delegates from low-income countries is a framework convention with uniquely shallow procedural and institutional mechanisms.

In contrast, in the Code negotiations, the character of the state delegations differed markedly and was reflected in the negotiations and the final text. Delegations from developing countries, particularly sub-Saharan Africa, consisted of senior diplomats and highly experienced international lawyers. Such delegations came to the table with a keen understanding of what agreement was possible and targeted critical areas of negotiations. Unlike the FCTC negotiations, these delegations, recognising the realities of underlying politics of the negotiations, spent precious little time trying to hammer out deep substantive commitments to limit recruitment or create compensatory mechanisms. Rather, the skilled delegates and veteran negotiators, focused attention on the critical legal and institutional mechanisms of information exchange and monitoring and reporting that are necessary to maintain the legal regime and, perhaps, deepen it over time.

The differences in character of the negotiating teams at the FCTC and Code negotiations may reflect a deepening of interest in global health amongst Member States and an evolution of global health negotiations. As global health has risen on the political agenda, more and more states may be identifying global health negotiations as a priority and bringing more experienced diplomats and lawyers to the table. If this is the case, it is a welcome development to balance the negotiation dynamics and put high-income and low-income countries on a more even footing in terms of negotiating expertise although not, of course, negotiating power. However, the limited participatory scope of the Code negotiations may mean that it is too soon to draw a definitive conclusion of whether the Code negotiations reflect a genuine evolution in global health diplomacy.

Key Points

- Successful negotiation and adoption of the WHO Global Code was made possible due to a variety of factors, including the development of a single negotiating text, the staging and sequencing of the negotiations which included early input from Member States, recognition and engagement of political leadership throughout the process, an effective and constructive partnership between WHO, GHWA, and civil society, and nuanced understanding on the part of negotiating Members States of the value of non-binding instruments in global health governance.
- A comparison between the negotiation process of the Framework Convention on Tobacco Control and the WHO Global Code evidences an evolving legal capacity by WHO developing country Member States to engage in global health diplomacy.

Conclusion

The WHO Global Code of Practice, only the second of its kind promulgated by WHO, was adopted almost three decades after adoption of its predecessor, the International Code of the Marketing of Breast Milk Substitutes. The historic nature of the WHO Global Code adoption makes evident the gauntlet of a process associated with promulgating global health 'law' at the WHO. Without the range of factors identified in this case study, including recognition of the value of non-binding instruments, development of a simple negotiating text, appropriate staging and sequencing, strong civil society engagement, political leadership, and support for the negotiation capacity of developing countries, work toward development of the Code could very easily have resulted in a failed effort.

The WHO Member States have however, come together to make available a powerful and unique instrument to begin addressing the challenges associated with health worker migration. Long ignored, the issue of health worker migration is and, thanks to the Code's reporting requirements, will remain on the global health agenda for the foreseeable future. As one African government representative at the Health Assembly stated, the issue of health worker migration long "under the table, is now squarely on the table."

References

1. Organisation for Economic Co-operation and Development (2007) Immigrant Health Workers in OECD Countries in the Broader Context of Highly Skilled Migration. In: OECD. International Migration Outlook, OECD, Paris: 161–228.
2. Robinson, M., Clark, P. (2008) Forging Solutions to Health Worker Migration, *The Lancet* 37 (9613): 691–693.
3. World Health Organization (2010) WHO Global Code of Practice on the International Recruitment of Health Personnel, WHA 63.16.
4. Dhillon, I., Clark, M., Kapp, R. (2010) Innovations in Cooperation: A Guidebook on Bilateral Agreements to Address Health Worker Migration. The Aspen Institute.

5. Willets, A., Martineau, T. (2004) Ethical international recruitment of health professionals: Will codes of practice protect developing country health systems?, Liverpool School of Tropical Medicine, United Kingdom.
6. Taylor, A.L. (2008) The Proposed WHO Code of Practice on Health Worker Migration: Issues of Form, Substance and Negotiation. Paper presented at: Health Work Migration Global Policy Advisory Council Meeting, May 18, 2008.
7. Taylor, A.L. (2008) The Draft WHO Code of Practice on the International Recruitment of Health Personnel, Am. Society of Int'l Law Insights 12 (23).
8. World Health Organization (2010) Sixty-Third World Health Assembly Provisional Agenda Item 11.5. International recruitment of health personnel: draft global code of practice, Report by the Secretariat, WHA A63/8.
9. World Health Organizations (2010) Sixty-Third World Health Assembly Provisional Agenda Item 11.5. International recruitment of health personnel: draft global code of practice, A63/INF.DOC./2.
10. Roemer, R., Taylor, A., Lariviere, J. (2005) Origins of the WHO Framework Convention on Tobacco Control. *Am J Pub Health* 95 (6): 936–938.
11. World Health Organization (2001) Framework Convention on Tobacco Control, Document A/FCTC/INB2/2.
12. Taylor, A.L., Global Health Law, in Textbook on Global Health Diplomacy. Kickbush, I. *et al.*, (eds). Forthcoming 2011.
13. Taylor, A.L., Bettcher, D.W., Peck, R. (2003) International law and the international legislative process: The WHO Framework Convention on Tobacco Control. In: Smith, R., Beaglehole, R., Woodward, D., Drager, N. (eds.), *Global Public Goods for Health*, Oxford: 212–230.

7

Negotiating Issues Related to Pandemic Influenza Preparedness: The Sharing of Influenza Viruses and Access to Vaccines and Other Benefits

John E. Lange[i]

Abstract

What began as the Government of Indonesia's insistence on transparency in the Global Influenza Surveillance Network and its assertion of control over pandemic influenza viruses became much broader once the matter was brought to the multilateral forum of the World Health Assembly. Intriguing negotiation processes evolved as the complex debate over virus sample sharing and benefit sharing attracted ministries of health, foreign affairs, and trade. This case study describes the dynamics from literally thousands of hours of discussions in multilateral, bilateral, formal, and informal forums as diverse stakeholders sought a common way forward along a critical divide. Whilst developed countries focused on the importance of rapid and unencumbered virus

[i] Ambassador Lange (Retired) served as Special Representative on Avian and Pandemic Influenza at the US Department of State from March 2006 to February 2009.

sharing to benefit global public health, many developing countries emphasised their need for assured access to vaccines in the event of a human influenza pandemic.

The Problem

In 1997, the first human cases from a new influenza strain, influenza A (H5N1), arose in Hong Kong. By 2005, the world had witnessed the continuing spread of the virus (known as avian influenza, or "bird flu") in poultry and a high mortality rate amongst the small number of humans who had become infected. This led to fears that the virus could evolve to allow for sustained and efficient human-to-human transmission leading to a severe global human influenza pandemic. There had been three such pandemics in the twentieth century, and the worst, in 1918 (known as the "Spanish flu"), had killed an estimated 20–40 million people worldwide.

Governments and international organisations took action to combat the spread of avian influenza and to prepare for a possibly catastrophic human pandemic. Dr. Margaret Chan was appointed Representative of the Director-General for Pandemic Influenza at the World Health Organization (WHO) in June 2005. In September 2005, Dr. David Nabarro joined the office of the United Nations Secretary General as Senior Coordinator for Avian and Pandemic Influenza. US President George W. Bush formed the International Partnership on Avian and Pandemic Influenza (IPAPI) that first met in Washington, D.C., in October 2005, and the US Department of State appointed a Special Representative on Avian and Pandemic Influenza. The European Union led the effort to organise a ministerial-level conference in Beijing, China in January 2006 and hosted a senior officials meeting in Vienna, Austria in June 2006. The International Conference on Avian Influenza, organized by the African Union and the European Commission and hosted by the government of Mali, took place in Bamako in December 2006.

The WHO Global Influenza Surveillance Network (GISN), which serves as a global alert mechanism for the emergence of influenza viruses with pandemic potential (in addition to its work on seasonal influenza), had a key role to play. Since 1952, the GISN has been based on the free flow of influenza virus samples for the benefit of global public health. Its main components are WHO, National Influenza Centres (which sample patients with influenza-like illness and submit representative virus samples), and WHO Collaborating Centres (which analyse the samples). The Collaborating Centres are located in Australia, Japan, the United Kingdom, and the United States.[1]

During this period much attention was focused on countries such as Indonesia, Thailand, Vietnam, China, Egypt, and others where avian influenza was spreading in poultry. Most observers considered Indonesia to be the key country of concern. The decentralised nature of Indonesia's governmental structure, varying levels of competence and cooperation amongst ministries, and the geographic and cultural diversity of the country presented challenges to effectively combating the spread of avian influenza in poultry in the archipelago.

Dr. Siti Fadilah Supari, Indonesia's Minister of Health, was concerned that Indonesia was providing viruses for analysis but would not have ready access to lifesaving vaccines if a human pandemic began. She noted that WHO Collaborating Centres had been forwarding samples of the Indonesian strain (and other strains) of avian influenza viruses to companies in developed countries. The latter, in turn, were in a position to develop the viruses into vaccines, but then sell them — commercially and expensively — on terms unfavourable to developing countries (including those that had initially provided the viruses). She believed that, under the GISN, the free flow of virus samples that originated in Indonesia served to benefit developed countries and threatened the sovereignty of her country. "Since around 50 years ago, the system of the world health management has been very exploitive. It has been controlled by inhumanly [sic] desires, based on the greediness to raise capital and to control the world."[2] To stimulate a change in the system, the Government of Indonesia decided in December 2006 that it would no longer share influenza viruses with WHO Collaborating Centres.

This action generated great consternation amongst those concerned with monitoring mutations in the virus that could lead to a pandemic. The WHO Executive Board met in January 2007 and adopted Resolution EB120.R7 recommending that the 60th World Health Assembly (WHA60) in May 2007 adopt a resolution that, inter alia, would urge Member States "to continue to support the WHO Global Influenza Surveillance Network."[3]

In an attempt to resolve the crisis, WHO worked with the Indonesian Ministry of Health to organise a March 26–27, 2007, high level technical meeting in Jakarta on Responsible Practices for Sharing Avian Influenza Viruses and Resulting Benefits. At the conclusion, WHO welcomed Minister Supari's statement at a joint news conference that Indonesia would resume sharing of H5N1 avian influenza virus samples "immediately."[4]

This was followed the next day by a high-level meeting involving Ministers of Health and senior health officials from 27 countries who adopted the "Jakarta Declaration." The Declaration noted that health ministers assembled "to explore the modalities of a framework that strongly emphasizes the need for developing countries to share in the benefits resulting from the open and timely and equitable sharing and dissemination of information, data and biological specimens related to influenza, and especially the development and production of influenza vaccines that are accessible and affordable for all countries in order to accelerate local, regional and global preparedness and response to the threat of pandemic avian influenza." They called upon WHO Member States to discuss the matters at WHA60.[5]

On April 25, 2007, WHO hosted a meeting in Geneva on Options for Increasing the Access of Developing Countries to H5N1 and other Potential Pandemic Vaccines. Thailand, Switzerland, and other governments described plans for production of pre-pandemic H5N1 vaccine (which could be produced in advance and, it was hoped, would be effective when the real pandemic virus emerged) and pandemic vaccine (which would be based on the actual pandemic virus but would take many weeks to produce). But the discussions indicated there was no ready solution to increasing developing countries' access to vaccines. Dr. Supari said on April 30 that Indonesia was ready to resume sharing specimens but had postponed doing so after the talks in Geneva on technical details "ended in deadlock." She told the Associated Press, "I am afraid to send (the samples) because we have not seen WHO's commitment assuring not to hurt us."[6]

This set the stage for a major confrontation at WHA60 and in the intense negotiations in formal and informal meetings that followed. It came at a time when many in the world feared that a devastating influenza pandemic could begin at any moment.

Key Points

- A global health scare galvanized action by international organisations and governments.
- One key governmental official, the Minister of Health of Indonesia, was able to use that scare to lead a challenge to the status quo which, she argued, favoured developed countries.

The Players and Their Roles

The complex debate over sample sharing and benefit sharing involved many players in governments and international organisations, as well as many others. Within governments, officials included those representing offices of heads of government (demonstrating highest-level fears about a global pandemic), health ministries (since the essential concern was human health), foreign ministries (due to potentially far-reaching foreign policy implications), trade ministries (considering the trade-related aspects of intellectual property rights, or TRIPS, issues), agriculture ministries (since the origin of the concern was avian influenza in poultry), and others.

Developing countries

Indonesian Minister Supari, supported by officials in the health and foreign ministries, led the effort to raise the issues of sample sharing and benefit sharing on the world stage. Numerous countries co-sponsored Indonesia's resolution on sample sharing and benefit sharing that was introduced at WHA60, including Malaysia, Vietnam, Cambodia, Bhutan, Laos, Algeria, Brunei, North Korea, Cuba, Solomon Islands, Myanmar, Maldives, Peru, Qatar, Saudi Arabia, Sudan, East Timor, Iran, and Iraq. A delegate from Thailand chaired a drafting group at WHA60, and as time went on Brazil, India, Egypt, Nigeria, Bangladesh, and other developing nations were active in the negotiations.

Developed countries

The United Kingdom and the United States co-chaired a Pandemic Influenza Working Group that discussed sample sharing and benefit sharing under the auspices of the Global Health Security Initiative involving Canada, the European Commission, France, Germany, Italy, Japan, Mexico, the United Kingdom, and the United States. Separately, the United States (led by the Department of State) chaired periodic meetings of officials from health ministries and foreign ministries from other like-minded countries — Australia, Canada, the European Union Presidency and European Commission, Japan, and the United Kingdom — that together comprised the IPAPI "Core Group."

World Health Organization and World Health Assembly

The Director-General of WHO is responsible for providing leadership on global health matters, and WHO had a vested interest in the results of the negotiations. Dr. Margaret Chan, who was appointed to be Director-General in November 2006, and Dr. David Heymann, Assistant Director-General for Communicable Diseases, initially led WHO's engagement. At a May 16, 2007 technical briefing on the International Health Regulations during WHA60, Dr. Chan made an impassioned plea: "You are tying my hands, muffling my ears, and blinding my eyes" by not sharing virus samples necessary for understanding the risk, assessing the effectiveness of stockpiled influenza vaccines, and developing seed strains for new vaccines. She also stated that developing countries need "equitable access to affordable vaccines" and said that WHO was working on mechanisms to achieve this. Despite her plea, the controversy had become highly politicised amongst Member States. Whilst the WHO Secretariat provided extensive legal and technical support throughout the negotiations, the Director-General had limited ability to forge a political compromise.

Jane Halton, the Secretary of Australia's Department of Health and Ageing, was a driving force chairing intergovernmental meetings called for under the key World Health Assembly resolution.

Non-governmental actors

Non-governmental actors also were very interested in the negotiations. The Third World Network, a non-profit international network of organisations and individuals involved in issues related to development and North-South affairs, was actively involved in generating support for Indonesia's efforts early in the discussions. The International Federation of Pharmaceutical Manufacturers and Associations (IFPMA), representing the global research and development pharmaceutical industry, was not a direct party to the negotiations but was active in trying to influence discussions through its Influenza Vaccine Supply international task force. The Developing Countries Vaccine Manufacturers Network also made its views known.

Key Points

- The immediacy of the problem, coupled with the complexity and potential wide-ranging implications of the issues, attracted actors from many different disciplines representing many different interests.

Challenges Faced And The Outcomes

World Health Assembly negotiations lead to Resolution 60.28

At the 60th World Health Assembly, May 14–23, 2007, the issues of virus sample sharing and benefit sharing were assigned to Committee A. Given the complexity of the subject, Committee A formed a separate, informal drafting group to discuss three resolutions: document EB120.R7 approved by the WHO Executive Board in January 2007; a resolution on responsible practices for sharing avian influenza viruses and resulting benefits (proposed by Indonesia and other countries); and a resolution on mechanisms to promote access to influenza pandemic vaccine for developing countries lacking sufficient influenza vaccine production (proposed by the

United States). The drafting group was chaired by Dr. Viroj Tangcharoensathien, Director of the International Health Policy Program in Thailand's Ministry of Public Health.

The fact that so many developing countries — including ones with active H5N1 outbreaks in poultry — supported Indonesia presented the very real possibility that they could follow Indonesia's lead and cease sharing viruses and cooperating with the GISN. The potential effect on global public health was heightened by the fact that the GISN was responsible not only for pandemic influenza surveillance leading to development of pandemic vaccines (a potential health threat and response), but also for seasonal influenza surveillance and seasonal vaccines (an on-going, actual health threat and response). Thus, a breakdown in the one system could very likely lead to a breakdown in the other.

Negotiations were difficult. Countries could not even agree on which of the three resolutions should serve as the basis for on-going discussions, and some countries (including Iran, which was active in the discussions) opposed linking the three. The debate divided primarily amongst the several co-sponsors of the Indonesian resolution, who sought to maintain a right to "prior informed consent" for virus sharing (which would allow countries sharing the virus to control its destiny), versus countries that felt such a stipulation would delay sharing of virus samples exactly when a rapid public health response was most necessary. On the fourth day of drafting group negotiations, the Chairman introduced his own draft resolution that included elements from the other three proposals and the group's discussions. By the end of the 11th session of the drafting group, a core group of interested parties agreed in principle to a "package deal" to be fully elaborated by the Chair in a new draft. Finally, after a week of negotiations, the drafting group achieved consensus on a draft and the Chair forwarded it to Committee A. In introducing the document, Dr. Viroj called the last week "one of the most difficult drafting groups I ever chaired." He estimated that the effort required 41 hours of deliberations and 3588 person-hours of negotiation. The final draft, which reflected major concessions by all parties involved, was accepted by Committee A and forwarded to the WHA Plenary. The compromise resolution, WHA60.28, was adopted by consensus on May 23, 2007, the last day of the World Health Assembly.

WHA60.28 did not bring the contentious issues to a conclusion, but instead created mechanisms intended to resolve them in the future. The resolution described a range of issues and requested that the Director-General convene an interdisciplinary working group (IDWG) to revise the terms of reference of components of the GISN and to formulate draft standard terms and conditions for sharing viruses "based on mutual trust, transparency, and overriding principles." It also requested that the Director-General convene an intergovernmental meeting to consider several reports to be produced by WHO, including the results of the IDWG deliberations.[7]

Countries with a vested interest in the subject subsequently used a multitude of forums to continue their efforts to generate support for their positions and to seek solutions to the problems posed.

Formal and informal meetings discuss sample sharing and benefit sharing

Health ministers and other senior officials of the Asia-Pacific Economic Cooperation (APEC) economies held a meeting June 7–8, 2007, on the theme, "Building on our investment: A sustainable and multi-sectoral approach to pandemic preparedness and emerging health threats." Indonesian Health Minister Supari, in a prepared presentation, said the current framework through which virus isolates were shared must be modified immediately. Australian Health Minister Tony Abbott and I (as head of the US delegation) made interventions on the importance of sharing of virus samples.

In an effort to move the negotiations forward, Indonesia and Thailand presented to the WHO Secretariat a proposal for global private-public influenza virus sharing and benefit sharing. On June 27, on the margins of a technical meeting in Rome on highly pathogenic avian influenza, WHO Assistant Director General Heymann met with the IPAPI Core Group to discuss the concept. WHO had put together a draft diagram of how such a system could work and asked if the idea was worth pursuing in advance of the WHO IDWG meeting. Under the proposal, viruses would be shared by countries with WHO Collaborating Centres without regard to any claims for patent rights or TRIPS issues. In return, WHO would assure the source countries that a system was in place whereby donors and third parties (vaccine manufacturers, research institutions, etc.) receiving the virus samples were required — as a condition for having access to the virus samples from the Collaborating Centres — to make contributions to a global influenza benefits-sharing mechanism for countries in need (through a vaccine stockpile, WHO's Global Pandemic Influenza Action Plan to Increase Vaccine Supply, technology access or transfer, training, or other mechanisms). IPAPI Core Group members asked questions but were not in a position to make commitments. As time passed, however, this concept did not gain support.

In July, in advance of the IDWG meeting, Indonesia invited countries from the WHO South-East Asia Region and certain others to a preparatory meeting in Jakarta. The United States, meanwhile, organised a conference call for the IPAPI Core Group and sent a demarche cable to all US Embassies asking them to inform host governments of US goals for the IDWG.

WHO Interdisciplinary Working Group meeting is unable to reach agreement

With this build-up, the IDWG meeting on Sharing of Influenza Viruses and Access to Vaccines and Other Benefits took place in Singapore July 31–August 4, 2007. Not surprisingly, the first day of the meeting was marked by a resumption of positions from the May WHA deliberations and substantive progress was slow in coming. The delegates were consumed with debate about whether or not discussion of mechanisms for benefit sharing should precede negotiation of the GISN's terms of reference and standard terms and conditions. The split amongst the countries remained roughly the same, and on the margins of the meeting the Third World Network, a non-governmental organisation, consulted actively with several delegations from developing countries.

Discussion next focused on the scope of WHO influenza activities and the current structure and function of the GISN. Some developing countries posed extensive questions on the mandate of the network and the specifics of ownership and control of samples. Indonesia tabled its own diagram of proposed revisions in the organisational structure that reflected its priorities. As part of the dialogue, France, the United Kingdom, and others pointed out that the IDWG could not debate intellectual property rights (IPR) because WHO Member States were awaiting a report on the issue from another body, and that discussion of technology transfer was inappropriate because governments were not in possession of most vaccine production technology. At one point, two proposals encountered substantial opposition: an Indonesian assertion that benefit-sharing should be "specific, mandatory, and binding;" and a US proposal that benefits should be reserved for GISN members in good standing. There were conflicting views on who owns a virus within the GISN until the Brazilian delegate proposed that WHO could own the virus. There was general support for the idea that countries could transfer viruses to the WHO, which would serve as the owner or custodian of all samples, but there was great disagreement about the details. Countries (and the WHO Secretariat) expressed concern about the implications of such a fundamental change to the GISN as it pertained to the development of vaccines and the status of any resulting intellectual property. Nothing was concluded, and participants could not even agree on which entities were part of the GISN (versus outside entities).

Negotiations over standard terms and conditions governing the transfer of virus samples evinced fundamental differences on issues such as signed consent for the movement of viruses, the requirement of developing country scientists to be included in research, and a proposed link between the sharing of viruses and royalties. Negotiations over the draft terms of reference for WHO Collaborating Centres were able to reach consensus on many issues, but differences persisted on prior informed consent for sharing samples with third parties, deposit of virus sequences into public databases, and terms for sharing samples with the network. As a result, the text of those sections was placed within brackets (i.e. not agreed to and requiring future reconsideration).

At the very end of the day, the Chair solicited views from attendees on the major outstanding themes: benefit sharing; ownership of viruses; and the rights of countries that share viruses. Most speakers said they trusted WHO to devise a compromise solution, but there were also many re-statements of well-entrenched positions. In his final statement, the Indonesian delegate said, "We are only discussing influenza viruses, but this will be a precedent for future agreements on biologic specimens and probiotics with regard to ownership, custodianship, and transfer of rights." Delegates were well aware that any decisions made through the WHO process could set precedents beyond the immediate issue at hand, and that prospect made delegates even more reluctant to compromise in the negotiations.

In the end, the IDWG ended its deliberations without finalising work on the major topics it was mandated to discuss. Although progress was made, it was evident that differences of opinion persisted on some fundamental principles of how the surveillance network should function. The group successfully defined the goals and objectives of an oversight mechanism for the GISN, as well as some of the core elements of a benefit-sharing scheme, but disagreements about specifics prevented the development of a full draft text. It was also increasingly evident that the complex nature of the negotiations involved IPR and other issues beyond the traditional domain of public health experts.

The IDWG forwarded the products of its deliberations to the WHO Secretariat, which worked to synthesise them into draft documents for deliberation at the Intergovernmental Meeting on Pandemic Influenza Preparedness: Sharing of Influenza Viruses and Access to Vaccines and other Benefits (IGM).

More formal and informal meetings discuss sample sharing and benefit sharing

Whilst governments continued to disagree, the threat from the H5N1 virus persisted. WHO released its annual World Health Report in which it described pandemic influenza as "the most feared security threat."[8] With the fear of a pandemic in mind, the WHO Secretariat hosted meetings to discuss the feasibility and utility of establishing a stockpile of H5N1 pre-pandemic vaccine for use at the beginning of a pandemic.

In this period, non-governmental actors tried to facilitate agreement. Chatham House, London, hosted a conference October 17–18, 2007, entitled, "Pandemic Flu: Towards an Effective Global Preparedness Policy." It included sessions on such contentious issues as Vaccines and Benefit Sharing and Intellectual Property Rights and Viruses.

Prior to the November 2007 IGM, Indonesia and the United States engaged in occasional bilateral discussions. On the margins of the Chatham House conference, David Hohman, Health Attaché at the US

Mission in Geneva and I met with Dr. Widjaja Lukito, Adviser to the Indonesian Minister on Health Public Policy, and Dr. Endang Rahayu Sedyaningsih, Director of Indonesia's Biomedical and Pharmaceutical Research Centre (who became Indonesia's Minister of Health in October 2009). US Under Secretary of State for Democracy and Global Affairs Paula Dobriansky, accompanied by US Ambassador Cameron Hume, met in Jakarta October 25 with Bayu Krisnamurthi, Secretary of the Indonesian National Committee on Avian Influenza Management and Pandemic Alert (known as KOMNAS). Dobriansky stressed Washington's concerns about the serious risks associated with not sharing viruses and the need to maintain private sector incentives for the development of vaccines by all nations, whilst Krisnamurthi described likely elements of an Indonesian package on sample sharing: access to vaccine during a pandemic; the long-term development of WHO reference-laboratory capacity; and the long-term development of Indonesian vaccine-production capacity. But none of these discussions led to an agreement on key issues that could then be taken to the broader group of interested countries at the IGM.

The intergovernmental meeting makes progress but cannot reach agreement

The WHO Intergovernmental Meeting on Pandemic Influenza Preparedness began its four-day meeting in Geneva on November 20, 2007. The meeting opened with another impassioned plea by WHO Director-General Margaret Chan recognising the real threat that avian influenza posed and the need for collective action to address it through the sharing of viruses for surveillance and the development of countermeasures. "Millions of people outside this hall depend on us to make progress," she told the delegates.[9]

Jane Halton, Secretary of Australia's Department of Health and Ageing, who had been well-respected for her leadership as President of WHA60,was elected IGM Chair. The first country to speak was Indonesia. Health Minister Supari recounted a series of incidents that she saw as indicative of an unfair and dysfunctional system, concluding that the GISN should be scrapped for a new system. She also asserted that viruses received through the GISN "might" be utilised for development of biological weapons. On behalf of the US Government, I later recounted the full range of elements that the US considered relevant to addressing the threat of a pandemic, including rapid response, community mitigation measures, humanitarian assistance, support for the GISN, and voluntary benefit sharing.

In an echo of the fundamental differences in the drafting group at WHA60 and the IDWG, delegates on the first day could not even determine the framework for negotiations and much time was consumed by discussion of which texts should be the working document and how the negotiations should proceed. By the second day, the Chair proposed a new method of work, resulting in a decision to begin substantive work by discussing principles of virus sharing. Delegates articulated several of these principles in a list, but did not negotiate them or reconcile conflicting principles. In an evening session, delegates broke into two groups — one to continue the discussion of guiding principles and one to discuss operational components of the GISN — but the operational group was hindered by the fact that there was no agreement on the principles. Making matters worse, all of the discussions were slowed by persistent disagreement on fundamental concepts, such as prior informed consent. Many groups contributed new documents for consideration, including a consensus document from WHO Member States from the Americas region stating the outcomes of a meeting they had held in Argentina, and a proposed standard terms and conditions document submitted by Nigeria on behalf of the Africa region.

Delegations able to include experts from different disciplines were in some respects at an advantage. However, they were negotiating with many governments that could not afford the financial cost, or did not have readily available expertise, to send a large delegation with experts in public health (particularly global influenza surveillance), international treaties, intellectual property rights, international trade, and diplomacy. As a result, basic misunderstandings occasionally arose that contributed to delays and deadlocks in the negotiations.

As is normal for international negotiations, a multitude of side discussions took place. David Hohman and I had a lengthy meeting with Indonesian Health Minister Supari and Ambassador to the UN in Geneva Makarim Wibisono. The Minister raised a series of familiar Indonesian issues and repeatedly insisted on equity, transparency, and fairness, including through such mechanisms as a materials transfer agreement (MTA) to govern the movement of viruses. I, in turn, reiterated US support for measures to ensure transparency in the GISN, such as an electronic tracking system for virus samples, as well as for benefits provided on a voluntary basis. But the two parties fundamentally disagreed on the concept of free and unencumbered sample sharing. I considered our meeting to be a frank and candid exchange of views, whilst Minister Supari later wrote, "It was the most violent argument I ever had."[10] In the end, we both agreed the two governments would continue our dialogue.

After extensive corridor discussions at the IGM, a document was brought to the plenary body on the last day of negotiations, November 23. Delegates agreed — pending subsequent approval by the African group on the consensus "Interim Statement" — to specific steps aimed at improving the GISN and to establish a way forward for further negotiations on unresolved issues. The Member States asked Director-General Chan to move forward on two immediate measures to improve transparency: (1) a "traceability" mechanism to track the H5N1 virus and other potential pandemic human viruses that are shared with the GISN; and (2) an advisory group, appointed by the Director-General, to monitor and advise on strengthening the network. Those two elements were chosen as actions on which there was agreement that would serve to enhance trust in the WHO system, possibly paving the way for the resumption of virus sharing by Indonesia. Countries agreed to resume sharing virus samples "in accordance with national laws" whilst discussions continued on a detailed framework for virus sharing and benefit sharing. Whilst the phrase "in accordance with national laws" can be found in other UN resolutions, Indonesia made an intervention at the end of the session making it clear that they interpreted the phrase to allow Indonesia to insist on an MTA (which could include a requirement for prior informed consent for uses beyond risk assessment) for the samples that it shared. Since developed countries had opposed application of the principle of prior informed consent, this meant that sample sharing was unlikely to resume.

In the IGM working groups on principles and operational elements, consensus had been reached on some paragraphs but large sections of text remained in dispute and therefore were bracketed (i.e. not agreed to).

Overall, the IGM had two key outcomes: Indonesia conceded that virus sharing continued to be important to global public health, and Member States generally acknowledged that WHO and the GISN could operate more accountably and transparently. But delegates left the intractable benefit sharing and virus sharing controversies for resolution at a later date. The Chair agreed to convene an Open-Ended Working Group with balanced representation, and that working group would report later to a reconvened IGM. The IGM finally concluded its exhausting session just before 11:00 pm.

More meetings discuss sample sharing and benefit sharing

Under the theme, "One World: United for Avian Influenza and Pandemic Preparedness," the Government of India hosted the New Delhi International Ministerial Conference on Avian and Pandemic Influenza December 4–6, 2007. The array of leaders in attendance indicated the world's continuing concern for the pandemic threat: India's Ministers of Agriculture and Health presided over an inaugural session that featured speeches by the Directors-General of WHO, the Food and Agriculture Organization, and the World Organization for Animal Health, as well as by the UN System Influenza Coordinator.

Ministerial interventions included a speech by Indonesian Health Minister Supari, who said that "fair, transparent and equitable" governance of virus sharing was more important than the issues on the conference agenda (which deliberately did not mention virus sharing, since that issue was being considered in the WHO forum). She said that benefits should be provided as a "right" rather than as "charity" and claimed that it was not known if viruses were used for research, vaccine manufacture, or "development of biological weapons." Other nations in general did not raise the issues of sample sharing and benefit sharing and focused instead on other elements of animal health and human health related to threats from the H5N1 virus.

At the January 2008 WHO Executive Board meeting, members discussed an information item with a lengthy annex containing the consolidated outcome of the official negotiations, including agreed text and bracketed text (on which consensus was not reached).[11] Director-General Chan told the board that the H5N1 avian flu remained a threat. "This season has again given us some stark reminders that the threat of an influenza pandemic has by no means diminished."

In light of the difficulties in reaching consensus on complex issues in a multilateral setting, two governments that had played leading roles in the negotiations — Indonesia and the United States — decided to meet bilaterally in negotiations facilitated by the IGM Chair. They met in Sydney, Australia in March 2008 to discuss the sharing of influenza samples and benefits and participation in the WHO influenza surveillance network. The meeting was hosted by Chair Jane Halton and facilitated by Australia's Assistant Secretary of Health and Ageing Simon Cotterell. In two and a half days of talks, participants successfully highlighted several areas for possible progress as well as some areas of persistent disagreement between the two countries. The meeting was conducted on an *ad referendum* basis, and a draft paper was then submitted for further consideration by officials in Jakarta and Washington with authority to make final decisions. Although some outsiders were suspicious that Indonesia and the United States were endeavouring to broker a bilateral deal on sample sharing and benefit sharing that would leave others out, the purpose of this and subsequent US-Indonesia meetings was to search for common ground and then advance those ideas through the existing IGM process.

On the day before the meeting of the IGM's Open-Ended Working Group, Health Minister Supari and other Indonesian officials met for two hours at the Indonesian Ambassador's residence in Geneva with William Steiger, Director of the Office of Global Health Affairs at the US Department of Health and Human Services, Health Attaché David Hohman, and me. That meeting served to consolidate understandings from the Sydney discussions but resulted in no breakthroughs. During the discussion of benefit sharing, the Minister raised a new issue: monetary benefits (such as a percentage of the sales of vaccine sold by a pharmaceutical company) should be provided to the country that provided the virus samples used by the vaccine manufacturer. US officials noted that this appeared to be like payment of royalties for viruses, which the US Government had opposed. Indonesian officials indicated the concept was still being refined.

The open-ended working group makes more progress

On April 3–4, the Open-Ended Working Group, chaired by Jane Halton, met in Geneva. Director-General Chan used the occasion to remind delegates that the danger of a pandemic had not dissipated – and there must be immediate international cooperation because a pandemic would be rapid in spread, global in impact, and potentially devastating in consequences.

The negotiations were less contentious than previous WHO gatherings, in part because the Chair urged delegates to focus first on areas of possible common ground. The group agreed on consolidated text on several issues: research and publication (authorship, acknowledgement and attribution); safe handling of materials; transparency and traceability; and the Director-General's Advisory Mechanism. Delegates also encouraged the WHO Secretariat to accelerate work on developing stockpiles of antivirals and vaccines.

It became clear that it would not be possible to conclude the negotiations in advance of the 61st World Health Assembly (WHA61). The group agreed to a timetable for the way forward, including distribution of a Chair's text (consolidating all elements of the sample and benefit sharing debate) for comments by Member States, resumption of the Working Group in late 2008, and resumption of the IGM in hopes of concluding the process that same week.

US-Indonesia discussions continue

During the same month US Secretary of Health and Human Services Michael Leavitt visited Indonesia, Singapore, and Vietnam and met with Minister Supari in Jakarta. The two discussed sample sharing and benefit sharing but were unable to resolve the issues. Leavitt wrote in his blog that the availability of vaccines and the sharing of samples are both legitimate issues, "And we must deal with them both, but we should not link [them]. World health should not be the subject of barter."[12]

In May, during WHA61, Secretary Leavitt and Minister Supari again held bilateral discussions. Minister Supari said her goal was to employ a 60-day roadmap for US-Indonesian discussions and to prepare a progress report for the two respective heads of state prior to the July 2008 meeting of G-8 countries. She emphasised this effort was not to impose US-Indonesian views on other countries, but was rather part of a multilateral process facilitated by Australia that would culminate at the November IGM session. Secretary Leavitt agreed to continue discussions to narrow differences and said the US Government continued to support and focus on the multilateral process led by Australia.

Later during WHA61 US and Indonesian representatives again met in discussions facilitated by Australia. The Indonesian delegation was led by Ambassador Makarim Wibisono and Dr. Widjaja Lukito. The United States presented the Indonesians with a proposal for elements and principles of a standard, non-negotiable MTA for viruses, and Indonesia subsequently responded with a counterproposal that accepted many of the US concepts but required further negotiations. Simon Cotterell, who facilitated the negotiations, agreed to take the discussions into account in the work on finalising the draft Chair's text that would eventually be debated at the IGM session later in the year.

Others try to influence the process

Other discussions on sample sharing and benefit sharing took place during WHA61 including amongst health ministers of the Non-Aligned Movement (the group of states considering themselves not formally aligned with or against any major power bloc), but the WHA did not pass another resolution on the subject.

As the fear of a pandemic continued whilst negotiators could not reach agreement, the dispute received greater international attention. Influential US commentators Richard Holbrooke and Laurie Garrett expressed alarm and were sharply critical of Indonesia and its allies:

> Here's a concept you've probably never heard of: "viral sovereignty." This extremely dangerous idea comes to us courtesy of Indonesia's minister of health, Siti Fadilah Supari, who asserts that deadly viruses are the sovereign property of individual nations — even though they cross borders and could pose a pandemic threat to all the peoples of the world. So far "viral sovereignty" has been noted almost exclusively by health

experts. Political leaders around the world should take note — and take very strong action....

A year ago, Supari's assertions about "viral sovereignty" seemed to be odd yet individual views. Disturbingly, however, the notion has morphed into a global movement, fuelled by self-destructive, anti-Western sentiments. In May, Indian Health Minister A. Ramadoss endorsed the concept in a dispute with Bangladesh. The Non-Aligned Movement — a 112-nation organisation that is a survivor of the Cold War era — has agreed to consider formally endorsing the concept of "viral sovereignty" at its November meeting....

The failure to share potentially pandemic viral strains with world health agencies is morally reprehensible. Allowing Indonesia and other countries to turn this issue into another rich-poor, Islamic-Western dispute would be tragic — and could lead to a devastating health crisis anywhere, at any time.[13]

Ambassador Makarim Wibisono responded in the English-language *Jakarta Post* by stating the Holbrooke-Garrett op-ed article contained "factual mistakes and misleading statements." He wrote that "the Global Influenza Surveillance Network is not transparent, just nor equitable. The system takes resources from developing countries and provides little to them in return while leaving developing countries all the more vulnerable to an influenza pandemic." He added that, contrary to their assertion, de facto "viral sovereignty" already exists because "...the Convention on Biological Diversity, among other international instruments, has recognized national sovereignty over genetic resources, including microbes." In the absence of a just MTA defining the rights of the parties, he said companies intend to profit from viruses obtained from Indonesia, Vietnam, and other countries "while Indonesia and many other resource donor countries will receive nothing from the proceeds."[14]

Another meeting between the US and Indonesia, again facilitated by Australia, took place in Manila in September 2008. By this time, the discussions had led to familiarity and greater appreciation for each delegation's viewpoints. Although the atmosphere was constructive, the meeting did not deliver a clear agreement that could be built on in the multilateral negotiations.

Over 120 countries attended the International Ministerial Conference on Avian and Pandemic Influenza place in Egypt October 25–26, 2008. Whilst the focus was on sustaining efforts to control highly pathogenic avian influenza and mitigating the impact of an influenza pandemic, Egypt's "Vision for the Future" included a paragraph highlighting the importance of expeditiously resolving the issues of virus and benefit sharing.

The Bill & Melinda Gates Foundation was active in supporting an analysis of the feasibility and costs of an H5N1 pre-pandemic vaccine stockpile, which was considered to be a tangible benefit that would help developing countries during a pandemic.

Meanwhile, governments prepared for the December 2008 session of the IGM. WHO released to Member States a key document for those negotiations: a revised Chair's text on sharing of influenza viruses and access to vaccines and other benefits. The text reflected comments submitted by governments on a previous version.

In advance of the IGM, US and Indonesian negotiators exchanged views in a December 1 conference call and met at the US Mission in Geneva in discussions facilitated by the Australian Chair. All agreed that US-Indonesian differences had narrowed, but key issues – including the degree to which benefit sharing would be mentioned in the MTA (Indonesia wanting a specific mention in the MTA), and Indonesia's desire for prior informed consent for onward transfers of pandemic influenza preparedness biologic materials that had already been transferred out of the network — remained unresolved.

On the first day of the IGM, Health Attaché David Hohman and I met with Indonesian Health Minister Siti Supari and Dr. Widjaja Lukito. Minister Supari said she was hopeful of "maximum progress" in Geneva and emphasised the importance that Indonesia placed on having mention of benefit sharing in the body of a standard MTA (which the United States opposed, in order to avoid explicitly linking sample sharing and benefit sharing). She repeated that concern in her speech later to the IGM plenary meeting. In that speech, she mentioned the discussions that had been ongoing between the United States and Indonesia, facilitated by Australia, and specifically thanked her "US colleagues, who have demonstrated good will to continuously engage in the discussion."

By now the bilateral track — US-Indonesian negotiations facilitated by the Australian Chair of the IGM — had continued periodically for many months. As the IGM began, the participants in those bilateral negotiations had generated good will but had been unable to reach agreement on fundamental issues that could be passed on to the multilateral IGM forum. The situation remained deadlocked.

Intergovernmental meeting makes progress but key issues remain

On the first day of the December 8–13, 2008, IGM negotiations — which took place nearly two years after Indonesia had decided to stop sharing influenza viruses with WHO Collaborating Centres — Director-General Chan reminded delegates of the pandemic threat and urged them to approach the meeting with a sense of urgency. In response to a query on the difficulty of maintaining preparedness in light of "flu fatigue" in some quarters (since the H5N1 threat had not yet materialised), she told the IGM, "Pandemic influenza preparedness is the first priority for the WHO."

Given the complexity of the issues and the deep divisions amongst governments, by the fourth day the negotiations were about to founder. One of the continuing sources of friction over the course of the multilateral negotiations had been Indonesia's persistent challenge to the concept that it was mandatory for countries to share virus samples but voluntary for countries to share the benefits (such as pandemic influenza vaccines) derived from those samples. A breakthrough on language proposed by the US delegation was to refer to both virus sharing and benefit sharing as "commitments" that were made by Member States rather than as "mandatory" or "voluntary" actions. In the debate, the commitments to share both viruses and benefits were then described as being on an "equal footing." The goodwill generated by the US-Indonesian discussions over the previous seven months then led to the joint submission of a key paragraph for a standard MTA, and that proved to be instrumental in changing the meeting dynamics. Although a few delegations had been critical because they feared a separate bilateral agreement had been in the works, by the closing session the Vice Chair for the African region, Dr. Abdulsalam Nasidi from Nigeria, specifically commended the US and Indonesian delegations "for making everything possible."

Delegates reached general agreement on guiding principles for development of terms of reference for laboratories in the WHO influenza surveillance network and terms of reference for the new Advisory Group. Two important principles were established at the meeting: (1) benefits should not be provided in a preferential manner to the country from which the virus had originated, but rather as a pooled benefits system based on public health risk and need (aimed at developing countries); and (2) the scope of the IGM negotiations was limited to influenza viruses with pandemic potential and did not extend to seasonal influenza viruses (thereby limiting one of the key strategic concerns regarding the entire negotiation).

Despite substantial progress on complex issues, however, delegates still were not able to bring the negotiations to successful conclusion. Unresolved issues before the IGM generally fell into two categories: attempts to re-define IPR (with Brazil leading the charge in cooperation with others); and various matters related to the connection between virus sharing and benefit sharing (with Indonesia and many other developing countries trying to create linkage whilst developed countries opposed such linkage).

It was agreed that the IGM would reconvene (again) for a final session in connection with the 62nd World Health Assembly (WHA62) in May 2009. In the meantime, interested governments would again engage in informal consultations facilitated by the Australian Chair and Vice Chairs from other regions. An informal meeting facilitated by Norway took place at the end of March 2009 in Montreux, Switzerland, to discuss IPR, a standard MTA, and other issues of contention. In the meantime, the WHO Secretariat prepared an informational report to WHA62.[15]

And then, in April 2009, global fears that a new pandemic would emerge became a reality. After early outbreaks in North America, a new "pandemic (H1N1) 2009 virus," known informally as "swine flu," spread rapidly around the world. It was not the H5N1 virus that had led to the initial international concern, but it generated an immediate response at the highest levels of governments. On April 27, WHO raised the level of pandemic alert to Pandemic Phase 4, moving to Phase 5 on April 29 and to Phase 6 (the maximum level) on June 11. By that time, a total of 74 countries and territories had reported laboratory-confirmed infections and, as time went on, most countries in the world confirmed infections from the new virus. The incremental increases in phases of pandemic alert reflected the geographical spread of the disease; WHO did not require a set level of severity as part of its criteria for declaring a pandemic (a matter for which it later received criticism from some quarters). Dr. Keiji Fukuda, WHO Special Adviser to the Director-General on Pandemic Influenza, noted in February 2010 that it appeared "to be on the less severe side of the spectrum of pandemics that we have seen in the 20th century."[16] Whilst the pandemic turned out not to be as severe as the planning scenarios for H5N1, it gave immediate relevancy to the negotiations at hand.

The IGM resumed in the days before WHA62. By this time, the fundamental differences were abundantly clear and there was little possibility that they could be overcome in a few days. The H1N1 pandemic gave an additional urgency to the negotiations but also served to sharpen differences in perspective: developed countries were focused on the importance, and success, of rapid and unencumbered virus sharing whilst developing countries were focused on their effective lack of access to any vaccine or vaccine production capacity. This sharpened the differences in perspective on the idea of having an MTA, the proposed link between virus sharing and benefit sharing, and, as a subset of that, IPR-related issues. Aside from these three core issues, the IGM settled a large amount of text in the framework document.[17]

WHO member states continue to negotiate and finally reach agreement

Over the course of two years, the negotiations process under WHA60.28 served to keep all Members States at the table (no other country, at least openly, followed Indonesia's lead in refusing to share virus samples with the GISN) and successfully prevented the pandemic influenza issue from affecting the seasonal influenza virus-sharing and vaccine-development system. In addition, the negotiators rejected the idea that future arrangements would include quasi-royalties or one-for-one benefits to countries from which viruses originated; the principle of pooled benefits distributed according to risk and need, particularly for developing countries, may be an important precedent for other diseases and pharmaceuticals. Importantly, the negotiations repeatedly highlighted for WHO and governments the importance of pandemic preparedness and the recognition of developing-country needs during a pandemic; this proved to be a contributing factor in the September 2009 decision by donor governments to contribute a portion of their H1N1 vaccine supply to developing countries.

Nevertheless, for anyone hoping the issues could be resolved after literally thousands of hours of discussions in multilateral, bilateral, and informal forums and huge sums of money spent to facilitate so many meetings around the world, the results were disappointing. After two years of negotiations on an issue of global health urgency which also involved trade, IPR, and political issues, far from the remit and expertise of public health experts, the best that the May 2009 62nd World Health Assembly could do was to pass a short resolution recognising "further work needs to be done on some key remaining elements" and requesting the Director-General:

(1) to work with Member States to take forward the agreed parts of the Pandemic Influenza Preparedness Framework for the sharing of influenza viruses and access to vaccines and other benefits as contained in the report of the outcome of the Intergovernmental Meeting;
(2) to facilitate a transparent process to finalize the remaining elements, including the Standard Material Transfer Agreements and its annex, and report the outcome to the Executive Board at its 126th session in January 2010.[18]

An Open-Ended Working Group of Member States on Pandemic Influenza Preparedness: Sharing of Influenza Viruses and Access to Vaccines and Other Benefits met in Geneva on May 10–12, 2010, and produced yet another report. The 63rd World Health Assembly later that month passed another short resolution, WHA63.1, that was very similar to the previous one and requested the Director-General:

(1) to continue to work with Member States and relevant regional economic integration organisations, on the Pandemic Influenza Preparedness Framework for the Sharing of Influenza Viruses and

Access to Vaccines and Other Benefits as decided in Resolution WHA62.10 and to convene the Open-Ended Working Group before the 128th session of the Executive Board; [and]

(2) to undertake technical consultations and studies as necessary in order to support the work of the Open-Ended Working Group in reaching a final agreement.[19]

The resolution was yet another signal of the importance that WHO Member States placed on resolving the issues at hand. Progress had been made, but fundamental differences remained. In an attempt to produce a framework agreement, Ambassador Juan José Gomez-Camacho (Mexico) and Ambassador Bente Angell-Hansen (Norway), who were now the co-chairs of the Open-Ended Working Group, worked tirelessly with WHO Member States, industry representatives, civil society and other organisations involved in influenza pandemic preparedness. Finally, after numerous consultations and a week of intense negotiations in Geneva, the working group reached consensus on April 16, 2011.

> The new framework includes certain binding legal regimes for WHO, national influenza laboratories around the world and industry partners in both developed and developing countries that will strengthen how the world responds more effectively with the next flu pandemic. By making sure that the roles and obligations among key players are better established than in the past — including through the use of contracts — the framework will help increase and expedite access to essential vaccines, antivirals and diagnostic kits, especially for outbreak areas.
>
> In addition, the framework will also put the world in a better position for seasonal influenza and potential pandemic threats such as the H5N1 virus, because some key activities will begin before the next pandemic, such as greater support for strengthening laboratories and surveillance, and partnership contributions from the industry....
>
> The new framework will help ensure more equitable access to affordable vaccines and at the same time, also guarantee the flow of virus samples into the WHO system so that the critical information and analyses needed to assess public health risks and develop vaccines are available.[20]

Nearly four years after the negotiations on sample sharing and benefit sharing had officially begun at WHA60, during a time of intense concern that a severe pandemic could kill millions, WHO Member States had finally reached agreement.

Key Points

- Whilst official negotiations took place under the auspices of a World Health Assembly resolution, the importance of the issue led to many other, parallel efforts to solve particular aspects of the complex issues under consideration. A bilateral negotiating track involving two of the main protagonists, Indonesia and the United States, at first generated suspicion among others not involved. Whilst these face-to-face negotiations served to build goodwill, they were unable to overcome fundamental differences between the two parties and, in the end, were limited in their ability to help advance the multilateral negotiations.
- Fundamental differences among the many governments negotiating in the WHO multilateral forum delayed for years the ability to reach consensus on a framework agreement, despite the negotiating timetables set forth in World Health Assembly resolutions and the very real threat of a global human influenza pandemic.

Lessons to be Learned

The negotiating process effectively began in December 2006, when Indonesia decided to stop sharing influenza viruses to pressure for a change in the Global Influenza Surveillance Network. Indonesia insisted on transparency in the GISN and asserted that it should retain control over influenza viruses that it shared in order to receive benefits such as pandemic vaccine.

To achieve its goals, Indonesia brought its concerns to the World Health Assembly in May 2007. At that point, the issue became broader and no one country could control the debate or the direction.

In contentious multilateral negotiations, the official debate on the floor virtually never reflects the true extent of serious dialogue amongst the contesting parties. In this case, bilateral negotiations between Indonesia and the United States often facilitated by Australia, at times provoked suspicion amongst their respective allies (as if a separate deal were being cut). The understandings and goodwill established through these bilateral negotiations however, proved beneficial and resulted in important compromises at particular points in the negotiations. Nevertheless, in the end those understandings and goodwill were not sufficient to bridge fundamental differences amongst WHO Member States.

The technical complexity of discussions about the GISN was difficult for many delegates to understand. Some non-governmental entities were engaged in the discussions, but due to the intricacy of the negotiations and the absence of relevant technical experts in most of those groups, their numbers were far fewer than for some other major health issues (such as HIV/AIDS). This stemmed in part from the fact that pandemics are infrequent occurrences (there were three in the twentieth century) and vary in their fatality rate, so the discussion was to some extent considered theoretical until the actual outbreak of the H1N1 pandemic virus in 2009. Some well-intended outsiders presented ideas to solve the impasse in negotiations but they did not take into account the range of national interests amongst the WHO Member States most interested in the negotiations, and as such, their suggestions did not significantly influence the deliberations.

The complexity of issues made it clear that negotiating teams required a mix of skills: public health experts who understood the GISN and the respective roles of National Influenza Centres, WHO Collaborating Centres, researchers, pharmaceutical companies and others; lawyers with expertise in health, IPR, trade law, and other fields; and diplomats who understood competing national interests and political motivations that dominated the negotiations.

Conclusion

In September 2009, when concern for the H1N1 influenza pandemic was at its height, Australia, Brazil, France, Italy, New Zealand, Norway,

Switzerland, the United Kingdom, and the United States announced that they were prepared to make up to ten per cent of their H1N1 vaccine supply available to developing countries through WHO.[21] Other nations later joined in making such a contribution.

This was a significant step in recognising the needs of people in developing countries to have access to life-saving vaccines during an influenza pandemic. It may have served to set a precedent for future pandemics. However, it must be recognised that this was a voluntary contribution on the part of certain donor governments and it was not a required benefit under a new sample sharing and benefit sharing regime.

With the needs of developing countries in mind, the Bill & Melinda Gates Foundation in 2009 proposed a set of principles to guide global allocation of pandemic vaccine that began, "The global community should take steps to protect all populations, including those without resources to protect themselves."[22] Developing-country access to vaccines will be enormously important at some undeterminable date in the future, when the world experiences what most experts consider inevitable: a severe human influenza pandemic capable of killing tens of millions of people. The April 2011 framework agreement, when fully implemented, has the potential to be a critical factor in mitigating the effects of such a pandemic. If that proves to be the case, the four years of negotiations will have been well worth the effort.

References

1. WHO Global Influenza Surveillance Network, http://www.who.int/csr/disease/influenza/surveillance/en/.
2. Supari, Siti Fadilah (2008) *It's Time for the World to Change*, pp. xi–xii, PT. Sulaksana Watinsa Indonesia, Jakarta.
3. EB120.R7, Avian and pandemic influenza: developments, response and follow-up, application of the International Health Regulations (2005), and best practice for sharing influenza viruses and sequence data, January 26, 2007, http://apps.who.int/gb/ebwha/pdf_files/EB119–120-REC1/p4-en.pdf
4. Indonesia to resume sharing H5N1 avian influenza virus samples following a WHO meeting in Jakarta, March 27, 2007, http://www.who.int/mediacentre/news/releases/2007/pr09/en/index.html

5. New Mechanism Needed for Virus Sharing Equity, April 10, 2007, http://www.indonesia-ottawa.org/information/details.php?type=press_releases&id=122

6. "WHO fails to assure bird flu samples not to be used commercially," Jakarta Post, May 1, 2007

7. WHA 60.28, Pandemic influenza preparedness: sharing of influenza viruses and access to vaccines and other benefits, May 23, 2007, http://apps.who.int/gb/ebwha/pdf_files/WHA60/A60_R28-en.pdf

8. The World Health Report 2007: A Safer Future: Global Public Health Security in the 21st Century, http://www.who.int/whr/2007/whr07_en.pdf

9. Opening remarks at the Intergovernmental Meeting on Pandemic Influenza Preparedness, Geneva, Switzerland, 20 November 2007, "Sharing of influenza viruses and access to vaccines and other benefits," Dr. Margaret Chan, http://www.who.int/dg/speeches/2007/20071120_pip/en/index.html

10. Supari, Siti Fadilah (2008) *It's Time for the World to Change*, p. 125, PT. Sulaksana Watinsa Indonesia, Jakarta.

11. EB 122/5, Pandemic influenza preparedness: sharing of influenza viruses and access to vaccines and other benefits — Intergovernmental Meeting: report of progress to date, January 17, 2008, http://apps.who.int/gb/ebwha/pdf_files/ EB122/B122_5-en.pdf

12. HHS secretary blogs on impasse with Indonesia, April 17, 2008, http://www.cidrap.umn.edu/cidrap/content/influenza/avianflu/news/apr1708asia-jw.html

13. "'Sovereignty' That Risks Global Health," Richard Holbrooke and Laurie Garrett, *The Washington Post*, August 10, 2008 http://www.washington-post.com/wp-dyn/content/article/2008/08/08/AR2008080802919.html

14. "The responsible virus and sharing benefits," Makarim Wibisono, *The Jakarta Post,* August 27, 2008, http://www.thejakartapost.com/news/2008/08/27/the-responsible-virus-and-sharing-benefits.html

15. A62/5, Pandemic influenza preparedness: sharing of influenza viruses and access to vaccines and other benefits — Report by the Secretariat, April 30, 2009, http://apps.who.int/gb/ebwha/pdf_files/A62/A62_5-en.pdf

16. "Transcript of virtual press conference with Dr Keiji Fukuda, Special Adviser to the Director-General on Pandemic Influenza," 24 February 2010, http://www.who.int/mediacentre/vpc_transcript_24_february_10_fukuda.pdf

17. A62/5 Add.1, Pandemic influenza preparedness: sharing of influenza viruses and access to vaccines and other benefits — Outcome of the resumed Intergovernmental Meeting — Report by the Director-General, May 18, 2009, http://apps.who.int/gb/ebwha/pdf_files/A62/A62_5Add1-en.pdf

18. WHA62.10, Pandemic influenza preparedness: sharing of influenza viruses and access to vaccines and other benefits, May 22, 2009, http://apps.who.int/gb/ebwha/pdf_files/WHA62-REC1/WHA62_REC1-en-P2.pdf

19. WHA63.1, Pandemic influenza preparedness: sharing of influenza viruses and access to vaccines and other benefits, May 19, 2010, http://apps.who.int/gb/ebwha/pdf_files/WHA63/A63_R1-en.pdf

20. "Landmark agreement improves global preparedness for influenza pandemics," April 17, 2011, http://www.who.int/mediacentre/news/releases/2011/pandemic_influenza_prep_20110417/en/index.html

21. "President Announces Plan to Expand Fight Against Global H1N1 Pandemic," Office of the Press Secretary, The White House, September 17, 2009, http://www.whitehouse.gov/the_press_office/President-Announces-Plan-to-Expand-Fight-Against-Global-H1N1-Pandemic/

22. Tadataka Yamada, M.D. (2009) Poverty, Wealth, and Access to Pandemic Influenza Vaccines, *The New Engl Med*, 361: 1129–1131.

8

Negotiating Equitable Access to Influenza Vaccines: Global Health Diplomacy and the Controversies Surrounding Avian Influenza H5N1 and Pandemic Influenza H1N1

David P. Fidler[i]

Re-printed with permission from: Fidler DP (2010) Negotiating Equitable Access to Influenza Vaccines: Global Health Diplomacy and the Controversies Surrounding Avian Influenza H5N1 and Pandemic Influenza H1N1. PLoS Med 7(5): e1000247. doi:10.1371/journal.pmed.1000247. *This article is part of the PLoS Medicine Global Health Diplomacy series.*
Academic Editor: Kelley Lee, London School of Hygiene & Tropical Medicine, United Kingdom.
This article is part of the PLoS Medicine Global Health Diplomacy series.

Abstract

Threats posed by both avian influenza (H5N1) and pandemic influenza (H1N1) have heightened the importance of equitable access to vaccines.

[i] Dr. Fidler is James Louis Calamaras Professor of Law and Director, Center on American and Global Security, Indiana University.

However, moving towards more equitable access through global health diplomacy has proved difficult and controversial. The limited results produced by negotiations have stimulated calls for a new global framework to improve equitable access to influenza vaccines. The prospects for such a framework are not, however, promising because the national interests of most developed states vis-à-vis dangerous influenza strains favour retaining the existing imbalanced, reactive, and ad hoc approach to vaccine access. This chapter examines why negotiating equitable access to influenza vaccines in the context of H5N1 and H1N1 has been, and promises to continue to be, a difficult diplomatic endeavour.

Introduction

One of the most controversial areas of global health diplomacy over the past five years has involved negotiations to increase equitable access to vaccines for highly pathogenic avian influenza A (H5N1) (HPAI-H5N1) and pandemic 2009 influenza A (H1N1) (2009-H1N1). The limited results produced by these negotiations have stimulated calls for a new global framework to improve equitable access to influenza vaccines. The prospects for such a framework are not, however, promising, because the national interests of most developed states vis-à-vis dangerous influenza strains favor retaining the existing imbalanced, reactive, and ad hoc approach to vaccine access. This article examines why negotiating equitable access to influenza vaccines in the context of HPAI-H5N1 and 2009-H1N1 has been, and promises to continue to be, a difficult diplomatic endeavor.

Influenza Vaccine Access Controversies: HPAI-H5N1 and 2009-H1N1

The re-emergence of HPAI-H5N1 in 2004 and its spread triggered fears that the world was on the brink of a potentially devastating influenza pandemic.[1] Preparations for pandemic influenza frantically began, and included plans to develop a vaccine for a pandemic H5N1 strain. These plans ran headlong into developing-country concerns that their populations would not have access to H5N1 vaccines. These concerns, and the lack of any mechanism to ensure equitable access to vaccines and other benefits from research on influenza viruses, prompted Indonesia, in 2007, to refuse to share H5N1 virus samples with the World Health Organization (WHO) that would be used for surveillance.[2] Supported by many developing countries, Indonesia's action questioned the legitimacy of WHO's Global Influenza Surveillance Network and forced WHO and its member states to begin negotiations to create a new system of influenza virus and benefits sharing.[4] Although WHO member states agreed to establish a stockpile of H5N1 vaccine,[5] the negotiations have, to date, failed to reach agreement.[6]

Concerns about equitable access flared again in 2009 when a novel strain of influenza A (H1N1) emerged and spread around the world. The speed and ease with which the 2009-H1N1 strain moved meant that a vaccine was the only practical means of preventing infection, and efforts to produce a vaccine began in the late spring and early summer.[7] Developed countries placed large advance orders for 2009-H1N1 vaccine and bought virtually all the vaccine companies could manufacture.[8,9] Developing countries and WHO identified the lack of equity in how developed countries were securing access to the vaccine.[10] WHO entered talks with manufacturers and developed-country governments to secure some vaccine for developing countries,[11] and WHO and the United Nations (UN) appealed for monetary donations to purchase vaccines and other supplies to help developing countries address the 2009-H1N1 virus.[12] These efforts yielded donation pledges from manufacturers[13] and developed countries,[14] but the donations still left the developing world with limited supplies[15] compared to developed countries, which would retain, even after donations, sufficient vaccine to cover their populations.

Feared and actual problems with 2009-H1N1 vaccine production, however, affected the amount and timing of vaccine available for developing countries. As of this writing, Canada had not joined other developed countries in pledging to donate vaccines, because of shortages within Canada,[16] and Canada awarded its vaccine contract to a Canadian company because it feared that foreign governments might restrict exports to Canada because of vaccine shortages within their territories.[17] The Australian government made it clear to the Australian manufacturer CSL that it must fulfill the government's domestic needs before exporting vaccine to the United States.[18] The United States pledged on September 17, 2009, to donate 10% of its vaccine purchases to WHO, but on October 28, US Secretary of Health and Human Services Kathleen Sebelius stated that the United States would not donate H1N1 vaccine as promised until all at-risk Americans had access, because production problems had created shortages in the United States.[19] These fears and actions reinforced the sense that the status quo concerning equitable access to influenza vaccines for developing countries was flawed.

Moving Beyond Strain-Specific Responses: The Call for a Global Access Framework

The unsatisfactory nature of vaccine access concerning HPAI-H5N1 and 2009-H1N1 has created interest in creation of a global framework for equitable access that would become operational *before* the next influenza crisis. In a presentation to the Forum of Microbial Threats of the Institute of Medicine in September 2009, WHO's lead influenza specialist, Keiji Fukuda, described the problems experienced with the negotiations on HPAI-H5N1 virus and benefits sharing and on obtaining donations from manufacturers and developed countries for 2009-H1N1 vaccine.[20] Fukuda emphasized that the process and outcomes of the negotiations were sub-optimal in terms of both public health and global equity and justice. Other experts have made similar claims concerning the moral and social justice issues at stake in equitable access to 2009-H1N1 vaccines.[21,22] In the interests of global health and global solidarity, Fukuda argued that a framework was needed to support global responses to influenza threats and ensure equitable access to vaccines for developing countries.[16] He asserted that improving access is the central global governance issue of our times, which gives the need for a global access framework importance beyond the world of public health.

Getting to Access: Negotiating Equitable Access to Influenza Vaccines

Negotiations to increase access to vaccines for HPAI-H5N1 and 2009-H1N1 have not proved successful for many reasons. In the Inter-governmental Meeting (IGM) on Pandemic Influenza Preparedness

Framework for the Sharing of Influenza Viruses and Access to Vaccines and Other Benefits, WHO member states failed to reach agreement because they could not agree on benefit sharing.[23] Developing countries want obligatory benefit sharing in return for virus sharing, with binding terms spelled out in a Standard Material Transfer Agreement (SMTA). In contrast, developed countries want to avoid binding obligations to provide benefits (e.g., vaccines, antivirals) in exchange for access to virus samples provided by developing countries. At least one news report indicated that developed countries wanted to avoid losing their ability to place advance orders for influenza vaccine because of a binding SMTA.[19]

Interestingly, the 2009-H1N1 outbreak was underway when the IGM negotiations concluded unsuccessfully, meaning that this latest influenza threat was not a "game changer" for the positions staked out by WHO member states. In fact, the manner in which the outbreak and vaccine development and use proceeded favored developed countries for two reasons. First, countries with cases of 2009-H1N1 shared virus samples with WHO for surveillance and vaccine development without a *quid pro quo* for benefit sharing. To date, Indonesia remains the only country that has refused to share virus samples; other developing countries, even those that have supported Indonesia, share their samples without requiring benefits in return. Second, developed countries were able, through advance purchase contracts, to access almost all the vaccine existing manufacturing facilities can produce[8,9] in order to ensure they would have 2009-H1N1 vaccine for their populations — precisely the option developed countries do not want the proposed SMTA to affect.

In terms of vaccine for 2009-H1N1, donations from manufacturers and developed countries were not the product of real negotiations, given that WHO and developing countries had little leverage to influence developed countries other than rhetoric about equity, justice, and solidarity. As experts noted, the donations from manufacturers were initially made without out a fixed delivery date, meaning that the donated vaccines might arrive too late to be of much benefit in developing countries.[24] Developed countries only agreed to make donations *after* (1) they learned, unexpectedly, that a one-dose regimen would immunize adults, which doubled the amount of vaccine available[25]; and (2) data from the Northern and Southern hemispheres revealed that the 2009-H1N1 virus was behaving as a mild virus and not as a killer strain,[15] which reduced the threat the virus posed. In addition, developed countries pledging donations made sure that they had enough vaccine to cover their populations or, as happened with the United States, postponed donations in order to address national needs. In essence, manufacturers and developed countries incurred minimal financial, national public health, or political costs in pledging and, if necessary, delaying vaccine donations.

Vaccine and Resource Access in International Law

What has transpired in the contexts of HPAI-H5N1 and 2009-H1N1 reflects patterns seen in other efforts to create equitable access for vaccines and drugs. Existing international legal regimes that support global health, such as the WHO Constitution, the "right to health" in human rights treaties, and the International Health Regulations 2005, do not contain specific, binding provisions on equitable access to vaccines and drugs for developing countries. WHO's interest in creating a new global framework rather than relying on existing legal agreements reinforces the lack of any specific equitable access regime. Efforts to generate equitable access are not operated through purpose-built international legal instruments, and these efforts include WHO's adoption of a nonbinding global strategy on public health, innovation, and intellectual property[26]; provision of vaccines and drugs by intergovernmental organizations (e.g., WHO, UNICEF); bilateral donation schemes (e.g., the President's Emergency Plan for AIDS Relief); and public–private and nongovernmental mechanisms that make vaccines and drugs more available to developing countries (e.g., the Global Fund to Fight AIDS, Tuberculosis, and Malaria; the GAVI Alliance; Clinton Global Initiative; Médecins Sans Frontières' Campaign for Access to Essential Medicines; the International Finance Facility for Immunization; UNIT AID; and Advance Market Commitments for Vaccines).

This reality provides insight into why negotiations on virus and benefit sharing in connection with HPAI-H5N1 have, to date, failed, and why negotiations on a global access framework in the wake of the problems surrounding 2009-H1N1 would face obstacles. In short, states have not agreed to binding arrangements on more equitable access but, rather, attempt to increase such access through ad hoc, reactive, and nonbinding activities that preserve national freedom of action while demonstrating some humanitarian concern.

Moreover, the situation concerning access to vaccines and drugs reflects how states generally allocate control of and access to resources. The central principles for allocating resources in international law are (1) sovereignty for resources found within a state's territory,[27] and (2) exclusive jurisdiction or control for resources found seawards from coastal states (e.g., the Exclusive Economic Zone in the law of the sea).[28] International relations provide few, if any, examples of states establishing a global framework to allocate resources, or the benefits derived from their exploitation, equitably. The most famous effort occurred in the negotiation of the UN Convention on the Law of the Sea (UNCLOS) in the 1970s and early 1980s and involved designating mineral resources found beyond 200 nautical miles from coastal states as the "common heritage of mankind," which would be exploited under jurisdiction of an International Seabed Authority, with benefits accruing to developing countries.[29] However, the United States and other developed countries opposed this aspect of UNCLOS, which, because of this opposition, has been revised to reflect what these developed countries prefer concerning exploitation of these mineral resources.[30]

The problems of equitable access to vaccines and drugs reflect these larger patterns in international law and international relations. As Indonesia's assertion of "viral sovereignty" demonstrates, states have sovereignty over biological samples isolated within their territories. Negotiations within the WHO[5] and the IGM[19] have re-emphasized that states have sovereignty over biological resources found within their jurisdictions. Similarly, states in which vaccines and drugs are manufactured have sovereignty over the manufacturing process and the products themselves, until they are exported. States that import vaccines and drugs then have sovereignty over such resources and, absent a binding obligation, may allocate them however they wish. Negotiations to create a global access framework that more equitably distributes influenza vaccines would need to navigate through triple claims of sovereignty — a very tall order, without even factoring in the divergence of national interests seen in the IGM negotiations on virus and benefit sharing and the access problems associated with vaccine for 2009-H1N1.

Conclusion

Increasing equitable access to vaccines for dangerous influenza strains represents a difficult challenge for global health diplomacy, a challenge this article has addressed in only a preliminary manner. Efforts to recalibrate virus- and benefit-sharing in connection with HPAI-H5N1 through intergovernmental negotiations have not, so far, been successful. The manner in which access to vaccine for 2009-H1N1 played out highlights why the interests of developed and developing countries diverge in this context, and the reasons behind this divergence deserve deeper study. Existing international legal regimes on global health provide no templates for negotiating the new global access framework that WHO and others perceive is necessary. Similarly, negotiations for equitable access to resources, or the benefits of their exploitation, have generally failed in other areas of international relations, dimming prospects that precedents for a global access framework for pandemic influenza vaccines can be found outside the global health context. The default rules for allocating resources in international law rely on the principle of sovereignty, and these rules hold in the context of virus samples and vaccine supplies, as demonstrated with HPAI-H5N1 and 2009-H1N1.

Even the emergence of the first pandemic strain of influenza in 40 years in 2009 did not break the pattern of state behavior with respect to equitable access to a valuable but scarce resource. The appearance of a more severe influenza strain will reinforce rather than overcome this pattern, because developed countries will prize their power and flexibility of action more in a severe pandemic than in a mild one, thus making hope for a crisis-sparked breakthrough misguided. The negotiating path that could lead to a new global access framework for influenza vaccines is not apparent, especially in a context in which aggregate global production capacity is woefully inadequate, the geographic location of production facilities is concentrated in developed countries, timelines for developing new vaccines create problems for rapid prevention strategies, and existing manufacturing technologies and distribution systems require improvements.

The need to increase global production capacity, diversify locales for manufacturing facilities, decrease the time from "lab to jab," and reduce production and distribution uncertainties, has been recognized for years without sufficient progress being made, as evidenced by the HPAI-H5N1 and 2009-H1N1 controversies. Further research is required on ways in which states and non-state actors can address these problems through negotiated collective action. The diplomatic environment may have been made more difficult by accusations made and hearings held by officials in the Council of Europe that WHO succumbed to pressure from the pharmaceutical industry to declare a "false pandemic" and support development and use of a vaccine.[31,32] In the environment that exists on these issues, diplomatic advances will not be made simply by repeated claims that an undefined "global framework" is required because more equitable access is the just and moral end all states should seek.

Author Contributions

ICMJE criteria for authorship read and met: DF. Wrote the first draft of the paper: DF.

References

1. Garrett L. (2005) The next pandemic? Foreign Affairs 84(4): 3–23. Find this article online.
2. Fidler DP. (2008) Influenza virus samples, international law, and global health diplomacy. *Emerging Infectious Diseases* 14(1): 88–94. Find this article online.
3. Garrett L, Fidler DP. (2007) Sharing H5N1 viruses to stop a global influenza pandemic. *PLoS Med* 4(11): e330. doi:10.1371/journal. pmed.0040330.
4. For documentation produced by the IGM, see Intergovernmental Meeting on Pandemic Influenza Preparedness: Sharing of Influenza Viruses and Access to Vaccines and Other Benefits, Documentation. Available: http://apps.who. int/gb/pip/. Accessed 5 February 2010.
5. World Health Assembly (2007) Pandemic Influenza Preparedness: Sharing of Influenza Viruses and Access to Vaccines and Other Benefits. WHA 60.28, 23 May.

6. Third World Network (2009) WHO: Negotiations to Continue on Influenza Virus and Benefit Sharing. Available: http://www.twnside.org.sg/title2/intelle_ctual_property/info.service/2009/twn.ipr.info.090507.html. Accessed 5 February 2010.

7. Collin N, de Radigues XWHO H1N1 Vaccine Task Force (2009) Vaccine production capacity for seasonal and pandemic (H1N1) influenza. *Vaccine* 27: 5184–5186. Find this article online.

8. Brown D. (2009) Vaccine Would be Spoken for; Rich Nations have Preexisting Contracts. Washington Post, 7 May. Available: http://www.washingtonpost.com/wp-dyn/content/article/2009/05/06/AR2009050603760.html. Accessed 5 February 2010.

9. Whalen J. (2009) Rich Nations Lock in Flu Vaccine as Poor ones Fret, Wall Street Journal, 16 May. Available: http://online.wsj.com/article/SB1242430-15022925551.html. Accessed 5 February 2010.

10. Chan M. (2009) Director-General of the World Health Organization, Strengthening Multilateral Cooperation on Intellectual Property and Public Health. Address to the World Intellectual Property Organization Conference on Intellectual Property and Public Policy Issues, Geneva, Switzerland, 14 July. Available: http://www.who.int/dg/speeches/2009/intellectual property_2009-0714/en/index.html. Accessed 5 February 2010.

11. Butler D. (2009) Q&A with Marie-Paule Kieny, the Vaccine Research Director of the World Health Organization, on Swine Flu. Nature News, 13 May. Available: http://www.nature.com/news/2009/090513/full/news.2009.478.html. Accessed 5 February 2010.

12. Evans R. (2009) More H1N1 Vaccines Likely for Poor Countries: U.N. Reuters, 25 September. Available: http://www.reuters.com/article/healthNews/idUSTRE58O4LG20090925?feedType=RSS&feedName=healthNews&pageNumber=2&virtualBrandChannel=0&sp=true. Accessed 5 February 2010.

13. WHO (2009) WHO Welcomes Sanofi-Aventis' Donation of Vaccine, 17 June. Available: http://www.who.int/mediacentre/news/statements/2009/vaccine_donation_20090617/en/index.html. Accessed 5 February 2010.

14. White House (2009) President Announces Plan to Expand Fight Against Global H1N1 Pandemic, 17 September. Available: http://www.whitehouse.gov/the_press_office/President-Announces-Plan-to-Expand-Fight-Against-Global-H1N1-Pandemic/. Accessed 5 February 2010.

15. Poorer nations get swine flu jabs. BBC News, 12 October 2009. Available: http://news.bbc.co.uk/2/hi/health/8302416.stm. Accessed 5 February 2010.

16. Branswell H. (2009) With H1N1 Vaccine Shipments Topping 20M, Canada Mulls Options for Leftovers. Canadian Press, 27 November. Available: http://www.google.com/hostednews/canadianpress/article/ALeqM5hzEQOdf AofKpIrKeqPuJqynx5WnA. Accessed 5 February 2010.

17. Branswell H. (2009) Fears that countries would hoard vaccine in pandemics behind single supplier. Canadian Press, 4 November. Available: http://ca. news.yahoo.com/s/capress/091104/health/health_flu_vaccine_single_supplier. Accessed 5 February 2010.

18. McNeil DG, Jr. (2009) Nation is Facing Vaccine Shortage for Seasonal Flu. N. Y. Times, 4 November. Available: http://www.nytimes.com/2009/11/05/ health/05flu.html. Accessed 5 February 2010.

19. Americans first before US gives H1N1 flu vaccine, Agence France-Presse, 29 October 2009. Available: http://newsinfo.inquirer.net/breakingnews/ world/view/20091029–232857/Americans-first-before-US-gives-H1N1-flu-vaccineexec. Accessed 5 February 2010.

20. Fukuda K. (2009) Influenza (H1N1) Pandemic: Lessons for Going Forward. Presentation at the Forum of Microbial Threats Workshop on the Domestic and International Aspects of the 2009 Influenza A (H1N1) Pandemic: Global Challenges, Global Solutions, 15 September. Available: http://www.iom.edu/ Object.File/Master/73/476/Fukuda%20revised%20for%20WEB.pdf. Accessed 5 February 2010.

21. Gostin LO. (2009) Global Goal for Swine Flu Vaccine Quest. The Australian, 8 August. Available: http://www.theaustralian.news.com.au/story/0,25197, 25896462-23289,00.html. Accessed 5 February 2010.

22. Yamada T. (2009) Poverty, wealth, and access to pandemic influenza vaccines. *N Engl J Med* 361: 1129–1131. Find this article online.

23. Third World Network (2009) WHO: Key Elements of Virus and Benefit-Sharing Framework Still Unresolved, 19 May. Available: http://www.twnside. org. sg/title2/intellectual property/info.service/2009/twn.ipr.info.090506.html. Accessed 5 February 2010.

24. Garrett L. (October 7, 2009) 12 p. Global Health Update.

25. Neuzil KM (2009) Pandemic influenza vaccine policy — Considering the early evidence. *N Engl J Med* 361: e59. Find this article online.

26. World Health Assembly (2008) Global strategy and plan of action on public health, innovation, and intellectual property, WHA 61.21, 24 May.

27. Brownlie I. (2008) Principles of Public International Law, 7th ed. Oxford: Oxford University Press. 784 p.

28. Churchill RR, Lowe AV. (1999) The Law of the Sea, 3rd ed. Manchester: Manchester University Press. 500 p.

29. United Nations Convention on the Law of the Sea (1982) 10 December, Part XI. Available: http://www.un.org/Depts/los/convention_a_greements/texts/unclos/closindx.html. Accessed on 5 Febru ary 2010.

30. Agreement Relating to the Implementation of Part XI of the United Nations Convention on the Law of the Sea (1994) July 28. Available: http://www.un.org/Depts/los/convention_agreements/texts/unclos/closindxAgree.html. Accessed on 5 February 2010.

31. Pollard C. (2010) Swine flu 'a false pandemic' to sell vaccines, expert says. The Daily Telegraph, 12 January. Available: http://www.dailytelegraph.com.au/news/world/swine-flu-a-false-pandemic-to-sell-v_accines-expert-says/story-e6frev00-1225818409903. Accessed 5 February 2010.

32. Fukuda K. (2010) Statement by Dr. Keiji Fukuda on behalf of WHO at the Council of Europe on Pandemic (H1N1) 2009, 26 January. Available: http://www.who.int/csr/disease/swineflu/co_ehearing/en/index.html. Accessed 5 February 2010.

9

Preparing for Health Diplomacy Negotiations — Global Governance and the Case of Taiwan, WHO, and SARS

Bryan A. Liang[i] and Tim Mackey[ii]

Abstract

Health diplomacy in global governance is an emerging concept, particularly as applied to health care issues and public health. Yet challenges to policy promotion during conflict between autonomous entities continue to arise despite forums to address some of these concerns. Principles from public policy analysis can provide guidance to assist those involved in global governance issues to better prepare for negotiations to resolve conflict on the international and cross-national levels. The case study of Taiwan and the World Health Organization during the

[i] Bryan A. Liang is Executive Director and Shapiro Distinguished Professor, Institute of Health Law Studies, California Western School of Law; Co-Director and Professor of Anesthesiology, San Diego Center for Patient Safety, University of California, San Diego School of Medicine.
[ii] Tim Mackey, MAS, is Senior Research Associate, Institute of Health Law Studies, California Western School of Law, and PhD candidate, Global Health Program, University of California, San Diego-San Diego State University.

SARS epidemic can provide an illustration and lessons of applying these principles to better obtain positive outcomes in health diplomacy and global governance negotiations.

Introduction

Health diplomacy in global governance is a key concept that addresses the realities of a modern world, where products, services, and other tangible and intangible materials cross geopolitical borders and have impact in other countries. Importantly, global governance is essentially using cooperative means to solve and resolve conflict.[1] These processes, which employ health diplomacy negotiations, can be formal and informal.[2]

Global governance and health diplomacy have applications in a wide array of settings. In particular, healthcare-related issues involving disaster preparedness, disease epidemics, and access to medicines often are pointed to as some of the key issues that illustrate the need for such systems.

However, despite increasing recognition of the importance of and the need to expand global governance and health diplomacy efforts, their impact has been questioned. Although there is a wide spectrum of potential concerns regarding why impacts have been negligible,[3] it is clear that at least some of the limited success has been sourced to inadequate assessments of key factors associated with policymaking science in preparation for health diplomacy negotiations.

We review below, some of the principles that might be useful in promoting the use and success of health diplomacy in global governance. These principles should be the starting point for analysis of health diplomacy negotiations strategies in a global governance forum. We then move to a case study of Taiwan and the World Health Organization (WHO) during the SARS epidemic to illustrate the application of these principles.

Principles of Policymaking Science in Health Diplomacy Negotiations

Although health diplomacy in global governance is sometimes thought of as a unique conception, in fact it simply represents another form of negotiated policy formulation. Because the key aspects of policymaking processes apply to health diplomacy in any global governance forum, it is useful at the outset to briefly outline an accepted model of decision making in policy formulation.

Kingdon open window model

One model of policy formulation provides a bit of insight and is a good introduction to influencing and making public policy. In the book *Agendas, Alternatives, and Public Policies*,[4] Kingdon presents a simple model of policy opportunity, known as the Open Window Model, that provides a reasonable overview of some of the characteristics of public policy formation.

Public policy can be created most straightforwardly when three "streams" come together:

1. The Problem Stream (when key policymakers recognise the problem and it requires their attention);
2. The Policy Stream (when stakeholders provide some potential policy solutions to the problem); and
3. The Political Stream (when the political and policy climate makes one alternative favourable, e.g., public sentiment, new leadership, special interest/non-governmental organisation (NGO) campaign).

Hence, three factors are important in formulating policy: ensuring political attention, providing potential and available solutions, and the presence of an environment suitable for policymakers to adopt a solution.

As a beginning model, this tripartite conception is adequate to provide the rudimentary skeleton for thinking about policy formulation in global governance. But clearly it does not provide much detail in just how to go about doing the job. To move from a theoretical description of streams to actual strategy to achieve policy formulation in global governance negotiations requires an assessment of other characteristics. These include "Venning," Perception, Available Forum, Anticipated Results, and Enforcement.

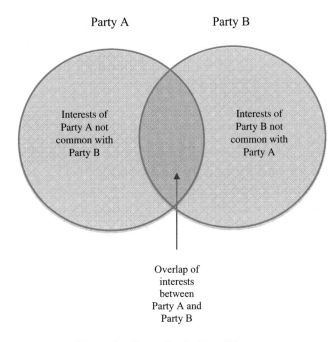

Figure 1.   Example of a Venn Diagram

"Venning"

For each conflict or issue, there will be a wide array of stakeholders that overlap in some areas and do not in others. The beginning of effective policymaking at any level requires identification of commonalities and differences between the parties. To do so, "venning," i.e. figuratively drawing Venn diagrams can provide awareness about these areas. Venn diagrams are diagrams often resembling circles that overlap, representing commonality, and areas that do not, representing areas of difference. An example of a Venn diagram is provided in Fig. 1.

Yet a key approach to understanding positions (that is posturing, or more precisely what parties say they want) and interests (what parties are willing to accept) requires a full and frank determination of expressed as well as underlying (disclosed and undisclosed) perspectives. Venning is an important tool to expressly think about and identify these contrasting and covert positions. This dynamic assessment is often the most critical for health diplomacy negotiations in global governance forums.

Two aspects of venning are a minimum assessment requirement when considering pursuit of a specific global policy. These are identification of resources, and identification of will.

Identification of resources

It is not costless to attempt to access global governance or other policy-making opportunity/desire in health diplomacy negotiations. Significant financial and human resources are essential for any successful effort. Hence, it is important to openly and frankly identify what resources are available to promote or challenge a position of policy. At a minimum, there are three resource questions that must be addressed in health negotiation efforts:

- Is there money to sustain the effort?
- Is there expertise?
- Is there an understanding of the forum?

Will for change

Beyond these resource-focused questions, we also need to evaluate the will for change. Five key questions that must be considered when addressing the will to promote a particular policy position in a global forum diplomacy negotiation are:

- What is the formal and informal political reaction?
- What is the political benefit?
- What is the internal/domestic/industry will for policy?
- What are the regulatory effects of the proposed effort?
- What are the international ramifications?

Here, the will for policy promotion or change is dependent upon downstream assessments of impact on parties. This analysis, then, will provide insight as to any overlapping political positions or interests. It is important to note that when little overlap exists, doing nothing is the best potential solution for at least some stakeholders, whose will to negotiate is limited by the potential negative impact of results that play poorly on a broad internal or external stage.

Perception

Once key aspects of stakeholders' positions and interests have been examined using venning, wherein the contexts for potential change are sketched for negotiation. The next essential step is to address how parties will be perceived.

Perceptions of direct and indirect actors should be included, and the dynamics of potential policy change or lack thereof must also be gleaned to determine what can and should be done to invest in the negotiated global governance process or to limit efforts at the present time.

One method to begin the assessment of perception is SWOT-BATNA analysis. This refers to identification of an entity's Strengths-Weaknesses-Opportunities-Threats (SWOT), and its Best Alternative To A Negotiated Agreement (BATNA). Strengths and weaknesses are internal to the entity; opportunities and threats are external. Evaluating a party's BATNA provides information on how far a party will go to obtain a negotiated agreement, or if the status quo renders more benefit.

Using the SWOT-BATNA analysis, how parties will be perceived by other parties and interested observers will provide significant guidance as to the potential for a negotiated health diplomacy resolution or promotion of a specific entity's perspective. The use of SWOT-BATNA analysis thus provides some additional information and perspectives on the usefulness and desirability of parties to move toward, or away, from a common, negotiated resolution.

It should also be noted that culture and, perhaps more importantly, cultural differences must be taken into account when performing this assessment. Because culture plays a key role in perceptions of individuals and institutions in a wide array of circumstances,[5] it behooves those involved in health diplomacy negotiations to expressly understand and be sensitive to differing cultural perspectives during this assessment.

Available forums

At this point stakeholder overlap, positions, interests, and perceptions have been assessed. However, the relevant forums (venues, policy realms, regulatory regimes, and other environments to advance agendas) for stakeholders to air and promote their positions and interests must also be analysed when considering global governance policy promotion efforts. Forums do not simply represent physical locations where parties meet; they also represent entities with their own positions, interests, and concerns regarding their own external perception.

Importantly, as any other entity involved in global governance negotiations, each forum is also a stakeholder, and has its own SWOT-BATNA, concerns, as well as culture. Hence, the forum or forums of interest must be assessed to ensure that the analytics of the stakeholders are also applied to each forum to best determine the advisability of using a specific one.

It is essential to note at this point that formal, organisational body processes need not be the only means to be considered for and by the parties. The analysis of the available forums for the parties to advocate their positions and interests should also always include informal approaches (such as informal meetings and approaches where discussions and agreements can take place) to determine what may be the most appropriate venue for obtaining a preferred outcome in health diplomacy negotiations.

Anticipated results

Understanding what the parties are interested in, their posturing, what they want, perceptions, culture, and forums provides significant amounts of insight as to how the issue will be framed for global governance negotiations. Yet from a policy formulation perspective, this analytic approach is insufficient to fully understand or resolve conflicts that require health diplomacy. What is missing is an assessment of the anticipated results.

The anticipated results are similar to BATNA, but represent the reverse of the same coin. Anticipated results that the stakeholders believe will occur must be reviewed to understand just how far an entity wishes to go in its policy negotiation. Hence, anticipated results represent the results each party perceives it will obtain from a negotiated agreement or adjudicated result.

Similar to other factors, anticipated results also should be assessed for the forum itself. Because global governance negotiations take place in a spectrum — from open formal discussions to closed informal reviews and agreements — anticipated results that a party wishes to achieve can very much have an influence as to the choice of an appropriate place and time for such efforts. It is therefore critical that those interested in global governance negotiations and policy formulation take into account what can happen from each stakeholder's point of view, including the influence and likely outcome in the forum that is utilised. This approach provides a level of comprehension of when and how negotiations may progress or become recalcitrant to agreement.

Enforcement

A final analytic focus is enforcement of the policy outcome. This factor is a key one in global governance analysis.

Traditionally, global governance does *not* mean global government. Rather, global governance relies on policy and global governance bodies (in most cases international organisations) as forums for negotiation. Hence, although agreements and systems processes may result in potential power to sanction and penalize as well as identify a "winner" as one party or another, there is generally no explicit enforcement power for any global governance body.

Consequently, for policy promotion, the goals of the entities and forum must be clear when considering negotiation outcomes and the impact of limited enforcement. Do these entities or forums want:

- A clear policy pronouncement that one perspective is correct?
- A clear policy pronouncement that the specific forum is the primary source for such decisions?
- World opinion favouring a specific position?
- Money/finances/greater profits?
- Sanctions or penalties?
- Something else?

Each of these considerations means different things relating to enforcement limitations.

Clear policy pronouncement favouring position

Policy pronouncements may be thwarted by lack of enforcement, yet still serve the entity that emerged victorious through provisions that outline implementation of the outcome of health diplomacy negotiations. Although there may not be a separate enforcement means, concrete steps that are set down can provide the basis for enforceable policies geopolitically and/or internationally.

Clear policy pronouncement favouring forum

Policy pronouncements that indicate a single specific body is the appropriate forum serves the winning party and the forum itself, in which the latter may have a vested interest in enforcement or pursuing enforcement as a legitimacy issue. In this latter case, the winning party and the forum become partners in attempting to promote the policy and its enforcement.

World opinion

If the goal is world opinion favouring a particular position, enforcement is a secondary concern. However, this is a typical dual-edged sword: bringing an action in a forum risks having world opinion turned against a position. In this case, if a victorious party can find means of enforcement, efforts to influence world opinion may be worse than a mere loss in the forum — the resulting loss may mean abdication of a position and opposing policy enforcement supporting opposing sentiments on a global scale.

Profits/Finances

Beyond public policy, another key goal to be considered in the context of enforcement is an underlying or overt desire of a party to maximize profits or financial benefit directly or indirectly. Sight of this goal should never be lost in global health diplomacy negotiations, since in many cases it is the primary driver of action. Yet what this also means, beyond assessing honest motives and desirability of a policy that is being promoted, is that enforcement is an important characteristic for the party promulgating the position. It may also mean that that party will be aggressive in attempting to influence the forum, media, and others, and may also enlist those who will obtain similar or derivative benefits. This potential lends itself away from negotiations and toward imposed outcomes. Particularly when the profit motive is involved, global health diplomacy efforts and outcomes must clearly ensure that stakeholder and forum interests are transparent.

Sanctions/Penalties

If parties want sanctions or penalties, this is a significantly difficult goal to accomplish given the lack of enforcement powers of global governance forums. Relying on an individual party or a geopolitical source for enforcement may or may not be feasible. Hence, this goal is, realistically speaking, one of the most challenging if a party or parties wish quick resolution and action on the issue. It also is generally the most highly resource-intensive goal to pursue.

Other issues

Finally, unique circumstances should be considered with respect to enforcement concerns. Environmental agreements may be laudatory, but irrelevant if unenforced. Intellectual property rights may be agreed to be important for economic development, but worthless if parties with "ends justify the means" philosophies expressly ignore or flout the agreements. Therefore, it is important to understand the nuances of the particular issue at hand and to consider how enforcement impacts (or not) the health diplomacy analysis.

Taiwan, WHO, and SARS

The problem: SARS and the need for WHO assistance

Background

In March 2003, the first case of the coronavirus infection known as Severe Acute Respiratory Syndrome (SARS) was identified in Taiwan. Taiwanese authorities acted aggressively to initiate a system that could respond to the potential spread of SARS resulting from these initial cases. However, though the initial outbreak was comparatively slow to extend to other affected countries, it quickly escalated and eventually led to the third largest outbreak of SARS on record, including 668 cases and 181 deaths.[6]

The SARS outbreak in Taiwan was rooted in the growing interdependence of health, economics, and international trade in an era of globalization. As an important business and cultural hub of Eastern Asia, Taiwan was closely connected with SARS epicenters of mainland China and Hong Kong. This is reflected in the estimated 4 million annual visits by Taiwanese to mainland China for business and tourism.[7] Given its close geographical proximity to the first reported cases of SARS, Taiwan faced many challenges including: (i) importation of SARS by travelers from other affected countries; (ii) identification, surveillance, isolation, and quarantine of SARS cases; (iii) containment of nosocomial infections (hospital acquired infections) and effectively implementing infection-control procedures; (iv) political challenges of the One China policy and associated cross-Strait relations;[8] and (v) exclusion from participation in international organisations, particularly WHO. These challenges were exacerbated by Taiwan's continued isolation from the international community due to a failure by both China and Taiwan to recognise the importance of shared benefit and conflict resolution through health diplomacy negotiations. This contributed to an exponential increase of SARS cases in Taiwan within a matter of months.

Initial SARS spread

The first SARS case in Taiwan was identified on March 14, 2003 and originated from a 54-year-old businessman who had traveled to Guangdong Province in China, where the earliest cases of SARS were confirmed to have occurred. By April 14, 23 individuals met WHO criteria for probable cases of SARS, with the vast majority (83%) reported to have traveled to mainland China and Hong Kong within 10 days prior to the onset of illness.[9] The remaining identified cases were 4 individuals representing secondary spread and a single healthcare worker, a physician who had been treating the wife of the initial case-patient. This represented a relatively small and confined outbreak.

Taiwan Department of Health authorities, through coordination between USA and Taiwan Centers for Disease Control (CDC) officials, quickly set up a task force to implement a framework for SARS control. This included review and reporting of all potential SARS cases, isolation of suspect or probable causes in negative pressure rooms, and implementation of infection control practices including protective equipment for healthcare workers. During the first 6 weeks of its introduction, the outbreak appeared to be limited to known imported cases and containment seemed to be within reach.

Expanding SARS infection

However, by the middle of May, SARS had spread rapidly with more than a six-fold increase to 680 cases and 81 deaths in less than a month's time.[10] A chain of local transmissions originating from unrecognised cases at Taiwanese hospitals led to rampant spread of the disease in healthcare settings and later to the wider community.[11] During this time, 4 hospitals discontinued emergency and routine services. This escalation occurred despite Taiwan's understanding of the epidemiology of the disease, initial precautions taken by Taiwan officials to isolate and limit the transmission of SARS to healthcare workers, and Taiwan's modern national healthcare delivery system.

Responding to this crisis, Taiwanese authorities upgraded their surveillance and reporting systems, tightened up their hospital procedures for infection control, initiated a massive public health education campaign to detect and report SARS, and implemented a logistics system to ensure efficient delivery of protective equipment.[12]

Global forum and negotiation

Taiwan also looked to the global community for help in dealing with the escalation of SARS. It requested formal assistance directly from WHO. However, due to its exclusion from membership in the United Nations (UN) and diplomatic pressure from China, WHO refused direct assistance. WHO, under UN auspice, adhered to China's claim that Taiwan was a rogue province and there was only one true China — the People's Republic of China, and thus it was bound by China's One China policy.

Hence, China effectively blocked Taiwan's efforts to obtain formal assistance. Taiwan was excluded from SARS meetings and conferences, was denied access to the global outbreak alert and response system of WHO, and was denied access to other important information and samples.[13] Taiwan health officials were told to contact Beijing directly for aid. This made it difficult for researchers to access SARS materials and up-to-date data necessary to combat the spread of the disease, whilst the death toll continued to rise. Further, Taiwan continued to be unable to participate in the WHO World Health Assembly (WHA) or achieve observer or "health entity" status in WHO during the course of the outbreak.

Late assistance

Finally at the beginning of May 2003, approximately two months after Taiwan's initial request for WHO assistance, China allowed a WHO advisory team, the first in 32 years, to visit Taiwan under the auspice of humanitarian aid. Later, 2 medical experts from WHO were also allowed to visit Taiwan for assistance. This represented a marked departure from WHO's longstanding policy of denying Taiwan access to direct contact with WHO. This occurred during a period in which China, Hong Kong, and Taiwan continued to struggle with bringing SARS under control.

Observers have questioned how the disease spread so rapidly after it had been already earlier identified by Taiwanese health officials and the global health community at large.[14] Taiwan's lack of expert assistance from WHO due to political discordance on the part of both China and Taiwan, not the health-related issues, was the key to this global governance outcome. This provides a compelling case study for illustrating the use of policymaking factor analysis. Below we analyse this case.

The Players and Their Roles: China, Taiwan, and WHO

Three players were key in the outbreak of SARS in Taiwan:

1. Taiwan: With a population of 22 million, and the 20th largest GDP in the world, Taiwan is one of the most influential state entities with its political sovereignty in question. Considering itself as an autonomous

nation-state, yet claimed as a province/territory by China, adverse cross-Strait relations made it difficult for Taiwan to seek formal help from the international community during the outbreak of SARS.

2. People's Republic of China: With one-fifth of the world's population and one-seventh of the world's disease burden when measured in years of health life lost, China plays a key role in global health and specifically in the health, economics, and security of its neighbors.[15] In the context of SARS, China was the origin of the earliest identified cases and the world's largest outbreak, with a total of 5327 cases and 349 deaths.[16]

3. WHO: As the international public health agency for the UN, WHO has the mandate of coordinating international efforts to control outbreaks of infectious diseases. WHO was an important source of expertise and coordination of global public health efforts in the SARS outbreak. However, since admission of China to the UN in 1972, WHO has denied Taiwan membership and avoided direct contact with its health authorities.

Challenges Faced and the Outcome

Venning (drawing Venn Diagrams identifying overlap of parties)

Overlap in interests

In assessing the potential for health diplomacy negotiations in this case study, it is important to identify where sufficient overlap exists in the key conflicts and interests of China and Taiwan:

1. Geographic Proximity: The three hardest hit areas in the SARS epidemic were China, Hong Kong and Taiwan, which share national borders. This close proximity in conjunction with economic and cultural interdependence of the regions provided the perfect climate for the cross-border transmission of this highly contagious disease. For this reason, China and Taiwan had a shared interest to contain the SARS outbreak in order to promote their own respective health and economic security. However, this opportunity to act out of a sense of shared responsibility and mutual reward was not leveraged.

2. Highly Impacted by SARS: China and Taiwan were the first and third most highly impacted areas in the SARS epidemic. The human and economic toll of the disease was especially devastating for these areas. Repercussions on society and national security were significant with many public services and institutions, including hospitals, public transit, schools, and borders being disrupted. Travel restrictions were put in place in both China and Taiwan to limit the spread of the disease, which had an adverse effect on financial growth and stability. In terms of economics, it has been estimated that SARS cost China up to US$25.3 billion and that it reduced China's gross domestic product growth rate by 1–2% for 2003.[17] Further, social upheaval in China regarding the government's handling of the outbreak was apparent. The SARS outbreak adversely affected many different social and industrial sectors that both China and Taiwan had a shared interest in stabilising.

3. Positions and Interests for Technical Assistance: Given their close geographical proximity and cultural ties, information sharing via an international public health agency such as WHO would have inured mutual benefits for both China and Taiwan. Both actors had an interest in providing and sharing technical information and assistance on anti-SARS activities to coordinate a comprehensive containment effort. This could have included leveraging respective strengths and weaknesses of health infrastructures, international partnerships and relationships, and economic resources.

4. WHO as Resource: The need for technical assistance and expertise through active participation of WHO for both China and Taiwan draws interesting parallels. Both actors, particularly China, relied on their own expertise and public health systems to deal with the onset of SARS. In the case of China, outbreak of the disease in late 2002 was largely controlled with a closed-door SARS policy and lack of transparency regarding the severity of the disease to the international community. This included initially denying WHO access to the Guangdong province, where the first cases of the disease were reported. However, failure to contain the disease and scrutiny from WHO, international monitors, and China's own medical establishment led to the dismissal of key officials, as well as a formal apology

from health officials regarding initial mishandling and concealment of SARS. In this admission, China was forced to confront the seriousness of SARS as a global health emergency with domestic and international consequences. This led to growing dependence on WHO and increased authority of WHO over China's domestic health policy actions in an effort to restore China's international standing and control the spread of the disease.[18] Taiwan also initially dealt with the SARS outbreak within its own system with help only from the USA CDC. However, when the disease rapidly spread, it became clear that direct involvement by WHO was necessary. Both actors realized the importance of utilising WHO expertise after failures and limitations of their own individual state actions and systems to control the outbreak.

5.   Interdependent Economies: Economic integration activities beginning in the late 1980s led to strengthening bilateral economic ties between China and Taiwan. This resulted in Taiwan becoming a major source of foreign direct investment for China and led to a robust trading partnership between the two neighbors.[19] This in turn led to greater disease transmission due to growing tourism, business travel, and financial investment with Hong Kong acting as an intermediary, and not surprisingly being adversely affected by SARS. Hence, both actors had an interest in the containment of SARS within its own borders and those of its major trading partner to maintain economic stability and to prevent the importation of the disease.

Importantly however, it is crucial to analyse areas lacking overlap of interests between China and Taiwan. Most notably were cross-Strait relations and the resulting conflict between China's policy goals of a One China framework, reunification, and authority over Taiwan, in contrast to Taiwan's own claims of national independence and autonomy. These stark, mutually-exclusive conflicting positions and interests made cooperation and positive health diplomacy negotiation outcomes during the SARS outbreak elusive. Both China and Taiwan viewed SARS in very different ways, both from opposing views of *political* opportunity instead of mutual policy promotion in the context of health.

Resources and will

Taiwan. From a financial resource standpoint, Taiwan had the means to sustain efforts to receive aid from WHO. Though a small country, Taiwan had a large population, robust economy, and even provided financial assistance for SARS projects in cooperation with China and Hong Kong. Taiwan also had limited participation in the World Trade Organization, providing an indication of its clout in the global economy. However, financial resources did not equate to understanding or expertise in actually getting SARS assistance from WHO. Though Taiwan had the financial resources and will, it did not have the appropriate status within the UN framework to request direct assistance, since it had not been a member of the UN or WHO for more than three decades. For this reason, it had few experts and limited experience. Hence, because of its own lack of understanding of the political challenges of navigating WHO publicly as an appropriate forum, initial requests for direct assistance were denied and Taiwan officials were predictably, if not helpfully, pointed to Beijing by WHO.

China. As the third largest and one of the fastest-growing economies in the world, China most certainly had the financial means to block Taiwan's efforts to gain formal WHO assistance. China also had the will to block WHO assistance given its political capital and clout within the international community. China's financial and political will was and has been committed to a One China policy. China viewed WHO assistance to Taiwan as incompatible with its One China policy under the doctrine of Chinese sovereignty and its representation of all Chinese territories (including Taiwan). Hence, despite the fact that Taiwan sovereignty was not relevant to WHO SARS help from a public health perspective, China strongly discouraged WHO direct, formal assistance. It did so on the premise that it was the "responsible state" to whom WHO should provide technical information and China would provide assistance directly to Taiwan.[20]

Formal and informal political reaction

From the standpoint of the various stakeholders, both formal and informal (express and underlining) reactions are important to recognise. In the case of China, the formal reaction was clear and predictable: intense resistance to direct, formal WHO assistance to Taiwan. This was despite other actors, including nation-states, international organisations, and the broader global community that were critical of this position. In the case of SARS, these international actors exerted open pressure on China to end Taiwan's exclusion from WHO participation on the basis of humanitarian need, but ultimately were limited in their ability to compel China to abandon this position. Though the international community and WHO were sympathetic to Taiwan, the formal politics of the UN dictated that Taiwan was not a member and that there was only one China. Informally, China's dominance as a major player in the global economy, politics, and military power, allowed it to maintain its entrenched position and prevent direct assistance from WHO unless provided within the context of its explicit authority and approval.

Political benefits

Taiwan. The immediate political benefit for Taiwan's position was obvious, that of direct assistance from WHO in combating an escalating outbreak of SARS with its dire public health consequences. Beyond this acute need for technical assistance, Taiwan's increased involvement directly with the international community would provide for increased autonomy separate from Beijing and also act as a bridge for future bids to achieve observer status or membership in WHO. This also had a downstream policy impact on nationalism, self-identification and independence, as well as possible political benefit in national elections.[21]

China. In successfully blocking WHO assistance directly to Taiwan, China could re-emphasise its authority and position of a One China policy to the international community. This could also act as a deterrent for Taiwan's efforts of becoming a more active and recognised participant in international meetings, conferences, and organisations. Successful containment of SARS within the framework of Chinese authority could have also invalidated claims of the necessity of Taiwan's membership status in WHO. Furthermore, perception of a responsible and cooperative China promoting cross-Strait relations through direct humanitarian aid with Taiwan could have lead to support of reunification factions in both China and Taiwan.

Internal/Domestic/Industry will for policy

For Taiwan, political support of WHO assistance, opposition for China's policies promoting Taiwan's isolation from the international community, and public perception of China's irresponsibility in dealing with SARS was widespread. This support grew from a national petition launched to promote WHO membership, vocal public criticism of China by Taiwanese officials, and national campaigns designed to influence public opinion.[22] First and foremost, all internal, domestic, and industry stakeholders had an immediate interest in ending SARS.

Conversely, political stakeholders, including high-ranking officials, such as then-China Premier Wen Jiabao, had a vested interest in maintaining a One China policy. In this effort, China remained steadfast in its insistence that SARS in Taiwan was an internal Chinese issue and that Taiwan's independent relationship with WHO would not and could not be entertained. Given the disposition of China's political regime, this policy position was supported by internal, domestic and industry stakeholders.

Regulatory effects of proposed efforts

Regulatory effects of obtaining direct, formal assistance from the WHO would be a watershed event for Taiwan. Direct involvement of WHO with Taiwanese health officials would allow mutual access to region-specific information and expertise in combating SARS and also represent landmark cooperation between the two public health agencies. There was no resistance to potential internal regulatory changes that would be required to share information.

For China, denial of WHO assistance to Taiwan would represent further confirmation that its unilateral One China policy would be appropriately recognised by international governing bodies. Importantly, this could result in a strengthening of internal political power.

It is clear that the potential regulatory effects were at odds with WHO formal standing, WHO formal decision-making processes that relied on UN policy, and potential WHO policy promulgation that could result in significant resistance from one of the world's most powerful countries. As such, China and Taiwan positions put it on a collision course with WHO potential regulatory outcomes, which may adversely affect WHO's legitimacy due to its independent inability to enforce its policy.

International ramifications

Analysis of the international ramifications regarding WHO direct, formal assistance to Taiwan showed a pragmatic need for Taiwan, China, and WHO to cooperate in needed public health exchanges. The world was at risk of a virulent, unknown disease in a global context. Hence, there was an overarching international concern for a global policy to effectively and efficiency share information to address SARS. Thus, little international resistance existed for WHO Taiwan assistance.

Taiwan appeared to believe that it could rely on this international support. Yet China, observing such perceptions, dug its heels in deeper and continued to resist direct, formal WHO assistance. In addition, China has previous experience flouting world opinion, and therefore has a culture that supports such perspectives and positions.

Perception

After identifying key aspects of conflicts and interests of the China and Taiwan with potential overlap, it is necessary to assess respective perceptions through the SWOT-BATNA analysis to determine the potential for negotiated health diplomacy resolution or policy promotion.

Taiwan

- **Strengths:** Taiwan's modern healthcare infrastructure and expertise of its health officials allowed it to initially respond positively to the SARS epidemic. In addition, regional technical information and data on SARS is essential in understanding the epidemiology of the disease, which would have benefited global health efforts in combating SARS.
- **Weaknesses:** Taiwan's citizen sensitivity to SARS and lack of experience in dealing with this novel infectious disease made it difficult for an appropriate containment. This is evident in the failure to control the surge of the disease after initial cases had been identified and necessitated the need for WHO assistance. Of special concern was the

lack of Taiwan's health structure to prevent the spread of nosocomial infections.

- **Opportunities:** Taiwan's handling of SARS provides opportunities in understanding the epidemiology of the disease, cross-border transmission, and necessary public health response to control the outbreak. These lessons could be shared with the broader international community for enhanced knowledge sharing and policy promotion.
- **Threats:** External threats of China's One China policy, its aggressive political stance of denying direct, formal WHO assistance to Taiwan, and China's political strength in the context of the global economy and authority within international organisations represented clear barriers to any global governance assistance for Taiwan.

China

- **Strengths:** China's large political and financial power bases, resources, and influence over other nation states and international organisations represented a tremendous set of strengths.
- **Weaknesses:** China's entrenched position and inflexibility regarding its One China policy as a success measure in the international forum was a key weakness, preventing any movement. In addition, China's initial mishandling of SARS within its own geographical boundaries, lack of cooperation at the onset, and international perception of it being the "exporter" of SARS, created internal challenges to defend its positions and status.
- **Opportunities:** By effectively blocking Taiwan's request for direct, formal WHO assistance, China could re-establish its authority over Taiwan and affirm international recognition and acceptance of its One China policy.
- **Threats:** International condemnation and accusation of China politics over public health and humanitarian aid could lead to further support of Taiwan's membership bid or observer status in WHO, which could undermine China's growing standing in the international community. From a cultural perspective, the threat of "loss of face" ("diu lian" 丢脸) in failing to maintain its policy position and historical authority over the region and more junior states would be a great political embarrassment.

Taiwan BATNA:

- Taiwan's BATNA was not favourable. In the absence of either direct or indirect help from WHO, it would face the SARS epidemic alone and be unable to deal with the continuing spread of the disease or advance its concerns and needs for SARS assistance in the global forum.

China BATNA:

- China's BATNA was highly favourable. Continued denial, delay, or lack of a final decision on direct, formal WHO assistance to Taiwan would continue to validate the One China policy and allow China to control the flow of international aid directed to Taiwan.

Available forum

With overlap of conflicts, interests and perceptions of China and Taiwan determined, it is clear that the appropriate forum for policy promotion was WHO. However, Taiwan sought direct, formal assistance whereas China resisted it. Although both parties seemed to understand WHO was the appropriate forum, they did not focus on alternative, informal means. Below, the assessment of formal versus informal SWOT-BATNA analysis indicates this approach would have been fruitful.

WHO Direct, Formal Assistance SWOT:

- **Strengths:** Importantly, direct, formal assistance would enable collection and sharing of global SARS data by WHO from an advanced, modern medical infrastructure that could be disseminated rapidly to Member States. Direct, formal assistance would also strengthen Taiwan's internal expertise and access to information, data, samples and participation in SARS conferences that would then feed back to WHO through established processes.
- **Weaknesses:** WHO was challenged by its inability to resolve conflicts formally and align interests of a public health mission for Taiwan with China. As well, any direct, formal assistance was politically untenable for WHO as part of the UN, given challenges of China's insistence on its longstanding One China policy.

- **Opportunities:** Worldwide sentiment supported WHO humanitarian aid and involvement in its public health mission to Taiwan in context of SARS. Calls for increased participation and recognition of Taiwan also were supportive of WHO direct, formal assistance.
- **Threats:** The largest potential threat to WHO of direct, formal assistance to Taiwan was possible retaliation by China against WHO and lack of cooperation/assistance from China in dealing with global outbreak of SARS. Downstream resistance to WHO in the future would also be a potential threat.

WHO Informal Assistance SWOT:

- **Strengths:** For WHO, informal provision to Taiwan of WHO resident expertise and data needed to combat SARS would be able to be provided without complications of political risk and alienation of a major superpower, China.
- **Weaknesses:** By relying on informal means, WHO's efforts would result in a lack of clear statement on global public health issues and undermine WHO's non-political stance. It also would represent a failure of WHO's ability to act autonomously on information from non-state actors in dealing with global disease emergencies.
- **Opportunities:** Through an informal process, WHO would be provided with timely and potentially life-saving access to and support of high infection SARS areas. This would provide the opportunity for international and other geopolitical actors to make better assessments of root cause and necessary containment measures to prevent escalation of outbreaks.
- **Threats:** A key, possible threat against WHO was retaliation by China, even given the informal nature of assistance. Yet this threat is much less intense than a threat posed by any direct, formal assistance to Taiwan by WHO.

WHO Formal Assistance BATNA:

- No agreement is generally favourable for WHO. WHO maintains good relations and cooperation with superpowers (specifically China, which has the largest outbreak and represents the highest public health risk) and avoids politicization of the issue. WHO can claim it has its "hands tied" and must work within the framework of the available international forum and can point to its parent organisation, the UN, for support. Note that by not providing direct, formal aid to Taiwan, other alternative forms of indirect or informal aid may still be available or negotiated.

WHO Informal Assistance BATNA:

*   Generally, lack of WHO informal assistance to Taiwan would not be favourable for WHO's standing and legitimacy in the international community. Lack of response by the pre-eminent world health agency to assist Taiwan in a humanitarian crisis even through informal channels would signal that WHO is in fact a political entity, contravening its purported public health mission. In addition, resources devoted to promoting informal aid to Taiwan are wasted if informal efforts fail and alternative channels (such as direct, formal aid) are not readily available. Lack of an informal agreement also results in the absence of a cogent, precedential policy for the appropriate forum to address public health emergencies arising from non-state actors. This creates issues for the international community, with timely sharing of important regional SARS information and data virtually impossible.

Anticipated results

Simply understanding what the interests, perceptions and appropriate forum was in the Taiwan SARS case is insufficient in resolving conflict as it arises in health diplomacy negotiations. Understanding what China, Taiwan, and WHO reasonably expected would be the outcome of their respective policy positions and interests is essential in understanding intent and motivation of key stakeholders in policy promotion.

China and Taiwan. For both China and Taiwan, respective anticipated outcomes were far apart. On one hand, China's expectation and predominant motivation during SARS was to deny direct, formal WHO assistance to Taiwan and control the flow of aid through cross-Strait interaction, thus reinforcing its authority and its One China policy. Conversely, Taiwan hoped to leverage support of the international community, particularly support from the USA, Japan, and the EU,[23] anticipating that it would receive formal direct assistance from WHO on the basis that humanitarian concerns, which would override political challenges of its lack of UN membership.

WHO. For WHO, understanding the limitations of the available forums resulted in assessments that focused on it being allowed to provide some level of assistance to Taiwan through negotiations with China within the existing political framework. The anticipated results, however, were clearly dominated by the political issues and positions of China in its One China policy. WHO, if providing direct, formal assistance, would anticipate retaliation by China in these circumstances.

Enforcement

The final key factor in assessing success in global health policy promotion is effectiveness of enforcement within the limitations of global governance. As in the analysis of anticipated results, expectations in the sphere of global governance and available forums were disparate. Both parties wanted a clear policy pronouncement that one perspective was correct, making formal enforcement a secondary concern beyond the act of WHO support for the position.

For Taiwan, the ultimate goal was a clear policy pronouncement stating that it was eligible to receive direct, formal public health assistance from WHO. It also would set the table for future health diplomacy negotiations with China and most likely allow Taiwan to receive direct, formal WHO aid. Further, global support of such a pronouncement could provide Taiwan the appropriate momentum for eventual observer status or membership in WHO.

For China, a clear pronouncement that WHO would respect and abide by China's One China policy, hence recognising China's sovereignty over Taiwan in public health matters by the international community, was its expected outcome. This would result in all formal aid being routed through Beijing and place it in a better position to aggressively pursue its policies and interests in health diplomacy negotiations involving Taiwan.

Lessons Learned and Conclusions

A common theme throughout this case study was the limited factor analysis by Taiwan in its efforts to obtain direct, formal aid from WHO. Each stage of assessment pointed more and more to *not* seeking direct, formal aid from WHO. Venning showed several important characteristics of the situation. First, the diametrically opposed policy perspectives became apparent: Taiwan believes it is independent, China believes Taiwan is a rogue province under the One China policy. But further, WHO, as a UN agency, recognised the One China policy. Indeed, it was apparent that whilst China has been at the UN/WHO table and hence has expertise and experience to engage the forum, Taiwan under the One China policy has been excluded from the UN/WHO for more than three decades, limiting its expertise and experience. Thus at the outset, Taiwan pushing for direct, formal aid from WHO — and implicitly if successful a recognition of Taiwan as a sovereign entity — was unlikely due to political and diplomatic concerns.

Importantly, using SWOT-BATNA analysis, party perceptions showed that Taiwan's BATNA was poor. Yet China's BATNA was excellent: long deliberations and delays supported the status quo of no formal WHO aid to Taiwan — exactly the goal of China. Add to this the "diu lian" culture and analytically it is apparent that this approach would be a strongly committed strategy by China. In combination with political realities, perception analysis adds weight to the likelihood that WHO would not provide direct, formal aid.

Furthermore, forum analysis of WHO as a discrete stakeholder provided significant insight as to formal versus informal efforts at assisting Taiwan. WHO formal aid to Taiwan would be highly likely to result in retaliation by China against, at a minimum, WHO. This stick of China retaliation was supported by the carrot of WHO's positive BATNA if it did not provide formal aid to Taiwan: WHO maintains relations with China — an economic and military superpower — and at most, upsets a small sovereignty unlikely to cause problems. Clearly, assessing the forum alone would have pointed to issues with Taiwan's attempting to obtain direct, formal WHO assistance. In combination with other factors, this conclusion is almost unassailable.

Yet when performing forum analysis and assessing WHO *informal* aid, many of the political challenges could be mitigated. Informal aid by WHO could have avoided political risks of contravening China in a key area. Even though there was the potential for China to retaliate, it would have been much less likely if WHO assistance was not seen as flouting the One China policy. Beyond the carrot of avoiding confrontation with China, WHO's BATNA if informal aid was not able to be provided was a stick that could have strongly pushed WHO to explore this alternative earlier if Taiwan had attempted to use this route at the outset.

Any room for negotiation when considering anticipated results was patently clear: there was none. Taiwan believed it would receive the direct, formal WHO assistance whilst China did not. Similarly, assessing party goals with respect to enforcement equally showed no room for negotiation on the formal level: Taiwan wanted a clear policy statement it could receive WHO direct, formal aid whilst China wanted the opposite: a validation of the One China policy and blocking WHO aid to Taiwan.

Hence, when assessing these policy factors together, it was highly unlikely that Taiwan would receive WHO direct, formal aid. The challenges for the forum, the political realities, and the emphasis on formal technical assistance rather than informal efforts with WHO created the perfect storm for failure.

Epilogue

After approximately two months of facing the SARS epidemic alone, Taiwan was finally sent two epidemiologists from WHO on May 3, 2003. China claimed credit for assembling a humanitarian team including WHO and USA personnel, although there was no evidence of this being the case.[24] Ultimately, during the time Taiwan faced the SARS epidemic alone, it had a sevenfold rise in the number of cases and infections during this period, which caused the lion's share of deaths there.[25] On July 5, 2003, WHO announced that SARS had been contained worldwide.

Recently cross-Strait relations between Taiwan and China have notably improved with the participation of Taiwan as an observer at the 62nd World Health Assembly under the name "Chinese Taipei,"[26] and a free-trade agreement signed between the two countries in June 2010.[27] Though such progress has allowed Taiwan the benefit of increased financial investment, economic growth, better access to the WHO, and strengthening of ties with the mainland, it is still a far cry from recognition of Taiwanese sovereignty and autonomy in the international community. Under the label, "Chinese Taipei," Taiwan has chosen to bypass the need for formal UN member status in exchange for improved participation in a more appropriate forum. Similarly, China has allowed limited WHO access to Taiwan within the boundaries of its One China policy. However, it remains to be seen whether both countries and WHO have gained some perspective from the global health diplomacy outcomes in SARS.

References

1. Thakur R, Weiss T. (2010) *The UN and Global Governance: An Unfinished Journey.* Indiana Univ. Press.
2. Karns M, Mingst K. (2004) *International Organizations: The Politics and Processes of Global Governance.* Lynne Rienner Pub.
3. Jacquet P, Pisani-Ferry J, Tubiana L. (2002) À La Récheche de la Gouvernance Mondiale [Online]: http://www.pisani-ferry.net/base/papiers/-re-03-REF-gouvernance.pdf.
4. Kingdon J. (1995) *Agendas, Alternatives, and Public Policies.* Longman.
5. *See,* e.g., Kong M & Jogaratnam G. (2007) The influence of culture on perceptions of service employee behavior. *Management Service Qual* 17 (3): 275–297; Timmerman G & Bajema C. (2000) The Impact of Organizational Culture on Perceptions and Experiences of Sexual Harassment. *J Vocat Behav* 57 (2): 188–205; Pillay N. (2005) Search the Y Drive or Simply Ask Sally: Staff Perceptions of Knowledge Creation in an Organisation. *Int'l J Know, Culture and Change Management* 5: 77–86; and Liang B & Liang A. (2001) Lies on the Lips: Dying Declarations, Western Legal Bias, and Unreliability as Reported Speech. *Law/Text/Culture* 5: 113–136.
6. Chen, *et al.* (2005) SARS in Taiwan: An Overview and lessons learned. *Intl J. of Infectious Disease* 9: 77–85. Note statistics vary based upon differences in cases which have been discarded in Taiwan. As of July 2003, a total of 325 cases had been discarded, including 135 discarded cases due to insufficient or incomplete laboratory information, of which 101 were deaths.

7. *Ibid,* Bureau of Immigration, Ministry of the Interior, unpub. Data

8. "Cross-Strait" relations generally refers to China-Taiwan relations, since they are separated by the Taiwan Strait.

9. Twu S-J, *et al.* (2003) Control measures for severe acute respiratory syndrome (SARS) in Taiwan. *Emerg Infect Dis* 9 (6): 718–720.

10. Hsieh Y-H, Chen CWS, Hsu S-B. (2003) SARS Outbreak, Taiwan. *Emerg Infect Dis* 10 (2): 201–206.

11. Center for Disease Control and Prevention. (2003) *Morbidity and Mortality Weekly Report* 52 (20): 461–466.

12. World Health Organization. (2003) Update 96-Taiwan, China: SARS transmission interrupted in last outbreak area. *Disease Outbreak News.* [online] http://www.who.int/csr/don/2003_07_05/en/.

13. Cyranoski D. (2003) Taiwan left isolated in fight against SARS. *Nature* 422: 652.

14. *Id* at 9. Indeed, issues at the local level including health infrastructure, hospital management, human error, and the nature of SARS as a newly emerging disease which is asymptomatic at onset, may have made it difficult to control the outbreak.

15. World Health Organization. (2002) China to study links between Sustainable Development and Investment in Health. *News releases.* [online] http://www.who.int/mediacentre/news/releases/pr96/en/.

16. World Health Organization. (2003) Summary of probable SARS cases with onset of illness from 1 November 2002 to 31 July 2003. *Global Alert and Response.* [online] http://www.who.int/csr/sars/country/table2004_04_21/en/index.html. China's handling of the SARS outbreak in its own borders, its cooperation with the international community, and its handling of SARS Taiwan diplomacy was the subject of much criticism and debate *see* Brown D. (2003) China-Taiwan Relations: The Shadow of SARS. *Comparative Connections,* [online] http://csis.org/files/media/csis/pubs/0302qchina_taiwan.pdf.

17. Hai W, *et al.* (2004) The Short-Term Impact of SARS on the Chinese Economy. *MIT Press* 3 (1): and other estimates show a decrease of up to 3% in GDP for calendar year Q2 quarter for China *see* 57–61; Brown M, Smith R. (2008) The economic impact of SARS: How does the reality match the predictions? *Health Policy* 88: 110–120.

18. Huang Y. (2010) Pursuing Health as Foreign Policy: The Case of China. *Indiana Jour of Glob Leg Stud* 17: 105–146.

19. deLisle J. (2003) SARS, greater China, and the pathologies of globalization and Transition. *Orbis* 47 (4): 587–604.

20. Shen S. (2004) The "SARS Diplomacy" of Beijing and Taipei: competition between the Chinese and Non-Chinese orbits. *Asian Perspective* 28 (1): 45–65. Ironically, China's miscalculation of potential backlash from the international community from a humanitarian perspective, and its own initial domestic mishandling of SARS, significantly diminished its ability to advocate this position.

21. Rich T. (2005) Taiwan in Crisis: The polticisation of SARS and Chen Shui-bian's re-election. *Grad J Asia-Paci Stud* 3 (1): 67–75.

22. This included a campaign linking number of SARS cases to communist spies in Taiwan and later claims in 2008 that China had used SARS as biological warfare.

23. This included a bill passed by the U.S. House of Representatives and a resolution passed by the European Parliament to support Taiwan's participation in the WHO, and Japan's support for Taiwan's bid for observer status.

24. Permanent Mission of the People's Republic of China to the United Nations. (2003) Speech by H.E. Madame Wu Yi Head of Chinese Delegation, Vice Premier and Minister of Health on Taiwan-Related Proposal at General Committee of 56th World Health Assembly. [online] http://www.china-un.ch/eng/zmjg/jgthsm/t85541.html.

25. Hsieh T-H. (2003) Politics hindering SARS work: Taiwan has been left to fight its outbreak with little help. *Nature* 423: 381.

26. deLisle J., Cozen SA. (2009) Taiwan in the World Health Assembly: A Victory, With Limits. *Brookings Northeast Asia Commentary* 29. [online] http://www.brookings.edu/opinions/2009/05_taiwan_delisle.aspx.

27. Prasso S. (2010) Taiwan-China trade agreement: A game changer. *Fortune.* [online] http://money.cnn.com/2010/06/29/news/international/china_taiwan_trade.fortune/index.html.

10

China's Engagement with Global Health Diplomacy: Was SARS a Watershed?*

Lai-Ha Chan[i], Lucy Chen[ii], Jin Xu[iii]

This article is part of the PLoS Medicine *Global Health Diplomacy series.*

Abstract

Growing interest in a wide range of global health issues makes China an increasingly important actor in the international health arena. This case

[i] UTS China Research Centre, University of Technology, Sydney, Australia. E-mail: Lai-Ha.Chan@uts.edu.au

[ii] Institute for Global Health, Peking University, Beijing, China.

[iii] Health Science Center, Peking University, Beijing, China

Citation: Chan L-H, Chen L, Xu J (2010) China's Engagement with Global Health Diplomacy: Was SARS a Watershed? PLoS Med 7(4): e1000266. doi:10.1371/journal.pmed.1000266

Academic Editor: Kelley Lee, London School of Hygiene & Tropical Medicine, United Kingdom **Published** April 27, 2010

Funding: The authors received no specific funding for this paper.

Competing Interests: The authors have declared that no competing interests exist.

Abbreviations: FCTC, Framework Convention on Tobacco Control; SARS, severe acute respiratory syndrome; WHO, World Health Organization

Provenance: Commissioned; externally peer reviewed.

study provides a closer look at the transitions in China's health policy after the epidemic of Severe Acute Respiratory Syndrome and yields insights into the wide-ranging consequences that can be observed both within and beyond the national borders. China now develops a higher profile of health on the political agenda and mechanisms to facilitate cross-ministry dialogues. Finanical injections (despite the legacy of the financial crisis) come along with active participation in global health governance, dynamic engagement on the regional level, and development of a vision for global health diplomacy. However, China's approach to global public health has yet to be fully in line with the norms of global health governance due to its concerns over state sovereignty.

Severe acute respiratory syndrome (SARS) was the first global epidemic of the 21st century. It not only caused mass panic but also generated a discourse on health insecurity around the world. Table 1 shows a chronological account of the disease outbreaks. Owing to China's belated response, particularly its obstruction in early 2003 of the entry of World Health Organization (WHO) assessment teams into the country for investigation of the virus, the subsequent mapping of the disease during the outbreak period kept global attention on China. In retrospect, there appear to be valuable lessons China can draw from its experience with SARS and several implications of SARS on China's engagement in global health diplomacy. This case study examines China's policy changes in the area of public health since the SARS outbreak. Using literature reviews, personal experience, and informal interviews with Chinese health officials, we provide insight into the extent of China's increased engagement in public health, at both the domestic and the international levels.

China Since the SARS Outbreak

We spoke with three high-ranking health officials in China's Ministry of Health in August 2009 who admitted that the SARS outbreak had alerted Chinese citizens as well as the government to the danger that public

---

The Policy Forum allows health policy makers around the world to discuss challenges and opportunities for improving health care in their societies.

health, particularly infectious diseases, could become a dire threat if not properly controlled. This perceived threat extended beyond their country to the world. In the face of criticism from abroad about China's handling of the SARS epidemic, the new Hu Jintao — Wen Jiabao leadership, taking office in early 2003, swiftly adopted a more open and proactive attitude to the WHO member countries and southeast Asian nations containing the disease.

Indeed, SARS appears to have prompted a national discourse on the interrelationship between infectious diseases and non-traditional security inside China. This is evidenced by the vast amount of literature on the subject of non-traditional security issues generated by Chinese scholars since the SARS outbreak. Using "非传统安全 (*fei chuantong anquan,* non-traditional security)" to search for articles contained in a database known as "China Academic Journals Full-text Database: Economics, Politics and Law (*Zhongguo qikan quanwen shujuku: jingji, zhengzhi yu falü zhuandang,* 中国期刊全文数据库：经济，政治与法律专档)," there are barely any "non traditional security" articles published before the SARS outbreak. However, subsequent to the outbreak it became a flourishing subject in China's scholarly world. Among the articles that include "non-traditional security" in their titles since the start of economic reforms in 1979, more than 95% of them were published after 2003 (see Figure 1).

At the domestic level, the SARS out break exposed a fundamental shortcoming of China's health care system. As such, China required a national health reform in order to improve its surveillance system and reorient its single-minded pursuit of economic growth since the late 1970s to a more balanced development between economic growth and social infrastructure building.[1-3] The health officials in Beijing were also of the view that SARS could be seen as a turning point for China's health reform because it provided a political rationale for the government to accelerate the reform. According to the Asian Development Bank, SARS cost China US$6.1 billion, or 0.5% of its GDP, in 2003.[4] This economic loss may seem insignificant, but for a regime that prioritizes economic growth and stability, the political repercussions of an economic decline caused by a health crisis cannot be underestimated. Indeed, SARS alerted the Chinese leadership to the pitfalls of a public health care system in disarray.[2] In order to maintain a sustained economic growth, the central government has increased its public health funding significantly since the SARS outbreak. For example, in 2003, the central and local governments altogether allocated 111 .69 billion yuan for public health, an increase of 23% over the previous year. Between 2002 and 2006, the government's public health spending grew by almost 100%. There was a further increase of 29.1% in 2007 to 229.71 billion yuan. The share of public health spending in the country's GDP was 0.89% in 2007, compared to merely 0.75% five years ago.[5,6]

Summary Points

- SARS not only exposed a fundamental shortcoming of China's public health surveillance system as well as its single-minded pursuit of economic growth since the late 1970s, but also forced China to realize that, in the era of globalization, public health is no longer a domestic, social issue that can be isolated from foreign-policy concern.
- Its ailing health care system, its aspiration to be seen as a "responsible state," and international demands for health cooperation have compelled China to be more proactive in the global health domain.
- There are signs that China is now using public health as a means to strengthen its diplomatic relations with the developing world, in particular the African continent.
- While China has embraced multilateral cooperation in a wide array of global health issues, its engagement remains "state centric" and therefore leaders attach primary significance to intergovernmental organizations, particularly the UN agencies.

External pressure has also impacted on the development of China's public health. During the SARS outbreak, the WHO directly told the Chinese government in its mission report in April 2003 that "[t] here was an urgent need to improve surveillance and infection control" in the country.[7] Two years later, the Chinese government officially admitted its health care system was ailing in a joint report issued by State Council's Development

Research Centre and the WHO.[8] The recent decision on a new rural cooperative medical system is one of its efforts to provide its rural residents by 2010 with more equitable and accessible health care[9–11] and improve its diseases surveillance system at the local level. In addition, both the "loss of face" in the SARS outbreak and its aspiration to be seen and respected as "a responsible state" have pushed China to enhance its

Table 1. The chronology of the SARS outbreak.

Date	Major Events
16 November 2002	The first known case of SARS occurs in Foshan, Guangdong, southern China.
8 February 2003	Guangdong government informs the central government in Beijing about the outbreak.
11–14 February	Vice-mayor of Guangzhou says that the city is coping with the outbreak of a typical pneumonia and that "no extraordinary measures are needed." On the 14th, the Ministry of Health officially tells WHO that the disease is under control in Guangdong.
21 February	Hong Kong index case arrives in the Metropole Hotel from Guangdong; the virus starts to spread globally.
11 March	The WHO Director-General, Gro Harlem Brundtland, raises member states' concern over the lack of information about the Guangdong outbreak to the WHO representative and asks him to convey it to Chinese Ministry of Health. On the same day, Hong Kong reports the Prince of Wales Hospital outbreak to WHO.
12–13 March	WHO issues global alert about atypical pneumonia; China's Health Minister accepts a WHO mission to examine the Guangdong outbreak.
15 March	WHO officially names the disease as "severe acute respiratory syndrome" (SARS).
17 March	China insists Guangdong's outbreak is "well under control."
2 April	WHO issues travel advisory for Hong Kong and Guangdong province.
3 April	The Guangdong government allows a WHO team to investigate SARS in the province; Health Minister Zhang Wenkang states that China is "safe."

(*Continued*)

Table 1.   (Continued)

Date	Major Events
8 April	Jiang Yanyong, a retired Chinese surgeon, exposes the under reporting of SARS cases in Beijing to *Time* magazine.
17 April	After a Politburo meeting, Beijing announces a national "war" on the virus.
20 April	Health Minister Zhang Wenkang and Beijing's Mayor Meng Xuenong were sacked for negligence in dealing with the disease. The Ministry of Health announces confirmed cases of SARS, which are at 9 times as the day before.
22 April	A major outbreak in Taiwan begins.
23 April	The SARS Control and Prevention Headquarters of the State Council is established with Vice-Premier Wu Yi as commander-in-chief; WHO issues travel advisory for Toronto, Beijing, and Shanxi province.
27 April	Xiaotangshan SARS hospital is completed in 8 days, involving 7,000 workers in Beijing.
29 April	WHO sends three officials to Taiwan with Beijing's consent.
3 May	WHO sends three officials to Taiwan with Beijing's consent.
8 May	WHO issues travel advisory for Tianjin, Inner Mongolia, and Taipei.
14 May	WHO team meets Wu Yi.
15 May	The Chinese government passes a new law against those who break SARS quarantine and deliberately spread the disease.
23 May	WHO lifts travel advisory for Hong Kong and Guangdong.
27 May	Delegates to the World Health Assembly approve a resolution on SARS and revising the International Health Regulations.
5 July	WHO announces that SARS is under control worldwide.

From [39].
doi:10.1371/journal.pmed.1000266.t001

cooperation with international institutions in dealing with other pressing health issues.[12]

One of the prominent examples is the problem of HIV/AIDS. China is now working with multiple actors, including UN agencies (i.e., UNAIDS, WHO, UNICEF, the International Labour Organization, and World Bank), international non-governmental organizations (i.e., The Global Fund to Fight AIDS, Tuberculosis and Malaria, Bill & Melinda Gates Foundation, and Clinton Foundation), other states (i.e., United States, United Kingdom,

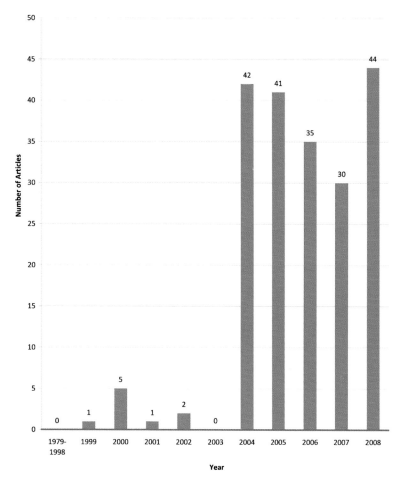

Figure 1. Number of Chinese journal articles per year on non-traditional security issues since 1979.
doi:10.1371/journal.pmed.1000266.g001

and Australia), as well as non-governmental organizations inside the country to combat the disease. However, while Beijing calls for and welcomes involvement of multiple actors in combating the disease inside its territory, it maintains little tolerance of anyone or any activity that would attenuate its absolute control over the country or threaten the supreme authority of the government. A major feature of China's multilateral public health engagement, then, is that of "state-led health governance."

Nevertheless, compared to its initial handling of SARS, China now reacts in more timely fashion in releasing information on contagious diseases, despite implementation problems that include sluggish responses to disease outbreaks on the part of local officials and technical incapacity to detect sudden outbreaks at the local level. In addition, China has shown increased willingness to engage with international organizations on a wide array of global health issues. For example, in order to align with international interests in tobacco control, Beijing signed the WHO Framework Convention on Tobacco Control (FCTC) treaty in December 2003. It was ratified in 2005 by the Chinese National People's Congress and its legislature and took effect in 2006.[13] Being the largest producer as well as the largest consumer of tobacco in the world, Chinese tobacco policy has long been influenced more by economic concerns than by public health.[14] Its ratification of the FCTC came as a surprise for many.

China's recent responses to the 2009 outbreak of swine flu (influenza A/H1N1) give an impression that the dreadful effect of SARS six years ago has taught China a lesson. As soon as the WHO raised its pandemic alert phase from 3 to 4 on 28 April 2009, Premier Wen Jiabao convened a cabinet meeting to discuss a set of response measures designed to deal with the disease, although there was neither any reported case of swine flu in China at that time nor a similar virus found in the pigs in the country. Two days later, the Communist Party of China (CPC) General Secretary Hu Jintao convened a meeting of the Standing Committee of the Politburo. That the holding of the highest level meeting was announced immediately after its adjournment was regarded as unusual by many China watchers.[15] China's aggressive and visible approach towards swine flu appears to demonstrate the government's determination in tackling the disease. However, this aggressive or even excessively stringent measure against swine flu, as some observers have said, aroused international debate. The WHO asked China to justify its decision to keep travelers from Mexico in quarantine. The Mexican government criticized China's response as "unjustified," threatened to take retaliatory action, and sent an airplane to Shanghai on 5 May 2009 to repatriate its quarantined citizens.[16–18] In contrast, others including health experts reportedly praised China for exercising extra vigilance against the virus.[19,20]

A More Proactive Stance in Global Health Diplomacy

At the international level, there have been signs since the SARS outbreak that public health is high on China's foreign policy agenda. First, Beijing has become more proactive in participating in global health governance. China had for a long time played a passive role in the WHO since gaining its membership in the organization more than three decades ago. The SARS outbreak let China experience the power of the WHO, which has become increasingly more influential while other international organizations, such as the United Nations Security Council, International Monetary Fund, World Bank, G8, and the World Trade Organization, are facing legitimacy, accountability, and representativeness challenges. WHO's authority in dealing with disease outbreaks is still widely recognized.[21] Without China's prior consent, the WHO issued a travel advisory against unnecessary travel to Guangdong province, putting China under the global spotlight for spreading infectious disease to other countries. Perhaps this lesson has prompted the Chinese government to realize the political importance of the WHO and to increase its participation in global health governance.

In the WHO Director-General election in 2006, China, for the first time since it gained its membership in UN agencies in 1971, nominated and supported a Chinese national, Margaret Chan, as a candidate for the top post. It is widely believed that Chan's success was a diplomatic triumph both for her and for China. Wang Yizhou, then with the Chinese Academy of Social Sciences, Beijing, told one of the authors (LHC) in March 2008 that Margaret Chan's nomination as the Director-General of the WHO was not a fortuitous incident. The health officials we spoke with in Beijing concurred with Wang's view and explained that China has recently realized and valued the increasing importance of the WHO at the world stage. It is also a source of national pride to have a Chinese national at the top post of the global health organization.[22] Chan was the Director of Health of Hong Kong during the SARS outbreak in 2003. Her nomination could be seen as a case of China's smart play and rising clout at the global stage, displaying its confidence in her managing of Hong Kong affairs and the successful implementation of China's "One Country, Two Systems" policy.[23] Furthermore, China's WHO role politically could be regarded as a pre-emptive measure to block Taiwan's attempts to seek WHO member-ship.[23] On the other hand, with improved relations with the Ma Ying-jeou administration in Taiwan, China has become more flexible in seeking cross-strait cooperation in health. For example, as a consultant for the Chinese Medical Association, Chinese Vice Minister of Health Huang Jiefu attended a conference on "Cross-Strait Cooperation in Preventing H1N1" in Taiwan in january 2010. During the meeting, Huang emphasized an extensive cross-strait collaboration in the area of public health, includ-ing disease notification and food safety.[24] In addition, Beijing dropped in 2009 its objection to Taiwan's application for an observer in the World Health Assembly. That being said, Taiwan's participation is allegedly required to be in line with Beijing's "One China" policy.[25]

More Public Health Assistance and Diplomacy

The second sign that China has put public health high on their foreign pol-icy agenda since SARS is their provision of development assistance and global public goods for health. As such, China is now using public health as a means to strengthen its diplomatic relations with the developing world, including African countries. China began in the 1960s to send "angels in white" and "barefoot doctors" to the sub-Saharan region to provide some of the poorest African countries with medical services. However, as argued by Huang Yanzhong of Seton Hall University, China's health diplomacy was "flimsy, passive, and asymmetric," at least until the 1980s.[3] After the SARS outbreak, in spite of its own failing health system, the Chinese government reiterated in its China's African Policy, published in early 2006, the nation's commitment to improving Africa's public health service.

To balance the criticisms that its energy and resource extraction in Africa grab the scarce resources there and that it shields disreputable regimes in such countries as Sudan and Zimbabwe from international opprobrium, China has stressed "win-win" relations in its deepening engagement with African countries. In response to the claims of exploitation in the natural resource sectors,[26,27] China emphasizes a no-strings-attached policy in offer-ing financial aid and technical support to less developed countries, including those in the African continent. In contrast, donor countries in the West and international financial institutions often attach conditionalities to their foreign aid programs, which are linked to market and political liberalization and good governance.[28] China has expanded its public health initiatives, such as in infrastructural building and health practitioner training, in Africa in recent years,[29] as well as commitment to cooperation with many African countries to help prevent and treat infectious diseases, particularly HIV/ AIDS and malaria.[30–34] In his African visit in June 2006, Chinese Premier Wen Jiabao asserted that China would promote sustainable development and help African countries tackle their burning social problems, of which public health was one of the top priorities.[35] Again in November 2009, during the fourth ministerial meeting of the Forum on China-Africa Cooperation in Egypt, Wen announced eight new measures to strengthen China-Africa cooperation in the following three years, including a 500 million yuan (US$73.2 million) assistance package that allows China to build 30 hospitals and 30 malaria prevention and treatment centers and to train 3,000 practitioners in the continent.[36]

Undoubtedly China has been learning from itself as well as from other developed countries the importance of providing sustainable development and global public goods for improving one's reputation on the world stage. At the "First International Roundtable on China-African Health Collaboration — New Health Initiative" in December 2009 in Beijing, one of us (LC) observed representatives from the WHO, World Bank, and the Bill & Melinda Gates Foundation praising China's development packages for their positive contributions to African development.

In addition, China's State Council has established in recent years a coordinating mechanism to facilitate cross-ministry dialogues and cooperation in global health and foreign aid initiatives. Chinese scholars have noted that a State Council "Global Health Diplomatic Coordination Office" (*quanqiu weisheng waijiao. xietiao bangongshi*, 全球卫生外交协调办公室), led by a senior official at vice-Premier level, is crucial to effectively coordinating and developing policies of health diplomacy.[37] In order to increase the capacity of China's health diplomats to deal with global health challenges, a training course, the first in a series, for Chinese officials, including officials from the Ministries of Foreign Affairs and Health, was held in August 2009 in the Institute for Global Health at Peking University.[38]

Was SARS a Watershed?

Following the Chinese government's acknowledgement of a SARS outbreak in the country, it began to acknowledge the importance of public health to national development and to accordingly strengthen its multilateral cooperation in combating contagious diseases inside and beyond its borders. For example, in the midst of the recent global economic downturn, the Chinese government announced in 2009 an injection of 850 billion yuan (US$125 billion) into its health care system to improve its operation. Since the SARS outbreak, it has not only deepened its engagement with other nations and international organizations, and cooperated with a variety of actors in dealing with its own fledgling health care system including the problem of HIV/AIDS, but China has also developed a vision for global health diplomacy. A ground-breaking implication of the SARS outbreak for China is that it was struck to realize that public health is not simply a domestic, social issue that can be isolated from foreign-policy and security concerns. In a globalizing world, the Chinese government appears to have learned that its health policy will be scrutinized by the world, and hence, it has become more open to and actively participates in global health governance. The government is now learning from such European countries as the UK, France, and Switzerland in the provision of the global public goods for health. Its substantial health assistance to sub-Saharan Africa in building hospitals and training health practitioners forms part of its health diplomacy and contribution to global health governance. It has also been proactively engaging with both regional and global health institutions since 2003 and set up different health surveillance networks with its ASEAN partners as well as other intergovernmental organizations, such as the Asia-Pacific Economic Cooperation (APEC) forum.[12]

Despite its increasing engagement with global health governance since the SARS outbreak, China's approach remains, however, fundamentally *state-centric,* contrary to the essence *of global* health diplomacy and governance. With grave concern about the loss of national sovereignty to external or nongovernmental actors, Chinese senior leaders have therefore attached primary significance to intergovernmental organizations, particularly the UN agencies. In evaluating the impact of SARS, Andrew Price-Smith has put the same point succinctly: "while the SARS epidemic may have generated moderate institutional change at the domestic level ..., it resulted in only ephemeral change at the level of global governance."[2] In other words, national sovereignty is still of paramount importance for the Chinese leadership. Because of its sensitivity to foreign interference into its internal affairs, the Chinese government has not yet formally or officially endorsed the notion of "human security." Under the umbrella concept of national security, "human safety," instead of "human security," is discussed throughout all of China's five white papers on national defense since 2000 (i.e., 2000, 2002, 2004, 2006, and 2008). Taiwan's participation in the World Health Assembly is predicated on the condition that it is considered part of China, not an independent entity. Having no tolerance in ceding its supreme authority, the central government has adopted a multi-faceted attitude towards its civil society organizations. While Beijing shows its willingness to cooperate with a wide array of actors inside China, it refuses to let its domestic NGOs and activists establish direct links with their counterparts overseas.

It is still uncertain whether this sovereign concern will trump the provision of global public good for health. Nevertheless, in a highly globalizing world, infectious diseases know no border. While China is seeking to adhere as much as possible to the underlying norms and rules of global health governance (and sometimes even applies them to their extremes), as evidenced by its handling of the recent swine flu outbreak, the major step forward is perhaps to reframe health as a *global* public good that is available to each and every individual of the world, rather than merely as an issue of concern to nation-states.

Acknowledgments

We are grateful to Dr. Pak K. Lee for his perceptive comments on earlier drafts of this article. Our thanks also go to Richard Scott Hutchinson for his technical support in producing the figure. We are, however, solely responsible for any remaining errors.

Author Contributions

ICMJE criteria for authorship read and met: LHC LC JX. Wrote the first draft of the paper: LHC. Contributed to the writing of the paper: LHC LC JX. Enrolled interviewees: JX.

References

1. Gu X (2004) Healthcare regime change and the SARS outbreak in China. In: Wong J, Zheng YN, eds. The SARS epidemic: challenges to China's crisis management., Singapore: *World Scientific*. pp. 123–155.
2. Price-Smith AT (2009) Contagion and chaos: disease, ecology, and national security in the era of globalization. Cambridge: *The MIT Press*. pp. 139–158.
3. Huang YZ March 2009 China's new health diplomacy. In Freeman CW, Lu XQ eds China's capacity to manage infectious diseases: global implications. Washington DC: centre for Strategic & International Studies. pp. 86–92.
4. (15–16 December 2003) speech by Dr Henk Bekedam, WHO representative in China at the International Forum on SARS Prevention and Control. Available: http://www.wpro.who.int/china/media_centre/speeches/speech_20031215.htm. Accessed 4 October 2009.
5. Zhongguo tongji nianjian (China Statistical Yearbook). Beijing: Zhongguo tongji chu ban she. The chapers on culture, sports and public health, various years.
6. (2005) Zhongguo weisheng nianjian (Yearbook of Public Health in China). Beijing: Renmin weisheng chubanshe. 565 p.
7. Schnur A (2006) The role of the WHO in combating SARS, focusing on the efforts in China. In: Kleinman A, Watson JL, eds. SARS in China: prelude to pandemic? Stanford: Stanford University Press. pp. 31–52.
8. (30 July 2005) Medical reform 'basically unsuccesful'. *China Daily*. Available http://www.chinadaily.com.cn/english/doc/2005–07/30/content_464795 htm. Accessed 14 August 2009.
9. Wang SG (July 2009) Adapting by learning: the evolution of China's rural health care financing. *Mod China* 35(4): 370–404.

10. Yip W, Hsiao WC (2009) Non-evidence-based policy: how effective is China's new cooperative medical scheme in reducing medical impoverishment? *Social Science & Medicine* 68: 201–209.

11. Brown PH, Brauw de A, Du Y (June 2009) Understanding variation in the design of China's new co-operative medical system. *China Q* 198: 304–329.

12. Chan LH, Lee PK, Chan G (January 2009) China engages global health governance: processes and dilemmas. *Global Public Health* 4(1): 1–30.

13. (29 August 2005) China ratifies WHO convention on tobacco control. Available http://www.highbeam.com/doc/1G1-135593920.html. Accessed 11 July 2009.

14. Hu T-W, Mao Z, Ong M, Tong E, Tao M, *et al.* (2006) China at the crossroads: the economics of tobacco and health. *Tob Control* 15(Suppl 1): i37–i41.

15. Bradsher K (1 May 2009) China's leaders take visible approach to swine flu. The New York Times.

16. Bezlova A (5 May 2009) China swine flu response criticized as 'unjustified' The Huffington Post.

17. Anderilini J. Jack A (4 May 2009) Mexico hits at China's quarantine policy. Financial Times.

18. Jack A. Hille K, Thomson A (5 May 2009) WHO tackles China on swine flu measures. Financial Times.

19. Cha AE (29 May 2009) Caught in China's aggressive swine flu net. The Washington Post.

20. Wong E (11 November 2009) China's tough flu measures appear to be effective. The New York Times.

21. Chan LH (January 2010) WHO — the world's most powerful international Organizations? *J Epidemiol Community Health* 64(2): 98–99.

22. Chan WY, Ma SY (2009) The making of a Chinese head of the WHO: a study of the media discourse on Margaret Chanis contest for the WHO Director-Generalship and its implications for the collective memory of SARS. *Int J Health Serv* 39(3): 587–614.

23. Shen S (Fall 2008) Borrowing the Hong Kong identity for Chinese diplomacy: implications of Margaret Chan's World Health Organization election campaign. *Pac Aff* 81(3): 361–382.

24. (20 January 2010) Cross-strait talks agenda urged to include healthcare. Taiwan Today. Available http://www.taiwantoday.tw/ct.asp?xItem= 92376& CtNode=413 Accessed 21 January 2010.

25. (30 April 2009) A healthy development. The Economist.
26. Brooks P (9 February 2007) Into Africa: China's grab for influence and oil. *Heritage Lectures* 1006: 1–5.
27. Klare M (2008) Rising powers, shrinking planet: how scare energy is creating a new world order. Oxford: Oneworld Publication.
28. Smith BC (2007) Good governance and development. Basingstoke: Palgrave Macmillan. pp 1–3.
29. Morrison JS (4 June 2008) China in Africa: implications for US policy. Washington DC: Centre for Strategic and International Studies: 6–10. Available http://csis.org/files/media/csis/congress/ts080604morrison.pdf. Accessed 16 February 2010.
30. Ministry of Foreign Affairs of the PRC (January 2006) China's African policy. Beijing: Ministry of Foreign Affairs of the PRC. Available http://www. fmprc.gov.cn/eng/zxxx/t230615.htm. Accessed 12 August 2009.
31. (1 June 2005) Guochan Atziyao chukou Nanfei (Chinese-made AIDS drug exports to South Africa). Ta Kung Pao (Hong Kong).
32. (18 January 2007) Chinese scientists take malaria fight to Africa. Reuters AlertNct. Availalble http://www.alertnet.org/thenews/newsdesk/B155919.htm. Accessed 12 August 2009.
33. Lague D (5 June 2007) On island off Africa, China's tries to wipe out malaria. The New York Times.
34. Tan EL (5 November 2009) China-adopts 'malaria diplomacy' as part of Africa push. Reuters. Available http://www.reuters.com/article/idUSSP503140. Accessed 16 February 2010.
35. Stamp G (26 June 2006) China defends its African relations. BBC News. Available http://news.bbc.co.uk/2/hi/business/5114980.stm. Accessed 17 February 2010.
36. (9 November 2009) Chinese premier announces eight new measures to enhance cooperation with Africa. People's Daily Online. Available http://english.peopledaily.com.cn/90001/90776/90883/6807055.html. Accessed 8 December 2009.
37. Chen L, Xu WZ (2009) Bianhua de Feizhou xuyao woguo xinxing de waisheng waijiao celue (The changing Africa necessitates our country's new health diplomatic strategies). Beijing: The Institute for Global Health, Peking University Unpublished report.

38. Ministry of Health (12 August 2009) Quanqiu weisheng waijiao peixunban zai jing juban (Global health diplomacy training course held in Beijing). Available http://www.moh.gov.cn/publicfiles/business/htmlfiles/mohgjhzs/s7952/200908/4233).htm. Accessed 16 February 2010.

39. World Health Organization (2006) SARS how a global epidemic was stopped. *Geneva: World Health Organization*, pp. 3–48.

11

Destruction of the Smallpox Virus Stocks: Negotiating for Consensus in the World Health Organization

Jonathan B. Tucker[i]

Abstract

More than three decades after the eradication of smallpox, a debate continues among the member states of the World Health Organization over whether or not to destroy the known stocks of the smallpox virus, which are held at two WHO-approved repositories in the United States and Russia. Defence and counterterrorism officials from developed countries believe that secret caches of the virus may exist that could be used for biological attacks and want to retain the known stocks for the development of medical countermeasures. Public health officials from developing countries, in contrast, oppose devoting scarce resources to combat an eradicated disease when they face current threats from AIDS and other scourges. The emerging ability to synthesize the smallpox virus from scratch has further complicated the debate.

---

[i] Jonathan B. Tucker, Ph.D., is a Senior Fellow in the Washington, D.C. office of the James Martin Center for Nonproliferation Studies of the Monterey Institute of International Studies.

The Problem

One of the most contentious and enduring policy debates in the field of international health has swirled around the fate of the last known stocks of variola virus, the causative agent of smallpox, which are preserved at two World Health Organization (WHO)-authorised repositories in the United States and Russia. After a global vaccination campaign under WHO auspices eradicated smallpox in the late 1970s, it was expected that the remaining stocks of variola virus would be destroyed. But US policy-makers became concerned in the early 1990s that some countries might have retained undeclared samples of the virus for biological warfare purposes. Because a smallpox outbreak anywhere on the globe would trigger a public health emergency, in 1999 the World Health Assembly, the annual policy-making meeting of WHO member states, approved the 'temporary retention' of the variola virus stocks at the two authorised repositories to develop improved medical defences against smallpox. In 2002 the destruction of the virus stocks was postponed indefinitely pending completion of the research goals, but today international pressures are growing once again to set a new deadline for virus destruction. This case study examines the negotiations over smallpox that occurred in the policy-making forums of the WHO from 1999 to 2007, focusing on the role of the US government. The chapter concludes by assessing the prospects for resolving the ongoing debate over destruction of the variola virus stocks.[1]

Background

Smallpox was a contagious viral disease that infected only humans and killed about a third of its victims, claiming hundreds of millions of lives over the course of history.[2] In 1966 the WHO launched an intensified global vaccination campaign that, over the next 11 years, eradicated smallpox from the planet in one of the greatest public health achievements of the twentieth century.[3] Even before the last natural outbreak of smallpox was contained in Somalia in 1977, the WHO sought to limit the number of facilities holding stocks of variola virus in order to prevent an accidental release that could reintroduce the disease. In 1975 the WHO conducted a survey of biomedical laboratories around the world, of which 74 reported possessing variola virus. Although China did not respond to the survey, an institute in Beijing held the virus at the time, bringing the total number of possessor-labs to 75.[4] It also appeared likely that other countries or individual scientists might have knowingly or unwittingly retained undeclared samples of the virus in their strain collections.

The hazards of continued research with live variola virus became clear in 1978, when an accident in a pox virology laboratory at the University of Birmingham in England resulted in two cases of smallpox, one of them fatal. In response, the World Health Assembly adopted a resolution in May 1980 urging all countries that possessed samples of variola virus either to destroy their stocks or transfer them to one of four designated WHO collaborating centres. Because the WHO had neither the authority nor the capability to verify the destruction and consolidation of the virus stocks, these steps took place on a good-faith basis.

By early 1984 the consolidation process had progressed to the point that the WHO named two government-owned facilities in the United States and the Soviet Union as the sole authorised repositories of the smallpox virus: the US Centre for Disease Control in Atlanta (CDC, renamed in 1992 the Centres for Disease Control and Prevention) and the State Research Institute for Viral Preparations in Moscow. These sites were chosen because they had served as the WHO reference laboratories during the smallpox eradication campaign and thus possessed the world's largest collections of variola virus isolates, obtained from outbreaks in many parts of the world. In 1994 the poor physical security at the Moscow institute, combined with political unrest following the break-up of the Soviet Union, prompted fears that the virus stocks might be at risk. Thus, without seeking permission from the WHO, the Russian government transferred the authorised smallpox repository from Moscow to the State Research Centre of Virology and Biotechnology "Vector" in the remote Siberian town of Koltsovo, near Novosibirsk. At the CDC and Vector laboratories, the variola virus stocks are stored in liquid-nitrogen freezers and protected with elaborate security measures. As of late 2008, the CDC held 451 samples of 229 different isolates, while Vector had 691 samples of 120 different isolates.[5]

In 1990 a WHO scientific advisory committee recommended that the authorised stocks of variola virus be destroyed by 31 December 1993, after the DNA sequences of representative strains had been determined for scientific and forensic purposes. But protests from the scientific community and delays in the DNA sequencing effort led the WHO to postpone the date of virus destruction. Meanwhile, a high-level Soviet official named Kanatjan Alibekov (aka Ken Alibek) defected to the United States in 1992 and revealed shocking details of the vast Soviet biological warfare programme, which had peaked during the 1980s. This top-secret programme was a clear violation of the 1972 Biological Weapons Convention, a multilateral treaty to which Moscow was a party. Alibek told his CIA debriefers that during the Cold War, the Soviet Union had developed a highly lethal strain of variola virus as a strategic weapon and had produced and stockpiled it in multi-tonne quantities for potential delivery against US cities in the event of World War III. Particularly alarming was Alibek's claim that the Vector laboratory — now one of the two WHO-authorised repositories of variola virus — had been involved in illicit military development work on smallpox.[6] At the time, however, the CIA kept this information highly classified and did not share it with the health-related agencies of the US government.

In May 1996 the United States, represented by the Secretary of Health and Human Services (HHS), supported a resolution in the World Health Assembly calling for the destruction of the authorised stocks of variola virus at the CDC and Vector on 30 June 1999, provided that the Assembly voted in May 1999 to confirm this decision. Over the next two years, however, the US Department of Defense became increasingly concerned about the potential use of smallpox as a military or terrorist weapon, the possible existence of undeclared stocks of the virus in hostile countries, and the lack of effective medical defences against the disease. Alibek's revelations suggested that Russia might have retained hidden caches of variola virus outside the official repository at Vector, contrary to WHO policy. The CIA also obtained circumstantial evidence that undeclared stocks of the virus might exist in other countries of proliferation concern, possibly including but not necessarily limited to Iraq, Iran, and North Korea.[7] (In the aftermath of the 2003 Iraq War, the US-led Iraq Survey Group deployed a "Team Pox" that searched for — but failed to find — conclusive evidence that the Saddam Hussein regime had possessed a secret cache of variola virus.) A few scientific research centres also reported discovering and destroying vials of the virus that had been retained inadvertently in laboratory freezers, sparking fears that other poorly secured samples might exist that could fall into the hands of terrorists.

In view of these reports, US national security policy-makers became increasingly concerned about the possible existence of undeclared stocks of variola virus and the growing vulnerability of the civilian population to smallpox infection. In the United States the mandatory vaccination of children at school entry had ended in 1972 and most other countries had halted the routine vaccination of their civilian populations soon after the WHO certified the global eradication of smallpox in 1980. Because the protection provided by the smallpox vaccine wanes over time, those vaccinated once in childhood would retain only partial immunity a few decades later. Moreover, most Americans born after 1967 (with the exception of those who served in the armed forces, travelled to endemic countries or did poxvirus research) were never immunized against smallpox and hence would be unprotected in the event of an outbreak.

The diminishing percentage of the US population with protective immunity against smallpox, the lack of physician familiarity with the disease, and the limited supplies of protective vaccine all stoked fears that a deliberate release of variola virus by a rogue state or terrorist organisation would spawn a rapidly spreading epidemic, threatening international health and security.[8] In 1998 the US government asked the Institute of Medicine (IOM), a policy-analysis arm of the US National Academy of Sciences, to assess the scientific need for further research and development work with the live variola virus. The terms of reference for the study instructed the IOM not to consider the possible benefits of destroying the virus stocks nor the risks associated with their continued retention and manipulation.

In March 1999 the IOM expert committee released its report, which recommended further work with live variola virus for the development of improved diagnostic tools, a safer vaccine and at least two antiviral drugs that could treat smallpox by different mechanisms.[9] The rationale for the development of antivirals was that in the event of a bioterrorist attack with variola virus, the disease might spread widely before large-scale vaccination could begin. In that case, therapeutic drugs would be needed to treat the first generation of cases and to help contain the epidemic.[10] Critics of the IOM report argued that the US government's charge to the committee had been intentionally biased with the aim of obtaining a preordained result: a set of scientific arguments supporting a decision to retain the variola virus stocks at the CDC indefinitely for defensive research.[11]

In late March 1999, drawing on the findings of the IOM study, a US government Interagency Working Group proposed a major shift in policy on smallpox. The agency representatives agreed that at the upcoming World Health Assembly in May, the United States should seek to delay indefinitely the planned destruction of the variola virus stocks at the CDC and Vector in order to develop improved defences against the potential use of the virus as a bioterrorist weapon. This unanimous recommendation was forwarded to President Bill Clinton, who decided that as head of state he could not forgo the development of new measures to protect the US population against a smallpox attack, however low the chances of such an event might be. On 22 April 1999, an official White House statement announcing the decision explained, 'While we fervently hope smallpox would never be used as a weapon, we have a responsibility to develop the drug and vaccine tools to deal with any future contingency — a research and development process that would necessarily require smallpox virus.'[12] Before the proposed research programme could move forward however, it had to be approved by the other WHO Member States at the World Health Assembly in May 1999. Thus, the United States faced the challenging diplomatic task of winning consensus support for an indefinite delay in the planned destruction of the variola virus stocks.

Local and External Players and Their Roles

The main players in the smallpox destruction debate are the 193 Member States of the WHO, which vary considerably in their views on this issue. As the host-countries for the two authorised repositories of variola virus, the United States and Russia both favour continued research with the live virus to develop more robust medical defences against the disease, and several dozen predominantly Western states support them in this effort. In contrast, the developing countries of Africa and Asia, which suffered disproportionately from the ravages of smallpox during the decades prior to eradication, fear an accidental release of variola virus and thus view the ongoing smallpox research at the CDC and Vector as a potential threat to their well-being. A third group of WHO Member States do not feel strongly about the issue and have remained on the sidelines.

Because the smallpox question lies at the nexus of public health and international security, a unique aspect of the debate in the World Health Assembly has been the involvement of officials from ministries of defence and other security-related agencies that do not normally participate in global health negotiations. The resulting "clash of cultures" between the public health and national security communities has increased the complexity of the talks, which also have a north-south dimension. Whereas defence and counterterrorism policy-makers from Western industrialised countries view the smallpox issue chiefly through the prism of national security concerns, public health officials from the developing world object to allocating scarce financial and scientific resources for research on an eradicated disease at a time when they face serious threats from current scourges such as AIDS, malaria, and drug-resistant tuberculosis.

Also participating in the smallpox destruction debate are several dozen substance-matter experts in virology, infectious diseases and public health, who are outspoken and highly opinionated. These individuals advocate positions on either side of the debate and seek to influence government policy-makers. Experts favouring the prompt destruction of the variola virus stocks, known as 'destructionists,' are mostly public health practitioners who believe that the danger of smallpox bioterrorism has been exaggerated and that the safety risks of continued research with live variola virus outweigh the potential benefits in terms of new therapeutic drugs and next-generation vaccines. In contrast, experts who favour retaining the known stocks of the virus for defensive research, known as 'retentionists,' are mostly virologists and national security officials who believe that the risk that smallpox could be used as a bioterrorist weapon is significant and increasing. These individuals stress the importance of developing improved medical countermeasures against smallpox as an insurance policy for — and a deterrent against — the threat of a bioterrorist attack. Although both destructionists and retentionists wrap themselves in the mantle of scientific objectivity, major differences in values and threat perceptions underlie their opposing positions.

Finally, a few small civil society groups have tried to influence the smallpox destruction debate. Before major discussions of the issue at the WHO policy forums, two left-leaning non-governmental organisations — the Sunshine Project and the Third World Network — have issued reports, given briefings, and created a dedicated website in an effort to persuade WHO Member States from the developing world to support the prompt destruction of the variola virus stocks. In addition, a small advocacy group in the United States called the Council for Responsible Genetics has lobbied against the US proposal to genetically engineer the smallpox virus by inserting a "reporter gene" to facilitate drug-screening studies.[13] Such pressure groups face an uphill struggle however, because they operate on an uneven playing field in which only WHO Member States have the power to make decisions and the consensus rule usually applies.

Challenges Faced and Outcomes

From 1999 through 2007, the international debate over whether or not to destroy the known stocks of variola virus played out in a series of meetings in Geneva, Switzerland, of the two policy-making bodies of the WHO: the Executive Board, which meets every January to set the agenda of the organization, and the World Health Assembly, the annual forum in May of WHO Member States.

Decision to launch the smallpox research programme

The initial debate over the US proposal to delay destruction of the variola virus stocks at the CDC and Vector and launch a programme of defensive research with the live virus took place at the 52nd World Health Assembly in May 1999. Although HHS Secretary Donna Shalala led the US delegation to the meeting, the point man on the smallpox issue was Dr. Kenneth Bernard, a special assistant to the president on the National Security Council staff who focused on international health and security issues. During a long career with the US Public Health Service, Bernard had served on several delegations to the World Health Assembly, but now he faced his most challenging assignment. Before he left for Geneva, several of his colleagues had predicted that the developing world would rise up in fury against the United States for seeking to delay the long-planned destruction of the smallpox virus.

After arriving in Geneva, Bernard made the rounds of the delegates' lounge at the Palais des Nations, conferring informally with various delegations and explaining the merits of the US position. Most of the developing country representatives he spoke with made clear that they wanted the variola virus stocks destroyed on schedule, but they listened with growing concern as he described the possible terrorist use of the virus as a biological weapon. Bernard's strategy was to build a broad base of support for a defensively oriented smallpox research programme at the CDC and Vector by proposing to subsume it under an international framework that included scientific oversight by the WHO. To pursue this objective, he organised an informal drafting group of some 30 countries, chaired by a Swiss delegate who was seen as a neutral mediator.

On 20 May 1999, drawing on a straw-man text that Bernard had written, the drafting group prepared an alternative resolution authorising the indefinite retention of the variola virus stocks at the two authorised repositories for the purpose of developing medical countermeasures against smallpox, including diagnostic tests, antiviral drugs, and improved vaccines. The draft resolution called for restricting all research with the live virus to the CDC and Vector, and funding it outside the regular WHO budget with voluntary contributions from Member States. To minimise the risk of an accidental release, all work with live variola virus would take place in hermetically sealed Biosafety Level 4 laboratories, where scientists work in full-body 'space suits' equipped with individual air supplies to protect them from infection.

The draft resolution also established a WHO scientific oversight body, the Advisory Committee on Variola Virus Research, to review and approve all proposed experiments with the live virus and monitor their execution. The research projects would have to be 'outcome-oriented and time-limited' and offer clear public-health benefits, so that experiments could not be justified merely on the grounds of 'interesting' science. To enhance transparency, the results would have to be published in the scientific literature or summarised in abstracts posted on the WHO website. Finally, WHO Member States would be guaranteed equitable access to the benefits of the research, including antiviral drugs, vaccines, and diagnostic tools.[14]

As a result of Bernard's informal consultations, 26 countries pledged to co-sponsor the draft resolution, while a few others agreed to provide passive support by not objecting to it. An important exception was the delegation of India, which made clear that it was under strict instructions from New Delhi to press for the immediate destruction of the virus stocks and could not accept the open-ended research programme proposed in the draft resolution. On the morning of 21 May, Bernard met for coffee in the delegates' lounge with two members of the Indian delegation and tried to work out a mutually acceptable formula. The Indians proposed amending the draft resolution so that research with live variola virus could continue only up to a specified date, after which the World Health Assembly would assess the situation and decide either to extend the research programme for an additional period or order the destruction of the virus stocks. Bernard agreed in principle to this approach and proposed a period of five years before the next decision-point. The Indian delegates however, insisted on three years.

Because India was a leader of the G-77 group of developing countries, New Delhi's opposition to the smallpox resolution might well doom it to failure, giving the United States a strong incentive to make a deal. Bernard told the Indians that he would consult with Washington and get back to them soon with a response. He first met with other members of the US delegation representing government agencies with a major stake in the issue, such as HHS and the Department of Defense. Although the Pentagon officials wanted more time for defensive smallpox research before the issue was sent back to the World Health Assembly for decision, they understood that the United States had to demonstrate that it was acting in good faith to address its legitimate security concerns and did not have a hidden agenda.

Bernard then consulted with the group of senior US officials back in Washington who were 'backstopping' the Geneva negotiations and received authorisation to accept the Indian proposal for a three-year smallpox research programme with the option of renewal. In return for this concession, Bernard asked the Indians to accept a small but significant change in the text of the draft resolution. He proposed modifying the sentence request-ing the WHO to 'appoint a new group of experts which will establish what research, if any, must be carried out to reach global agreement to destroy existing variola virus stocks' so that the second part of the sentence now read: 'to reach global consensus on the timing for the destruction of exist-ing variola virus stocks.' This minor change in wording — from 'global agreement' to 'global consensus' — later proved critical because it meant that the World Health Assembly could not decide to destroy the virus without the concurrence of the United States and its allies.

Having worked out a negotiating formula that was acceptable to both India and the United States, Bernard was fairly confident that the other WHO Member States would approve the draft resolution, but there was still the possibility of unanticipated objections. On the afternoon of 21 May 1999, Committee A (the subsidiary body of the World Health Assembly dealing with technical matters) took up Resolution 52.10 to establish an open-ended programme of applied smallpox research at the CDC and Vector. Early in the floor debate, the Indian representative, H. K. Singh, proposed an amendment to the resolution authorising the 'tempo-rary retention up to but not later than 2002' of the stocks of variola virus at the two WHO-authorised repositories 'for the purpose of further inter-national research into antiviral agents and improved vaccines, and to permit high-priority investigations of the genetic structure and pathogen-esis of smallpox.' Over the next hour, delegates from 25 countries took the floor, most of them endorsing the draft resolution as amended by India. Only Iran, Nicaragua, and Zambia opposed any further delay in destroy-ing the virus stocks.

By the end of the debate, it was clear that a broad consensus had emerged in favour of the resolution, which passed by acclamation. Final approval by the WHA plenary the next day was considered a mere for-mality.[15] Bernard was delighted that the smallpox resolution had been adopted by consensus rather than by a politically divisive vote. Over the next three years, the Member States would monitor the progress of the smallpox research programme at the CDC and Vector and determine in May 2002 whether they had reached consensus to move forward with the destruction of the variola virus stocks at the end of the year; if not, the virus would receive another stay of execution.

Indefinite extension of the smallpox research programme

By December 2001 it was clear that despite significant progress in the smallpox research programme since May 1999, the investigators at the CDC and Vector would not complete some key tasks by the end of 2002. The unfinished projects included the development of an animal model of smallpox in a non-human primate and the screening of additional antiviral drugs for their ability to inhibit the replication of variola virus in the test tube. Given the promising initial results of the research programme, the WHO variola advisory committee called for postponing the destruction of the virus stocks at the CDC and Vector to permit the completion of 'essential, goal-oriented research.'[16] WHO Director-General Gro Harlem Brundtland endorsed the committee's recommendation, while urging that all studies requiring access to live variola virus be completed as quickly as possible and that a new destruction date be set when the research results made it possible to reach an international consensus on timing.[17]

Dr. Brundtland's support for retaining the variola virus stocks beyond the planned destruction deadline of December 2002 angered some smallpox experts. In an interview with the *British Medical Journal*, Dr. Kalyan Banerjee of India expressed the view that allowing additional work with the live virus would enable the US military to develop it into a biological weapon behind the façade of defensive research, much as the Soviet Union had done in the past. 'The people of the world and the WHO worked hard to eradicate smallpox, only to leave the most potent bioweapon in the hands of the two custodial powers,' he warned.[18] Banerjee's views reflected a deep suspicion of US and Russian intentions on the part of many people in the developing world. Given this attitude, the success of the US bid to extend the smallpox research programme was far from certain.

On 14–21 January 2002 the WHO Executive Board, the 32-country body that sets the agenda for the annual World Health Assembly, convened in Geneva. That year the United States, Russia, and China were not members of the Board; according to a complex formula, they were off one year out of every four. Even so, delegates from nonvoting countries could attend as observers and make interventions after the voting members had spoken. Bernard represented the United States at the meeting. In his statement he described the potential hostile use of smallpox as 'a critical national and international security issue.' Referring to the horrific attacks of 11 September 2001, he added, 'The recent terrorist events in the US have regrettably confirmed that we cannot assume that the intentional release of smallpox is too remote a circumstance. A case of smallpox anywhere in the world is a case everywhere. Only developing and deploying both antiviral drugs and modern vaccines will protect all of our countries from the risk of unreported virus stores being released by terrorists.'

The Russian representative, Yuri Fedorov of the Ministry of Health, endorsed the US call to retain the live variola virus stocks at the CDC and Vector for additional defensive research. But Chinese ambassador Sha Zukang strongly opposed any extension of the smallpox research programme, warning that 'a most devastating biological catastrophe' could result if the virus stocks were not destroyed in a timely manner. 'A final date for destruction should be determined, and no excuses should be given for further delay,' he said. Because China was not a voting member of the WHO Executive Board in 2002 however, Ambassador Sha could not block the proposal to delay virus destruction. Cuba, a voting member of the Board, also called for setting a firm date to end all research with the live virus but did not attempt to prevent consensus. Despite the fact that India had been one of the strongest advocates of virus destruction at the May 1999 World Health Assembly, the Indian representative remained silent throughout the discussion.[19] Developments since 1999, including the 11 September attacks in the United States and an upsurge in Kashmir-related terrorism, had apparently caused a change of heart in New Delhi on the issue of smallpox research. After the discussion, the voting members of the Executive Board endorsed the WHO Director-General's recommendation to delay destruction of the live virus stocks until the agreed research objectives had been achieved.

During preparations for the 55th World Health Assembly in May 2002, the WHO Secretariat prepared a draft resolution based on the Executive Board decision. Noting that important smallpox research goals could not be completed by the end of December 2002, the draft resolution proposed to 'authorize the further, temporary, retention of the existing stocks of live variola virus at the current locations . . . for the purpose of enabling further international research, on the understanding that steps should be taken to ensure that the research should be completed as quickly as possible and a proposed new date for destruction should be set when the research accomplishments and outcomes allow consensus to be reached on the timing of destruction of the variola virus stocks.'[20] The draft resolution also called for maintaining the oversight role of the WHO variola advisory committee, ensuring that the research programme was open and transparent, conducting regular biosafety inspections of the smallpox repositories at the CDC and Vector, and submitting a progress report to the World Health Assembly no later than 2005.

Although US officials were satisfied with the draft resolution as written, they were concerned by the statements of the Chinese and Cuban representatives demanding a firm deadline for completing work with the live virus. In the weeks leading up to the 2002 World Health Assembly, the State Department cabled talking points on the smallpox research programme to US embassies in all WHO Member States, for delivery to the ministries of health and foreign affairs. This *démarche* (diplomatic note conveying an official position) elicited generally positive responses from governments around the world and provided grounds for cautious optimism in Washington. State Department officials were still worried about Dr. Banerjee's published remarks critical of smallpox research, but the Indian government reassured them that Banerjee's views were his own and did not reflect New Delhi's official position.

Although Russia was one of only two countries that hosted a legal repository of variola virus, the Russian government played a surprisingly passive role in the WHO smallpox debate. Prior to key decisions in the Executive Board or the World Health Assembly, Russian officials were not proactive, sending *démarches* to other states in their sphere of influence only when the US government specifically requested them to do so. According to Bernard, "We had to push the Russians frequently to speak out at meetings and talk to their allies. They did so each time we asked, using talking points not much different from ours but delivered by relatively junior officials. It was clear that no one in Russia took the issue as seriously as they should have, if the outcome made as much difference to them as it did to us."[21] Moscow's passivity led Bernard to suspect that the Russian military retained secret caches of variola virus and thus had less of a stake than the United States in preserving the WHO-authorised stocks. One suspect facility in Russia was the Centre of Virology, a Ministry of Defence laboratory near the city of Sergiev Posad (formerly Zagorsk) that had conducted offensive smallpox research during the Cold War and still remained shrouded in secrecy and off-limits to Westerners.

When Bernard arrived in Geneva in May 2002 for the World Health Assembly, he was apprehensive that China and Cuba might derail the smallpox resolution by insisting on a firm date for destruction of the virus stocks. If they did so, they might gain the support of countries that had poor relations with Washington, such as Iran, Libya, and Syria. But any demand to destroy the virus by a date-certain would make the resolution unacceptable to the United States. Bernard also worried that Taiwan's bid for WHO observer status would complicate negotiations with the People's Republic of China over the smallpox research programme. While adhering rhetorically to a one-China policy, Washington was a strong supporter of Taiwanese security and autonomy. Even so, backing WHO observer status for Taiwan might anger the Chinese authorities and reduce their willingness to cooperate with the United States on retention of the variola virus stocks. It was therefore essential to 'de-link' the two issues. On 13 May, HHS Secretary Tommy Thompson had a cordial bilateral meeting in Geneva with his Chinese counterpart, Minister of Health Zhang Wenkang. The two officials discussed the smallpox issue and agreed to instruct their respective delegations to work out a mutually acceptable solution. In a speech the next day to the World Health Assembly, Secretary Thompson made no mention of Taiwan's bid for WHO observer status, a diplomatic gesture that improved the atmosphere for cooperation with the Chinese.

Over the next few days, Bernard negotiated the specific wording of the smallpox resolution with an informal drafting group made up of delegates from China, Japan, Russia, Australia, and a few European countries. The draft resolution called for extending the smallpox research programme at the CDC and Vector for an indefinite period and delaying a decision on destruction of the virus stocks until all of the research goals had been achieved. To Bernard's surprise, the Chinese and Japanese delegations proposed amendments that were largely compatible with the US position. Chinese officials, while deferring to the US demand that the resolution not specify a firm deadline for destruction of the virus stocks, sought to insert the phrase that all approved research must remain 'outcome-oriented and time-limited and periodically reviewed.' The Chinese also considered inadequate a provision in the draft resolution requiring a progress report on the research by 2005, so Bernard agreed to language calling for annual reports. Finally, the Japanese delegation, responding to concerns by some countries that the United States and Russia might try to keep the benefits of smallpox research for themselves, inserted a phrase requesting the WHO Director-General 'to ensure that research results and the benefits of this research are made available to all Member States.'

The revised Resolution 55.15 was now acceptable to all delegations participating in the informal consultations, but it was not yet clear if the World Health Assembly would adopt the resolution by consensus. Bernard was pleased to learn that the Chinese delegation was actively lobbying some wavering states to support the amended text. In the late afternoon of 17 May 2002, toward the end of the week-long meeting, the smallpox resolution finally came up for discussion in Committee A.[22] Twenty-three country representatives took the floor and endorsed the resolution as amended by China and Japan. Even Iran, Cuba, and Libya, which normally opposed US-sponsored initiatives, praised the 'excellent' Chinese amendments.

During his intervention, Bernard stated that the events of 11 September 2001 had shown that terrorists were prepared to inflict mass casualties and that the danger that smallpox might be used as a weapon was "small but growing." He concluded, 'We support the recommendation of the Director-General that any new date for destruction be fixed when the research accomplishments and outcomes allow consensus to be reached on timing.' The Russian delegate also endorsed the proposed extension of the smallpox research programme and briefly summarised the work taking place at Vector. After the discussion, Committee A approved the smallpox resolution by acclamation. When the 2002 World Health Assembly came to a close, the United States had achieved its goal of retaining the stocks of live variola virus for an indefinite period until all of the research goals had been achieved.[23]

Growing opposition to smallpox research

After several years had passed without a clear effort by CDC and Vector scientists to complete the research tasks requiring access to live variola virus, many developing countries became impatient with the lack of movement towards a new decision to destroy the virus stocks. Although the smallpox research programme had yielded a useful collection of diagnostic tools and candidate antiviral drugs, the United States and Russia claimed that further work with the live virus was needed to screen additional antiviral compounds and develop a model of smallpox in a non-human primate, a requirement for regulatory approval by the US Food and Drug Administration (FDA) under the so-called Animal Efficacy Rule.[24] Although unlicensed antiviral drugs could be administered to the civilian victims of a smallpox attack under an Emergency Use Authorization from the FDA, the US military is only allowed to procure and stockpile licensed medical countermeasures.

Controversy also flared over a US proposal to genetically modify variola virus by inserting a gene coding for a "reporter" protein that would make the virus particles glow green when viewed under a fluorescence microscope, facilitating the drug-screening process. Opponents of smallpox research claimed that there was no longer any scientific rationale to retain live variola virus for the development of diagnostics, vaccines, or antiviral drugs. The critics also argued that after several years of failed efforts to create a realistic model of human smallpox in monkeys, the project should be terminated because the limited scientific returns did not justify the significant biosafety risks.[25]

By January 2006, when the WHO Executive Board reviewed the status of smallpox research, the tide of international opinion was shifting against the programme. According to the meeting minutes, 'Many speakers confirmed the need to ensure that all approved research remained essential, outcome-oriented, and time-limited. Some Board members felt that it was time to consider whether the benefits of destruction of the remaining stocks might not far outweigh those of continued research.'[26] This discussion led the Executive Board to request the WHO Secretariat to draft a new smallpox resolution for consideration by the 59th World Health Assembly in May 2006. The Board also approved the creation of an Intergovernmental Working Group on Smallpox Eradication, open to all WHO Member States, to discuss the draft resolution and make any necessary amendments.

At the first meeting of the working group in Geneva on 5 April 2006, the 46 member countries of WHO's African Regional Group made a number of suggestions for strengthening the draft resolution. These proposals included withdrawing approval to work with the live virus for the purposes of DNA sequencing, diagnostics and vaccine development; setting a new deadline for destroying the variola virus stocks at the CDC and Vector by 30 June 2010; and ensuring that all WHO Member States had access to the benefits of smallpox research, including any new antiviral drugs. The African countries also called for reforming the membership of the WHO Advisory Committee on Variola Virus Research, which consisted largely of virologists from Western countries, to include more experts from the developing world and the field of public health. The United States and Russia, however, were in no mood to make concessions and rejected most of the African proposals. As a result, the draft resolution was forwarded to the 59th World Health Assembly in May 2006 with many sections of text set off in square brackets, indicating a lack of consensus.[27]

When Committee A convened on the evening of 25 May 2006 to discuss the draft resolution, more than two dozen countries made interventions. The representative of Namibia, speaking on behalf of the African Regional Group, said that the time had come for WHO Member States to set a new deadline for destruction of the variola virus stocks, ban the genetic engineering of the virus, and reform the structure and procedures of the WHO variola advisory committee, which he claimed had been lax in performing its oversight role. Representatives from several other countries took the floor to endorse the African proposals, including Cameroon, Iran, Jordan, South Africa, and Thailand. The South African Minister of Health, Dr. Manto Tshabalala-Msimang, was particularly strident in her criticism of the smallpox research programme. When US officials expressed concern about her hard-line positions, the South African government reassured the State Department that, in the end, she would be flexible. The United States, for its part, continued to oppose setting a new deadline for virus destruction but acknowledged the need to

reform the WHO variola advisory committee and was prepared to negotiate on this issue. Canada, Israel, and the Marshall Islands endorsed the US
positions, while Australia and Japan offered more qualified support.[28]

To conduct further negotiations on the draft resolution, the World
Health Assembly established a working group chaired by Thailand, which
met twice on 26 May 2006 and once more the next morning, a few hours
before the final plenary. During the working group debate, which became
heated at times, the US delegation resisted demands to set a new destruction deadline. As the basis for a possible compromise, the United States
proposed a 'major review' of the smallpox research programme in 2010.
The working group also made some progress on reforming the membership of the WHO variola advisory committee to increase the number of
experts from developing countries and with a background in public health.
Even so, when the African Regional Group asserted that it was a conflict
of interest for US and Russian smallpox researchers to serve on the oversight committee and review the scientific merit and biosafety risks of their
own proposals, the United States demurred.[29]

During the final negotiating session in May 2006, the African countries offered a compromise formula in which they would drop their
demand for a new destruction deadline in return for a broad set of 'transparency measures,' including a comprehensive review of all smallpox
research completed, undertaken, and planned at the two repositories and a
detailed report on the results.[30] The United States however, refused to
move beyond its earlier proposal for a 'major review' of the smallpox
research programme in 2010, and Russia supported this position. Given
the negotiating deadlock, the World Health Assembly referred the draft
resolution for consideration at the next session of the WHO Executive
Board in January 2007, intending to conduct informal consultations during the intervening period.

In May 2007 the 60th World Health Assembly finally agreed to a
watered-down smallpox resolution affirming 'the need to reach consensus
on a proposed new date for the destruction of variola virus stocks, when
research outcomes crucial to an improved public-health response to an
outbreak so permit.' To help build international consensus on the destruction issue, the Member States requested the WHO Director-General to
conduct 'a major review in 2010 of the results of the research undertaken,

currently under way, and the plans and requirements for further essential research for global public health purposes.'[31] Based on this review, the 64th World Health Assembly in May 2011 will strive to reach consensus on the timing of virus destruction.

Whether the largely normative debate over variola virus destruction can be resolved through international negotiation remains to be seen. In general, the World Health Assembly prefers to act by consensus because WHO resolutions do not have the legally binding status of treaties but are instead largely hortatory, 'urging' rather than obligating Member States to take certain actions. On a few occasions in the past however, the World Health Assembly has taken important decisions by a majority vote rather than by consensus. The 1966 decision to launch the intensified smallpox eradication campaign, for example, was approved by a margin of only two votes.[32] It is therefore possible that if a consensus solution to the smallpox issue cannot be reached, the Member States may resort to a voice vote or a roll-call vote. In that case the United States and Russia could face a difficult choice among three unpalatable options: comply with the decision and proceed to destroy their virus stocks, refuse to accept the decision as legally binding and pursue open smallpox research, or claim to have destroyed their stocks but continue working with the live virus in secret.

Lessons Learned

Because of the contentious nature of the smallpox destruction debate, the US efforts in 1999 and 2002 to delay destruction of the variola virus stocks and pursue a programme of defensive research ran contrary to the preferences of many WHO Member States. For this reason, the US delegation faced a major diplomatic challenge in persuading the World Health Assembly to adopt these decisions by consensus. Dr. Kenneth Bernard shepherded the smallpox resolutions through the process by making effective use of the following negotiating tactics:

- He made sure that he had the trust and support of the public health and security agencies of the US government, as well as other key political constituencies in Washington. Having secured this backing, he was able to speak with confidence on behalf of the United States.

- He conducted preliminary consultations with other delegations to solicit their views and concerns, and created an informal group chaired by a neutral mediator to draft an alternative resolution based on a straw-man text that he had prepared.
- He conducted bilateral negotiations with a key developing-country leader (India in 1999, China in 2002) to secure its support for the resolution, in the expectation that other WHO Member States would follow that country's lead.
- He made strategic concessions on secondary issues where the US government had a policy preference in order to achieve the primary objective of retaining the variola virus stocks. Issues on which the United States was prepared to compromise included the length of the authorised smallpox research programme, the composition of the WHO variola advisory committee, and Taiwan's bid for observer status in the organization.

Although the smallpox destruction debate continues in the policy forums of the WHO, rapid advances in biotechnology are changing the context for decision-making.[33] Until recently, all discussions of eliminating the authorised stocks of variola virus were predicated on the belief that destruction would be final and irrevocable, yet that assumption may not be valid much longer. The development in the early 1980s of automated DNA synthesizers capable of producing customised strands of genetic material from off-the-shelf chemicals, and the steady refinement of this technology, have made it possible to synthesise infectious viral genomes in the laboratory — a feat that has already been accomplished for the polio, influenza, and SARS viruses. As DNA synthesis technology continues to advance, it will soon be possible for scientists to re-create by artificial means any virus whose genetic sequence is known, including variola virus. Although published WHO guidelines prohibit any laboratory outside the two authorised repositories from possessing segments of variola virus DNA that represent more than 20 per cent of the viral genome, or individual fragments more than 500 base pairs long, the WHO has no way of enforcing these rules.[34] Thus, when it becomes possible for a technically proficient laboratory to synthesise variola virus from scratch, the risk of hostile use will expand beyond any illicit stocks of the virus that may still exist to include an artificially created weapon.

Advocates of continued research with live variola virus contend that the impending capability to synthesise the virus by artificial means renders the destruction debate effectively moot. Even if all known stocks of variola virus had been destroyed in 1993 as initially planned, the availability in public databases of complete DNA sequences for several strains has made it possible to reconstitute the virus by chemical synthesis at some point in the future.[35] Retentionists also warn that within a decade, the technologies, skills, and know-how needed to synthesise variola virus from scratch may proliferate widely, making the need for effective medical countermeasures against smallpox bioterrorism more urgent than ever. Destructionists counter that the risk of viral synthesis makes it all the more important to prohibit the possession of variola virus in any form, either natural or artificial. In the destructionists' view, eliminating the WHO-authorised stocks would make it possible to brand any possession, synthesis, or hostile use of the virus as a crime against humanity, punishable with the most severe economic, political, and military sanctions. In contrast, allowing the two WHO-authorised repositories to continue doing research with live variola virus would seriously weaken the normative power of any attempt to ban its re-creation by artificial means.[36]

Some policy analysts have advocated a return to the universal smallpox vaccination of civilian populations as a way to foil a potential terrorist attack with the virus, thereby making it possible to destroy the authorised stocks without undue risk. (The smallpox vaccine is based on a different virus called vaccinia, a close but relatively benign relative of variola virus that protects against the much more lethal disease.) The proposal for universal vaccination is unrealistic, however, because the standard smallpox vaccine is medically contraindicated for individuals suffering from eczema, impaired immune function or HIV infection, in whom it can cause severe and even life-threatening complications. In addition, the smallpox vaccine is associated with a small but significant risk of adverse side effects in otherwise healthy people, including one or two deaths per million.[37] When smallpox was still endemic in large regions of the world, the danger of contracting the disease far outweighed the risks of vaccination, but that situation no longer applies.

Indeed, the US government's attempt to vaccinate health workers against smallpox in 2003 provides a cautionary tale. Responding to heightened fears of bioterrorism in the months preceding the US-led invasion of Iraq, the George W. Bush administration launched a three-stage smallpox vaccination campaign in December 2002. Stage 1 involved the voluntary vaccination of some 500,000 first-line health workers over a 30-day period, with the goal of creating Smallpox Response Teams around the country that would administer the vaccine in the event of a bioterrorist attack. Stage 2 called for a major expansion of the vaccination programme to 10 million first-responders, while Stage 3 involved the vaccination of members of the public upon request.[38] Nevertheless, the programme ended only six months into the first stage after fewer than 40,000 health workers had been vaccinated. The reasons why the campaign fell far short of its goals included the US government's failure to persuade health workers of the need for smallpox vaccination, the lack of a federal compensation plan in the event of adverse side effects, and the fact that 21 healthy people who were vaccinated against smallpox developed unexpected cardiac complications. After this troubling side effect appeared, a federal body called the Advisory Committee on Immunization Practices (ACIP) recommended against expanding the vaccination programme to additional health workers.[39]

Conclusion

Over the past three decades, the WHO debate over destruction of the variola virus stocks has dragged on with no obvious solution. The intractability of this issue can be attributed to four main factors. First, the smallpox question lies at the nexus of public health and international security, with implications for critical national interests. Second, the circumstantial evidence for the existence of undeclared stocks of variola virus is based on sensitive US intelligence sources and methods and thus cannot be widely shared with WHO Member States. Third, the smallpox negotiations involve atypical actors such as officials from ministries of defence, who have a different set of priorities and preoccupations than their counterparts in the field of international health. Fourth, the advocates and opponents of variola virus destruction are equally passionate and articulate, but their positions reflect fundamentally incompatible world views and risk perceptions. Given these complicating factors, finding a negotiating formula that can satisfy all parties has been a tall order.

In considering the fate of the variola virus stocks, a key challenge for US policy-makers will be to determine what additional medical defences against smallpox are truly essential. Although no antiviral drugs have yet been licensed to treat the disease, the United States already possesses some 300 million doses of the standard smallpox vaccine, or enough to protect all of its citizens. (In 2010, the US government supplemented this stockpile with 20 million doses of an attenuated smallpox vaccine called Modified Vaccinia Ankara, which is safer to use in individuals for whom the standard vaccine is contraindicated.[40]) Given these facts, US officials will have to weigh the extremely low probability of a deliberate attack with variola virus against the potentially catastrophic consequences, assess the feasibility of developing a realistic animal model of smallpox that can support the FDA drug-approval process, and weigh the benefits of continued research with the live virus against the safety, security, and political risks.[41] Another consideration is that in the unlikely event that the United States and Russia agree to eliminate their respective repositories, verifying the total destruction of variola virus stocks in each country will be an exceedingly difficult task.

References

1. Portions of this chapter are drawn from two of the author's previous works: Tucker JB. (2002) *Scourge: The Once and Future Threat of Smallpox*. Grove Press, New York; and Tucker JB (2006). Preventing the misuse of biology: lessons from the oversight of smallpox virus research. *International Security* 31(2): 116–150.
2. Hopkins D. (2002) *The Greatest Killer: Smallpox in History*. University of Chicago Press, Chicago.
3. For a first-person history of the smallpox eradication campaign, see Henderson DA. (2009) *Smallpox: The Death of a Disease*. Prometheus Books. Amherst, NY.
4. Fenner F, *et al.* (1988) *Smallpox and Its Eradication*. World Health Organisation, Geneva, p.. 1340.

5. World Health Organisation, Advisory Committee on Variola Virus Research (2008). Report of the ninth meeting, Geneva, Switzerland, 29–30 November 2007, WHO/HSE/EPR/2008.1, p. 2; World Health Organisation, Advisory Committee on Variola Virus Research (2009). Report of the tenth meeting, Geneva, Switzerland, 19–20 November 2008, WHO/HSE/EPR/2008.9, p. 1.

6. Alibek K, Handelman S. (1999) *Biohazard: The Chilling True Story of the Largest Biological Weapons Program in the World.* Random House, New York, pp. 107–122.

7. Gellman B. (2002) 4 nations thought to possess smallpox: Iraq, N. Korea named, two officials say. *Washington Post.* November 5, p. A1.

8. Henderson DA, Inglesby TV, Bartlett JG, *et al.* (1999) for the Working Group on Civilian Biodefense. Smallpox as a biological weapon. *JAMA* 281 (22): 2127–2137.

9. Institute of Medicine of the US National Academies (1999). *Assessment of Future Scientific Needs for Live Smallpox Virus.* National Academies Press, Washington, DC.

10. Miller J. (1999) Panel says smallpox stocks may be useful. *New York Times.* March 16, p. A8.

11. Hammond E for the Third World Network (2010) Update on smallpox (variola) virus destruction. *Briefing Paper No. 1,* 63rd World Health Assembly, 17–21 May 2010, Geneva, Switzerland, pp. 8–12.

12. The White House, Office of the Press Secretary (1999) White House statement on destruction of stocks of smallpox virus. April 22.

13. Council for Responsible Genetics (2004). Plan to engineer smallpox virus causes alarm [press release]. November 12, http://www.councilforresponsiblegenetics.org/ViewPage.aspx?pageId=145.

14. World Health Organisation (1999) Smallpox eradication: destruction of variola virus stocks. A52.A/Conference Paper No. 1, May 20.

15. Altman LK. (1999) Killer smallpox gets a new lease on life. *New York Times.* May 25, p. D3.

16. World Health Organisation (2002) Smallpox eradication: destruction of variola virus stocks. *Weekly Epidemiol Rec* 77 (5): 34–38.

17. World Health Organisation, Information Office (2001) Statement to the press by the Director-General of the World Health Organisation, Dr. Gro Harlem Brundtland. Statement WHO/16, October 2.

18. Sharma R. (2002) WHO dissenter warns against plans to retain smallpox virus. *Brit Med J* 324: 59.

19. Stone R. (2002) Smallpox: WHO puts off destruction of U.S., Russian caches. *Science* 295 (Jan 25): 598–599.

20. World Health Organisation (2002) Smallpox eradication: destruction of variola virus stocks. A55/21.

21. Bernard K. (2010) Personal communication to author, May 17.

22. World Health Organisation (2002) Smallpox eradication: destruction of variola virus stocks. WHA55.15.

23. Fowler J. (2002) World Health Organization reverses order to destroy smallpox stocks. Assoc Press, May 18.

24. Jordan R and Hruby D. (2006) Smallpox antiviral drug development: satisfying the animal efficacy rule. *Expert Rev Anti Infect Ther* 4 (2): 277–289.

25. Hammond E for the Third World Network (2010) Update on smallpox (variola) virus destruction, 63rd World Health Assembly, 17–21 May 2010, Geneva, Switzerland, pp. 6–7.

26. World Health Organisation (2006) Smallpox eradication: destruction of variola virus stocks. A59/10, p. 4.

27. *Ibid.*, pp. 4–7.

28. Hammond E for the Sunshine Project (2006) Smallpox update: WHA delays decision on smallpox virus stocks. E-mail listserv report from Geneva, May 30.

29. *Ibid.*

30. Government of South Africa (2006) Intervention on smallpox by the Minister of Health at the closing plenary of the 59th World Health Assembly, May 27.

31. World Health Organisation (2007) Smallpox eradication: destruction of variola virus stocks. WHA60.1, p. 2.

32. Henderson DA. (2009) *Smallpox*, p. 76.

33. McFadden G. (2004) Smallpox: an ancient disease enters the modern era of virogenomics. *Proc Nat Acad Sci USA* 101 (42): 14995.

34. World Health Organisation WHO (2008) recommendations concerning the distribution, handling and synthesis of variola virus DNA, May 2008. *Weekly Epidemiol Rec* 83 (44): 393–395.

35. In addition to various technical hurdles associated with the synthesis of variola virus, it is possible that errors in the DNA sequence of variola virus,

which occurred at a rate of about one per 10,000 base pairs at the time the virus was sequenced, could significantly reduce the virulence and infectivity of the synthetic virus.

36. Hammond E for the Third World Network (2010) Update on smallpox (variola) virus destruction, p. 15.

37. Fulginiti VA, Papier A, Lane JM, Neff JM, Henderson DA. (2002) Smallpox vaccination: a review, part II: adverse events. *Clin Infect Dis* 37: 251–271.

38. U.S. Department of Health and Human Services (2002) Protecting Americans: Smallpox vaccination program, http://www.smallpox.gov/VaccinationProgram.html.

39. Roos R. (2003) ACIP: Don't broaden smallpox vaccination program now. Center for Infectious Disease Research and Policy (CIDRAP), University of Minnesota, June 20, http://www.cidrap.umn.edu/cidrap/content/bt/smallpox/news/june2003smallpox.html.

40. Purt D. (2010) Bavarian Nordic begins Invamune deliveries. Vaccine News Daily.com, May 18, http://vaccinenewsdaily.com/news/213090-bavarian-nordic-begins-imvamune-deliveries.

41. A possible negotiating formula for breaking the deadlock over destruction of the variola virus stocks is proposed in Tucker JB (2009). The smallpox destruction debate: could a grand bargain settle the issue? *Arms Control Today* 39 (2): 6–15, http://www.armscontrol.org/act/2009_03/tucker.

12

Negotiating in the World Health Organization: The Intergovernmental Working Group on Intellectual Property, Innovation, and Public Health

Howard A. Zucker[i]

Abstract

Global health diplomacy is about much more than public health. This chapter describes the complex and dynamic process surrounding the contentious debates about the intellectual property rights of pharmaceuticals within the World Health Organization as a way to address the imbalance between demand and supply across developing and developed countries. Tracing the efforts of an intergovernmental working group and deliberations during the Executive Board and World Health Assembly over several consecutive years, the chapter highlights the challenges of responding to global health needs alongside persistent

[i] Howard Zucker, MD, JD, served as the Assistant Director-General for Health Technology and Pharmaceuticals and as Representative of the Director-General for Intellectual Property, Innovation, and Public Health at the World Health Organization from 2006–2008. He presently serves as Senior Advisor in the Division of Global Health & Human Rights at Massachusetts General Hospital in Boston, MA, as Adjunct Professor of Law at Georgetown University and as a pediatric cardiac aneothesiologist at Albert Einstein College of Medicine in NYC.

commercial interests. Long and arduous diplomatic processes, conducted through formal and informal meetings, demonstrate the need for
multidisciplinary expertise in global health negotiations. Specialists are
invaluable in areas such as medicine, public health, international treaty
law, trade, foreign affairs, and international security.

The Problem

Pharmaceuticals are a mainstay of medical therapy in the developed and
developing world. During the past 25 years new drugs have been developed for many ailments, from cancer to heart disease, diabetes to epilepsy.
Even though new anti-retrovirals for HIV/AIDS have flooded the market-
place, there are few incentives to develop medicines for many other
illnesses that disproportionately affect developing nations. With close to 5
billion people on the planet living in developing nations, and over 40% of
them living on less than $2 per day, it does not require rocket science to
realise that inadequate access to affordable medicines can hinder or extin-
guish any chance of therapy. Though humanitarian needs in this arena
may require difficult choices to be made, it is undeniable that the cost of
bringing a product from conception to market can cost upwards of $500
million and possibly as much as $2 billion.[1]

A paradox exists in that 90% of global pharmaceutical sales occur in
the developed world yet 90% of global deaths from infectious diseases
occur in the developing world. The challenge faced by creating medicines
for diseases with, at most, limited market appeal to those who manufacture them, has drawn much attention during the past fifteen years. Given
an imbalance between supply and demand, we are left with the task of
determining what is the cause and how best to resolve it. Many public
health experts direct their attention to the issue of intellectual property
rights (IPR) as the culprit of this inequity. However, others claim that it
involves inadequate governance and poor supply chain distribution. The
on-going controversy focused attention on many international agreements
including the Declaration on the TRIPs Agreement and Public Health
(Doha Declaration),[2] where Trade-Related Aspects of Intellectual
Property Rights (TRIPs) provides measures to promote access to medicines in developing nations. Subject matter experts working within the

public policy arena from across international organisations teased through many concepts in the hopes of finding a workable solution. Such discussions centred on the work of the World Health Organization (WHO), World Trade Organization (WTO), and World Intellectual Property Organization (WIPO). The WHO's engagement in this issue of intellectual property, innovation, and public health dates back many years. Resolutions addressing drug strategy were addressed at the 49th World Health Assembly (WHA) in 1996,[3] on access to essential medicines at the 53rd WHA in 2000,[4] and on intellectual property at the 56th WHA in 2003.[5] More recently it has come to the floor of the Assembly every year from 2006 through 2010 as Resolutions 59.24,[6] 60.30,[7] 61.21,[8] and 62.16,[9] respectively. These latter four resolutions all focused on the subject of this case study.

The Local and External Players and Their Roles

In May of 2003 the Fifty-sixth World Health Assembly adopted a resolution (WHA 56.27)[10] that established the Commission on Intellectual Property Rights, Innovation and Public Health (CIPIH, hereafter referred to as "the Commission"). The resolution requested the WHO's Director-General (DG) to "establish the terms of reference for an appropriate time-limited body to collect data and proposals from the different actors involved and produce an analysis of intellectual property rights, innovation, and public health including the question of appropriate funding and incentive mechanisms for the creation of new medicines and other products against disease that disproportionately affect developing countries."

Led by Ms. Ruth Dreifuss (former President of the Swiss Confederation) the Commission's report eventually recommended 60 action items. A progress report was initially presented in May 2004 to the 57th WHA. The final document was to be presented to the 115th session of the WHO's Executive Board (EB) but ultimately this was changed to the EB's 117th session in 2006.[11] Of note, in November of 2005, the Republic of Kenya submitted a draft resolution to the WHO EB (117th Session) for the establishment of a working group to look at prioritising research and development. Within this resolution were the many issues salient to the Commission's recommendations. Their ministry also provided a document signed by 285 scientists representing over 50 countries supporting their resolution. Included in this group were five Nobel Laureates.

Given the complexity of the issue and the need for additional time prior to presentation to the EB, the WHO hosted a special session in early 2006 to discuss the Commission's report. The Commission noted that intellectual property rights provide important incentives for the development of new medicines and medical technologies. However, they added that those rights do not provide an effective incentive if the patients are poor or the population in need is small in number. All WHO Member States ultimately would welcome the Report of the Commission.

Much transpired during the first half of 2006. After the Commission's report was presented to then-Director-General Dr. J.W. Lee there was a decision to have the recommendations reviewed internally within the WHO. Needless to say, many interested stakeholders from the public and private sector were busy dissecting the Commission's report. Those with a "pony in this race" included civil society groups, trade organisations, pharmaceutical companies, academia, and non-governmental organisations, to name a few. The Commission's report grouped its recommendations into 5 categories: discovery, development, delivery, fostering innovation in developing countries, and the way forward. Only a few recommendations created serious issues of contention. Most notably was the controversial subject of intellectual property rights, and under this umbrella rested the lightening rod issues centering on the TRIPs Agreement.[12] From the rights of governments to use compulsory licensing to the recommendation that companies adopt patent and enforcement policies that facilitate greater access to medicines in developing countries, it was clear that the debate would be electric when this subject came to the floor of the WHA that year.

In the lead-up to the 59th WHA in May 2006 there was preparation for the resolution recommending the establishment of yet another working group. The Kenya resolution (WHA 59.24), which was supported by Brazil, called upon the Director-General to establish an Intergovernmental Working Group (IGWG) to develop a global strategy and plan of action in response to the Commission's report. The WHO would serve as Secretariat. In the vernacular, the Commission's report was 'out there' and it required addressing. Though the WHO has excellent convening authority, its ability to enforce amongst its Member States strong recommendations — even those that have achieved consensus — is predominantly lacking [note: the one exception is within the arena of communicable infectious diseases where the International Health Regulations carry significant weight particularly in relation to disease reporting and quarantine].

Running almost in parallel to the Commission's report issues in 2006 was another controversial subject that would ultimately collide with IPR issues in the years to come. That topic was the ownership rights of biological specimens, particularly as it relates to a mutation in the Avian Influenza H5N1 virus (bird flu). The pot was starting to boil and it was going to be difficult to keep the lid on.

As final preparations were taking place before Monday's opening session of what was to be an engaging World Health Assembly, Resolution 59.24 was reviewed one last time by the WHO leadership. After years of experience, a very competent team of international civil servants had the practice of the WHA down to a science. Dr. Bill Kean (Director, Department of Governance), Mr. Denis Aitken (Advisor to the Director-General), Ms. Marjorie Dam (Director, Staff Services and formerly Director of Governing Bodies), and Mr. Gianluca Burci (Legal Counsel) were amongst the inner circle working closely with the Director-General to iron out any kinks before the gavel went down on Monday morning signifying the commencement of activities. However, no one ever could have predicted the events that would transpire over the weekend prior to the opening session of the 59th WHA in May 2006. Whilst Ministers of Health and their teams from 193 nations converged on Geneva for the annual gathering of international leaders in public health and public policy, a tragic event was soon to unfold.

Dr. J.W. Lee, Director-General of the WHO was truly at the centre of the World Health Assembly. As Director-General, he was the main actor in this orchestrated dance of the varying interests of multiple Member States. With avian influenza creating concerns, real and perceived, across the globe, Dr. Lee was involved in high-level discussions with ministers from many nations. Dr. Lee, originally from South Korea, was a highly distinguished public health expert whose career at WHO had spanned decades. He had the balance of public health expertise with political acumen — character traits that are extremely valuable when leading the world's most recognised international health organisation. His two senior advisors, Dr. Ian Smith and Dr. Kenneth Bernard served as proverbial wingmen to the distinguished Dr. Lee, as he navigated potentially stormy skies regarding divisive issues for the Member States, amongst which included the Commission's report. On Saturday, Dr. Lee attended a meeting at the Chinese mission in Geneva. For the casual "meet and greet" small talk visit Dr. Lee was accompanied by Dr. Margaret Chan (People's Republic of China), Assistant Director-General for Communicable Diseases. During lunch Dr. Lee developed a severe headache. The Director-General walked into a private room, collapsed to the floor, lost consciousness and was rushed to the hospital. Within 48 hours the Director-General was dead from a cerebral hemorrhage. Clearly, the focus of the World Health Assembly had changed before it had even begun. A whisper that was deafening circulated about the Palais des Nations as delegations gathered about for their last sips of cappuccino before the opening session where the news of Dr. Lee's death would be officially announced — for there was no deputy and no clear line of succession should the Director-General die suddenly in office.

A slim envelope left by Dr. Lee in a secure place over a year before was opened in front of all the Assistant Director-Generals and Regional Directors as they gathered together prior to the World Health Assembly. A note written by the now deceased Director-General appointed Dr. Anders Nordstrom (Sweden), Assistant Director-General for General Management, as the Acting Director-General in the event of his incapacitation or death. His temporary appointment was upheld by the WHO Office of Legal Counsel. The WHA would continue in the shadow of Dr. Lee's unexpected death, and the issue of next steps for the Commission's report now fell upon Acting Director-General Dr. Nordstrom.

One of the first tasks at hand in responding to the Kenya/Brazil Resolution 59.24 (which was signed by the all the Member States at the WHA in May 2006 requesting a strategy and plan of action), was to identify a "home" within WHO for these efforts. In addition, Dr. Nordstrom decided to create a position entitled Representative of the Director-General for Intellectual Property, Innovation, and Public Health. An undercurrent existed as to where within the complex organisation this issue would fall and who would lead it. The Acting Director-General was considering three venues: The Department of Ethics, Trade, Human Rights and the Law led by Dr. Nico Drager (Canada), The Special Programme for Research and Training in Tropical Diseases (TDR) led by Dr. Robert Ridley (UK), and the Office of the Assistant Director-General for Health Technologies & Pharmaceuticals (HTP), led by Dr. Howard Zucker (US) (author).

The issue of intellectual property rights was closely tied to the issues of access to medicines and as such fell within the HTP cluster of WHO. The Medicines Division within the HTP cluster had a tumultuous history and was divided into 2 teams: Department of Medicines Policy and Standards (HTP/PSM) and the Department of Technical Cooperation for Essential Drugs and Traditional Medicine (HTP/TCM), with the IPR issues falling under the aegis of the latter. TCM's objectives, as stated in its mission statement was to "support Member States in country, inter-country, and regional efforts to develop, implement, and monitor the effectiveness of national medicines policies, guidelines, strategies and plans that ensure the availability, affordability, and rational use of essential medicines…" Within the TCM department, led by Precious Matsoso (South Africa), was German Velasquez (Columbia), a polarizing figure, and frequently critical of the pharmaceutical companies.[13] Concerns were also replete amongst many in the cluster, as well as other professionals at WHO about the international pharmaceutical industry. Despite strong ideological opinions of many senior WHO staff, their institutional memory of the negotiations on this issue would be quite valuable so long as fair appraisal of the issues could be guaranteed. Dr. Nordstrom decided to place the IGWG within the HTP cluster.

Acting Director-General Nordstrom then charged Dr. Zucker, Director of the HTP Cluster, with the task of leading the Intergovernmental Working Group (IGWG) process. Dr. Zucker had been chosen by Dr. Lee to serve as Assistant Director-General of the Health Technology and Pharmaceuticals cluster and assumed his duties in January 2006. A physician, attorney, and former US Deputy Assistant Secretary of Health, Dr. Zucker's career had been in academic medicine until he entered the public sector, first as a White House Fellow (non-partisan programme on leadership and public service) and then as a civil service employee in the US Department of Health & Human Services. He had no professional or personal ties to the pharmaceutical or biotechnology industries but had worked with the US Food and Drug Administration (FDA), Centers for Disease Control (CDC), National Institutes of Health (NIH), and other agencies addressing public health issues. He would take on the responsibility of addressing the Commission's report recommendation of creating a strategy and plan of action. The challenge was as much a political tour de force as a public health task.

Within weeks of this appointment, Dr. Zucker met with Dr. Nordstrom and Mr. Aitken to discuss the next steps. To address all the nuts and bolts of the Commission's report, Dr. Zucker selected and brought Dr. Elil Renganathan (Malaysia) back to Geneva from Tunisia who had over a decade's experience within WHO to serve as Executive Secretary for this project. Dr. Renganathan's expertise and experience in the arena of prevention and control of endemic diseases in developing nations would be most beneficial to the Secretariat. The timetable was tight given the requirement that an update be provided to the WHO Executive Board (EB) in January 2007.

Though work within the WHO continued to progress, the uncertainty regarding who would be the new Director-General was palpable and put against that background, the IGWG needed to be quickly convened and functioning. Complicating the issue of succession was the global panic over potential spread of avian influenza. With this as a backdrop, posturing was beginning to occur as candidate names surfaced to replace Dr. Lee. The selection of a Director-General is through an election with each Member State casting one vote. The process has many of the nuances that go along with any campaign.

Despite external and internal focus on who will be elected as the next DG there was a growing unease about what would transpire at the first IGWG, with IPR issues being of most concern. Scheduling the first meeting required that several items jelled: lack of conflict between other long-scheduled meetings, an appropriate sized venue, enough time to prepare and distribute documents, follow-up time to synthesise all the information in time for the Executive Board meeting, absence of any overlapping religious holidays (primarily Christian, Jewish, and Muslim), and availability of the necessary interested attendees. Many without UN experience are surprised that issues such as these have significant impact on the work of these organisations. Luckily, December 4–8, 2006 was a clear window and met all the criteria. The wheels were in motion and the IGWG car was accelerating quickly.

Many stakeholders were bantering about the logistics to the meeting, from who would be invited, what would be the agenda, to who would chair the meeting. The issue of openness regarding the process was most important. To guarantee that as broad a net as possible for collecting information would be cast, the Secretariat opened a public hearing from November 1–15, 2006 to allow for as much input as achievable in the short time period.[14] Dozens of submissions were received from a vast array of interested parties: civil society, academia, governments, the pharmaceutical industry, and non-governmental organisations.[15]

It was clear that the IGWG negotiations would be tedious but the objective was to try to stay focused on the issues. To achieve this objective a Bureau was created which served as the representative governing body — a Board of Directors as it were — of the Member States to manage the process. Much discussion centred on who should chair the first IGWG with several candidate names proposed including representatives from the Ministries of Health of Australia, Canada, India, Kenya, and Switzerland. Dr. Peter Oldham (Canada) was elected as Chair of the IGWG; a noble task. The Vice Chairs included Mr. B. Wijnberg (Netherlands), Dr. H. Gashut (Libyan Arab Jamahiriya), Dr. A.E.O. Ogwell (Kenya), Mr. J. Ratnam (Singapore), and Mr. N. Dayal (India).

Challenges Faced and The Outcomes

The initial IGWG was a very complicated meeting. Though it was supposed to be technical in nature, it was fraught with political overtones that danced around the room without any particular style or grace. Among the many controversial issues was the role of industry in the sphere of public health. To provide some context to this subject was the fact that the Doha Declaration extended the transition period for least-developed nations for implementation of the TRIPs obligations from 2006 to 2016.[16] It related to the issues of enforcing patents and data protection for pharmaceutical products. The desire of many public health advocates and least-developed nations to have the ability to utilise the compulsory licensing or parallel importation components of TRIPs for as long as possible had major impact on the IPR issues that were apt to be debated at the IGWG.

Many organisations wanted a seat at the "table" for this discussion. From civil society groups to non-governmental organisations to trade associations, this was a meeting at which all stakeholders wanted to be present — if not to be heard then at least to be seen. It fell upon Dr. Zucker and his team to decide who else should be invited outside of Member States and those groups with formal WHO relationships allowing attendance already. Discussions within the Director-General's office centred on achieving a balance of interests between the two opposing viewpoints on how best to improve access to medicines in the developing world as well as increase research and development in the area of neglected diseases. The two sides of the coin were a) research and development for neglected diseases cannot progress without the incentives provided by patent protection and b) patents are a barrier to the access to affordable medicines.

The Commission's report touched upon so many topics that the field of talented individuals was quite broad. It was necessary that experts from numerous fields attend this meeting given the IGWG had much to accomplish and political generalities raised by the ministerial representatives often are assisted by interpretations of technical staff. Even the presumably simple task of noting who would be considered an "expert" raised eyebrows. With time constraints present, the WHO, serving as the Secretariat, decided that a broad representation was necessary and several experts were identified, although some had a political or legal bent, and others a technical one. They included: Mr. Dick Wilder (former Director of the Global Intellectual Property Issues Division at WIPO), Mr. Erik Iverson (Associate General Counsel for the Global Health Program at The Bill and Melinda Gates Foundation), Ms. Lila Feisse (Managing Director for Intellectual Property, Biotechnology Industry Organization), Dr. Bernard Pecoul (Executive Director, Drugs for Neglected Diseases [DNDi]), Mrs. Nicoletta Dentico (Policy and Advocacy Advisor, DNDi), Dr. Tido von Schoen-Angerer (Director, Campaign for Access to Essential Medicines, Medecins Sans Frontieres [MSF]), Ms. Ellen 't Hoen (Policy and Advocacy Director, MSF), Ms Benedicte Callan (Head of the Biotechnology Unit, Organization of Economic Cooperation and

Development [OECD]), and Ms Christina Sampogna (Biotechnology Division, OECD).

Despite this diverse group of exceptionally talented professionals, as well as the participation of senior leadership from WIPO, WTO, and UNICEF, there still were rumblings that the selection of experts was biased. Some criticised the lack of geographical balance and others questioned whether civil society and patient advocacy groups were consulted. For those critical of the IGWG, there was always a way to question the integrity of the team's work. By claiming bias it would raise doubt on the validity of the process. For those who were involved in the IGWG planning, the answer was simply to not bias the group in any way so far as possible, and then develop thick skin and recognise that everything was done honestly and with the best process. Mr. Aitken, a veteran of international negotiations, kept a calm sense about the disagreements, doing his best to balance all concerns, and quietly commented, "working groups always start out this way. We need to just keep our eye on the end product." His soothing words and all-knowing smile worked wonders.

The IGWG (December 2006)

The week long session opened with introductory remarks by Acting Director-General Anders Nordstrom, followed by an encapsulated summary presented by Dr. Zucker of the work performed to date by the WHO as it related to the sixty Commission's recommendations delineated in the five categories. Though some delegates complained that developing nations were not adequately represented amidst the 100 countries present, many Member States - both from developing and developed countries —spoke strongly on behalf of the poorest nations. Mr. Aitken, Dr. Renganathan, and Dr. Zucker handled on-going concerns regarding this issue, all trying to re-assure Member States that all points of view and WHO regions were fairly represented.

Dr. Renganathan had been in frequent conversations with the experts and interested parties in the lead-up to the IGWG and spent time with them prior to the opening session. The purpose of these discussions was to be sure that the brewing controversies about who was chosen for these roles were not creating "hard feelings" amongst them. Word circulated back to the Chair that the initial dissatisfaction was mostly mitigated. However, the real issue brewing was that of patents, and IPR would soon be the focus — and the nemesis of final consensus.

On the podium were the Bureau members (led by Mr. Peter Oldham), Mr. Denis Aitken, Dr. Zucker, Dr. Renganathan, Mr. Steve Solomon (Deputy Principal Legal Officer, WHO), Dr. Robert Ridley (from TDR), and Ms. Precious Matsoso and Dr. German Velasquez (from HTP). The negotiations began with a discussion on the best way forward on implementing the Commission's recommendations.

The voices of Member States echoed across the amphitheatre at the conference centre in Geneva. From the outset there was dispute over the six "big category" items presented to the representatives at the meeting (within the overarching six categories were the 60 recommendations). Negotiating this issue was a harbinger of things to come. Representatives from Brazil and Thailand advocated for removing two issues, "Application and Management of Intellectual Property," and "Transfer of Technology," from the original set of elements and making them separate topics for discussion. After much negotiation, it was agreed upon by the majority that these two subjects merited their own headings. The diplomatic negotiating process seemed as important as the substance.

It became clear that the technical issue of 'evergreening' (multiple patents on a single product) and access to medicines was sure to take centre stage when the IPR item was brought to the floor. How could it not? Negotiations on this issue had played out in years past in many other venues. TRIPs allows for the use of compulsory licensing for export purposes to countries without their own production capabilities for relevant medicines. With some claiming that this would enhance competition and reduce prices, others opposed this reasoning saying that IPR acted as an incentive for research and development of pharmaceutical and vaccine products, even those which are primarily intended for use in the developing world.

Despite the undercurrent of the controversial issues, there was a general agreement that the group was gathered in Geneva to try to do its best to come up with a workable plan for the Commission's recommendations. The distinguished representatives brought to the floor the issue of how the use of public-private partnerships could work towards implementing the

Commission's recommendations. Others raised the subject of how inadequate health systems contribute to the public health troubles in developing nations. No negotiation on innovation and public health would be complete without voicing one key topic: access to medicines and pricing regimes. This key topic was woven like a thread (although some Member States and interested parties would say — threat) into the fabric of the IGWG debate.

Controversy on how to tackle the elements consumed the Member States and was cast upon the Bureau Chair to help navigate. Mr. Oldham graciously received the suggestions of the delegates but also turned to the wisdom of Mr. Aitken for guidance. Denis Aitken, the consummate international public servant, could draw from his decades of experience to sail through any controversial issue. His toolbox of ideas of how to overcome obstacles, stalemates, and even difficulties with representatives from countries near and far was invaluable in the negotiating process. Moreover, his frighteningly accurate memory for historical events was most helpful. As the Member States spoke, the Bureau chair officiated, and the Secretariat listened, a plan was crystallizing during the course of the first few days. All believed that an outline regarding the strategic directions was necessary before a work plan was implemented. It was becoming evident that the first session of the IGWG would end with a framework of how to move forward. However, the specific details of the elements would not be tackled at this time. The IGWG international negotiations were living up to the standard United Nations process of a slow, steady, inclusive discussion with the inevitable conclusion that a future meeting will be needed to finish the work.

Eight elements for further work were identified: a) prioritising research and development (R&D) needs, b) promoting research and development, c) building innovative capacity, d) transfer of technology, e) management of intellectual property, f) ensuring sustainable financing mechanisms, g) improving access and delivery, and h) establishing monitoring and reporting systems.[17]

Though debate remained professional, it was clear that ideological lines had been drawn. No one doubted the need to prioritise R&D within government budgets as well as promoting such research, nor was there great disagreement in the areas of fostering innovation, providing the necessary technology transfer, or availing Member States of proper data-bases for monitoring and evaluation. These topics were outlined nicely and moved forward without much inertia. The challenge centred on the issue of patents and financing schemes. At times, the Secretariat and Bureau Chair commented that the IGWG was not the forum to re-open the debate of the TRIPs Agreement that had already concluded years before. During the first few days of the IGWG, TRIPs was the elephant in the middle of the room. The Doha Declaration from 2001 stated "the TRIPS Agreement does not and should not prevent members from taking meas-ures to protect public health."[18] It went on to say that the agreement should be interpreted and implemented in a fashion to protect public health and "promote access to medicines for all" referring back to the Ministerial Declaration.[19] Large, sucking up the oxygen, and with a great memory for past events, the "TRIPs Elephant" was hard to miss, even for those who tried to ignore it.

Ultimately, as the delineation of the elements reached number 5, intel-lectual property rights, the negotiators started to discuss what role WHO should play in this regard. The United States believed that IPR did not fall within the purview of the WHO, whilst others believed that the relation-ship between trade, health, and intellectual property was an important link for public health in developing nations. Though everyone claimed that there was a need to strike a balance with regard to IPR, the interests of the pharmaceutical trade organisations, particularly IFPMA (International Federation of Pharmaceutical Manufacturers Association), were diametri-cally opposite to the views of civil society groups, including the most outspoken of them, Knowledge Ecology International.

Though the WTO and WIPO were represented at the meeting, their voices were somewhat silent. In a moment of recess, Dr. Zucker asked their representatives whether they would like to have the floor. In their comments it was their view that the issues being raised had already been debated and agreed upon in resolutions, including the Doha Declaration and other Ministerial meetings in years past in their own agencies and fora. In fact, WHO had been working with WTO to develop a monitoring and reporting mechanism on the subject of availability of medicines for diseases that primarily affect the developing world. If there was one major advantage of the IGWG negotiation process it was the opportunity to bring all of the overlapping issues to the floor during one meeting. Sometimes debate needs to take place to avoid growing hostility about conflicting viewpoints.

After delegates of many Member States expressed their views, it seemed that the Commission's recommendations were coming down to ideological discussions on access to medicines in the developing world. Similarly, disagreements on financing mechanisms occurred. One organisation vehemently advocated for a prize mechanism awarded to the team that developed applicable medicines/vaccines for specific neglected diseases.[20] Another proposed the use of advanced market commitments.[21] Still another delegation questioned the need for a funding mechanism for neglected diseases given the presence of the Special Program for Research and Training in Tropical Diseases. Others suggested that the WHO look to other multilateral programs as models to use for addressing some of the Commission's recommendations. Examples cited included UNITAID (an international facility focused on the purchase of drugs against HIV/AIDS, Malaria, and Tuberculosis) and the International Finance Facility for Immunization (IFFIm) (a financing mechanism for vaccines through the issuing of bonds in the capital markets) as models for implementation of the Commission's recommendations.

At times even the greatest amount of tension was mixed with a sardonic levity. The delegate from Thailand said that he "might just be a small sparrow, but he was not afraid of the big eagle." Clearly, the eagle being a symbol of America, was a reference to the United States' position on intellectual property rights. Negotiations were occasionally cagey, mixing global public good, with financial self-interest. Some noted that that R&D fostered new drugs for neglected diseases. Others suggested that "enhanc[ing] access to the treatments [for] developing countries [occurs] through the transfer of generic drugs between developing countries [which] speeds up delivery of new technologies and medicines."[22]

Controversy centred on capacity building at the local level. No subject within the realm of IPR was intellectually far from Paragraph 7 of the Doha Declaration which stated that effective incentives should be in place in developed nations in order to encourage transfer of health technologies and pharmaceuticals to least-developed countries.[23] The "two sides of the aisle" had strong viewpoints — a) let countries decide for themselves about the use of TRIPs flexibilities versus b) Doha Declaration should be incorporated into all national legislation. It became evident that IPR issues would be tabled for further work at a later date.

Though seasoned veterans of international organisations anticipated this outcome, it was disappointing to some members of the Secretariat who naively believed that the week would conclude with actionable items — especially on IPR. But in the repeated words of all Director-Generals, the WHO is a Member State-driven organisation — Member States make policy at their governing bodies, the Secretariat then implements it.

The week of negotiations concluded with the ubiquitous smiles across the room, the congratulatory handshakes, and the celebratory reception, only to realise that the tough issues had been circumnavigated rather than tackled. In the Yoda-esque words of the wise Mr. Aitken, "great start, well done." But it was only the beginning. A report of the first session was provided to Member States.[24] A follow-up IGWG, quickly being coined IGWG2, was already being discussed. However, much was left to happen prior to that time. The WHO Executive Board was around the corner and the Secretariat needed to prepare a summary of the events that had transpired during IGWG1. After an end of the year holiday break the team re-assembled.

After IGWG1 and the WHO Executive Board meeting (January 2007)

The most visible change at WHO was that the year 2007 began with Dr. Margaret Chan assuming the role of the 7th Director-General, elected on November 9, 2006. She brought with her expertise in communicable diseases that was definitely a plus given H5N1 (avian influenza) was foremost on the minds of public health experts. The scientific issues involving risk of mutation and possible human-to-human transmission of H5N1 was hardly the only plague that this pathogen was playing on people's time, energy, and emotions. Indonesian officials were taking a hard stance on the sharing of influenza virus in the lead-up to a possible pandemic. They withheld the sharing of the H5N1 virus with the WHO and were challenging the WHO, claiming inequities within the system regarding influenza surveillance, management, and equity of access to vaccines and drugs. In essence, Indonesia wanted guarantees that their citizens would receive vaccinations if there were a mutant strain with high human fatality rates, isolated in their nation and where vaccines were developed by another country using their virus strain.

The subject of intellectual property rights of biological specimens opened a pandora's box of legal, public health, and political questions.[25] The IGWG issues were no longer just about pharmaceuticals for neglected tropical diseases. The IGWG was enveloping a greater issue. In fact, discussions within the Director-General's office focused on whether to tie the IPR issues of H5N1 into the IGWG or to leave the two separate. The workload of each of these subjects was so expansive that it seemed reasonable to continue on as separate teams but with frequent dialogue between the two. Moreover, these topics had so many politically explosive components to them that the merging of the two could set off a firestorm that would not be squelched even by the coolest of words from unbiased Member States.

To alleviate some of the on-going IGWG chatter centred on the question of whether all views on the Commission's issues received equitable hearing, the Secretariat decided to send two invitational circular letters to all Member States. These letters, dated January 12th and February 15th, 2007 asked for input into the IGWG strategy and plan of action. In response, the Secretariat received 22 submissions including one from the Presidency of the European Union on behalf of its 27 Member States, one from a group of Southeast Asian nations, and one from Kenya on behalf of Member States of the African Region. All the submissions were the work of talented individuals who were passionate about the issues central to the IGWG deliberations.

The request for a report on the IGWG was on the agenda for the January 22–30, 2007 World Health Organization Executive Board (EB) meeting.[26] The EB is comprised of 34 Member States that rotate off every three years and there was much interest in the IGWG at this year's gathering. Tensions were high as the IGWG concerned a controversial group of issues and many developing nations believed that their hopes of using the IGWG to promote research and development of new products to use for neglected diseases had not become realised in the past. Kenya and Switzerland tabled a draft resolution at the EB regarding early implementation of some of the

Commission's recommendations. The Brazilian delegate turned to Dr. Zucker and said that he believed the whole IGWG was "ridiculous." The genesis of this comment seemed to be that the IGWG was not focusing on the TRIPs issues and that the Secretariat should channel the attention towards that arena. Troubling to the Secretariat was the fact that it was believed that a member of the WHO had prompted the Brazilian delegate to speak those words.

Dr. Zucker provided the EB members a detailed summary of what transpired as well as a step-by-step process for the coming year. Many questions were raised by Member States at the EB on how best to move forward on the IGWG. Kenya, Brazil, Thailand, and the United States expressed disappointment with the IGWG progress and wanted a second meeting before the World Health Assembly in May 2008.

In response to their concerns, it was proposed that there would be a) Regional Consultations with identified experts, b) a second online "public hearing," and c) planning discussions during WHO Regional Meetings prior to IGWG2. In addition, background documents would be provided to all Member States in the months leading up to the next meeting. It seemed that the science and public health of these negotiations were more and more taking a backseat to the politics and optics of the issue. Many delegates at the EB believed that the WHO should be more focused on the process of the IGWG rather than the content. The procedural maturations of an international body were clearly consuming the IGWG and IGWG2. This was truly a paradox because there were Member States that wanted the WHO to weigh in if it would be consistent with their views. If not, then they wanted the WHO to just focus on the process. The fact remained that WHO is a Member State-driven organization, and the Secretariat could only move with clear directions from the Members — something not yet forthcoming.

The 60th World Health Assembly (May 2007)

The work of the Secretariat continued forward in preparation for the 60th World Health Assembly. Included in the efforts was an update report provided to the Member States six weeks prior to the WHA. Resolution 59.24 (from the 2006 WHA) was considered by all regional committees and some nations actually had their own IGWG regional discussions. Though the focus appeared to be on the substantive issues centred on the Commission's recommendations, there was much ideological chatter that filled the hallways in the lead-up to the 60th World Health Assembly.

It hardly seemed like a year had passed since the last World Health Assembly but the annual gathering of delegates was once again happening in Geneva. Dr. Chan, now at the helm of the organization, knew that two of the most difficult issues were: a) the Intergovernmental Meeting on Pandemic Influenza, and b) the Intergovernmental Working Group on Innovation, Public Health and Intellectual Property.

Unbeknownst to many, including the author, a plan was being conceived to disrupt the IGWG process. For some time, word had been circulating about in the rumour mill that there was going to be a new resolution before the Assembly on the issue of the IPR and public health, emphasising one side of the argument. The initial version of this rumoured resolution stated that there should be "unobstructed implementation" of the flexibilities found in the WTO Agreement on Trade-Related Aspects of Intellectual Property Rights as well as references to the use of patent pools. Rumbling also was heard that there was pressure being placed upon the Director-General by some countries to avoid a health vs. trade confrontation at the WHA that she would need to mention TRIPs and "health as a right" in her opening remarks.

Though the Director-General mentioned the need for "equitable access to quality, affordable medicines, and the long-term need to stimulate innovation"[27] she did not raise the subject of TRIPs that Monday morning in her opening speech to the WHA. Soon after, the delegate from Brazil introduced a resolution, entitled "Public Health, Innovation, and Intellectual Property." Sixty point thirty (Resolution 60.30)[28] as it was known, was introduced more for the political dialectic than for public health. It was primarily about the issue of TRIPs and would generate much debate, side meetings, private conferences, distractions, and discontent for the coming two weeks of the WHA.

By day two Mr. Suwit Wibulpolprasert, Thailand's Senior Advisor on Health Economics in the Ministry of Public Health, took the floor to criticise the IGWG stating, "in all my years I have not seen worse leadership from the Secretariat." It was clearly a personal attack. In the early morning meetings with the Assistant Director Generals (ADGs) and Regional Directors, the comment of the Thailand delegate was addressed. The Director-General said, "the Member State made unfounded comments and attacked personal integrity."[29] That being said, the Secretariat still needed to deal with the challenges confronted regarding any legitimate issues raised by Member States. Whilst this was playing out there was further debate over Resolution 60.30. In a separate committee, efforts were being made to work on the resolution but the United States delegation objected to many of the statements asking that they be bracketed (left for further negotiation). Moreover, the Brazilian delegation was meeting with Ministers from the African nations pushing for their support of 60.30. Interestingly however, word circulated back to the Secretariat that several Ministers from Africa questioned the need for 60.30 when Resolution 59.24 already existed.

By the fourth day of the WHA, the IGWG issue had become a subject of much discussion. As is common practice, when a subject requires discussion of a more in-depth nature, a technical briefing is scheduled during the WHA. The IGWG process had many technical "moving parts" to it and therefore such a briefing was scheduled for lunchtime. Dr. Zucker chaired the panel, and in collaboration with members of the Bureau, addressed questions regarding the process to date. The Chair and Vice-chairs of the Bureau presented up-to-date information on the IGWG process as it related to their specific regions. Mr. Santiago Alcazar, International Health Advisor Ministry of Health, Brazil, who introduced 60.30, was critical of the IGWG as was Mr. Suwit Wibulpolprasert from Thailand. The issue really focused on element number 5 of the Plan of Action — intellectual property rights as it pertains to pharmaceuticals.

Though there had been verbal criticisms which were simply personal in nature, there was one appropriate criticism which centred on the lack of documents available from the Secretariat for review prior to the IGWG negotiation. This was clearly a gaffe on the part of the WHO in not having provided enough information to the delegations. After much criticism from Brazil, Thailand, Kenya, and Indonesia as well as from non-governmental organisations, the United States stated that "the IGWG is us, the Member States, so don't criticize the Secretariat."[30] That being said, the WHO Secretariat had dropped the ball on being sure that all the technical material was available to the Member States. Needless to say, individuals representing interested parties from NGOs to industry that attended the WHA were quick to present their viewpoints about the IGWG issues.

There was however, some irony here. The resolution introduced by Brazil, 60.30, required negotiation. The United States delegation objected to major components of 60.30, and that itself created stalemates in reaching consensus on the wording of the resolution. At one point during an evening drafting group session (chaired by the delegate from Namibia), the US left the negotiation table altogether. The result was that there could then be forward progress from all the other delegations without any one particular Member State (the US) holding up the process. Whilst there were other Member States that shared the US position and which were still at the negotiating table, it seemed that the resolution had enough fatal flaws in it to result in support by the United States.[ii]

Behind the scenes there was much discord over this IGWG issue and the Director-General held a closed-door four-hour evening meeting with all members of the Secretariat. IGWG was causing unrest and the mechanics of the process, including document availability, had become as important, if not more important, than the substance. The negotiation process on 60.30 was troubling for all. Many Member States were questioning the need for this resolution in the first place. It had reached the point where back room deals were being brokered using the controversial Resolution 60.30 as a bargaining chip. For those who had never seen this kind of activity before it was puzzling and disappointing. Clearly, the political nature of international organisations – even the technical agencies like WHO, were not immune from the hidden components of negotiations that take place on the global stage, and the unlevel playing field. Though the Director-General refused any such deals, it did send a

---

[ii] For example, WHA 60.30 3 (4) "Requests the Director General to encourage the development of proposals for health-needs driven research and development for discussion at the IGWG that includes a range of incentive mechanisms including also addressing the linkage between the cost of research and development and the price of medicines, vaccines, diagnostic kits and other health products…"

chill through those who ultimately learned about the extent of the under-current that existed. Eventually, the content of the resolution was watered down to gain the support of many Member States other than the US.

The 60.30 Resolution continued to require negotiations and the drafting groups worked late into the evenings. Finally, a document was ready to be presented. When it came to the floor for a vote, all Member States present voted in favour, except for the United States who abstained because it had not viewed as acceptable the language regarding some of the contentious issues. It passed, but the United States' abstention would surely send a cloud over future negotiations at IGWG2. The Director-General commented at the closing session of the WHA about the work of the IGWG and the need to move quickly on this issue. By the time the 60th WHA ended there were many battle scars left upon the Secretariat leading the IGWG. Despite this, there was praise for the efforts of the World Health Assembly to advance the IGWG process by MSF and the Third World Network. But much preparatory work would be necessary before negotiating IGWG2.

IGWG2 (December 2007)

A second draft document of the strategy and plan of action was circulated to the Member States on July 31, 2007.[31] It incorporated the recommendations of the Member States from earlier discussions. It crystallised the strengths noted in the earlier document and improved on the weaknesses identified through formal and informal discussions. The issues raised in the Commission's report had not been prominent on the radar screen for many Member States but the sense from all Ministries of Health was that this is a significant subject that could impact their health systems. It was hard not to hear the cacophony that was turning from a soft murmur to a loud roar as the IGWG process continued to unfold. Many civil society groups and others were vocal about their perspective on how best to improve the development of medicines. Similarly, NGOs working in the area of international trade as well as intellectual property were expressing their own views. And of course the pharmaceutical and biotechnology industries had a vested interest in the outcome of the IGWG. From their vantage point, they did not want the perception that patents were the obstacle to affordable medicines/devices to become accepted as reality.

With the WHO Annual Regional Meetings "season" in swing, it seemed reasonable to foster regional and inter-country consultations organised through the WHO regional offices.

The Secretariat expanded its action items during the summer of 2007 and strategically held meetings in all regions attended by interested parties and Member States. Dr. Zucker and/or Dr. Renganathan participated in these discussions and provided the latest framework for the strategy and plan of action that would be addressed at IGWG2. This provided all stakeholders with an opportunity to express their views, concerns, and recommendations. To assure transparency of the process and avoid any accusations of bias, all reports from the consultations were available on the web. In addition, all WHO documents, submissions from stakeholders, and background articles were also easily accessible from the WHO website. A report on the work of the Secretariat since the first IGWG was circulated to all interested parties.[32] The elements of the Commission's report were also discussed at the Regional Meetings in the late summer and early autumn of 2007. An Ottawa Americas regional IGWG took place in late October prior to IGWG2 where all elements of the plan of action were addressed.[33] In preparation for further negotiations the Secretariat held a second web-based public hearing from mid-August through the end of September in 2007. Over 70 submissions were posted from various stakeholders. Responding to the concerns of the Member States after the first IGWG, the Secretariat provided all the necessary information requested in an effort to optimise the negotiation process at IGWG2. Lessons were learned from the initial IGWG and the WHA in preparation for the next steps.

In the evening of December 4th, 2007, one night before the opening of IGWG2 the Bureau and Secretariat gathered together at the home of Peter Oldham, Chair of the Bureau to discuss the latest information about the coming week. Though there were smiles on everyone's face as a buffet dinner was served, it was clear that much was at stake. Everyone was invested in the outcome.

The opening session of IGWG2 was uneventful and quickly the decision was reached that there should be two drafting groups to dissect the document. Negotiations regarding this issue resulted in two teams, one chaired by Dr. Tangcharoensanthien (Thailand) and the other by

Dr. Dayal (India). Of note, though Mr. Suwit Wibulpolprasert, Thailand's Senior Advisor on Health Economics, had been outspoken about the IGWG process, it was Dr. Tangcharoensanthien who chaired one of the drafting groups. Both groups would work through the Strategy and Plan of Action, and then report back to the Committee of the Whole. Though much was negotiated the most controversial areas - intellectual property, access to medicines, financing schemes - were still "hot potato" items that required much more diplomacy. Areas where overarching agreement existed resulted in quick consensus. This included the aims and strategies to promote research and development with a focus on Type II (diseases in rich and poor countries but primarily in the latter) and Type III (diseases overwhelmingly in poor countries) diseases.

Though all Member States agreed upon many issues in the strategy and plan of action that was negotiated at IGWG2, there was lack of consensus on the issues of IPR. At IGWG2 the Brazilian delegate put forth another document entitled the Rio Text Group. It was a white paper created by a group of 14 Latin American countries that proposed the following: "the right to health takes precedence over commercial interests."[34] The purpose was to counter the phrase: "the objectives of public health and the interests of trade should be appropriately balanced and coordinated" which appeared in the global strategy and plan of action. Furthermore, Kenya, on behalf of the 46 Member States of the African region, clearly stated that the needs of the poor have not been met by the current systems in place and that a clear funding scheme must be implemented if one wishes to view the IGWG process as a success. By week's end it was decided that IGWG2 would need to be suspended and resumed on April 28th 2008. Though much was negotiated and many components of the document were brought to closure, there still remained the thorny issues that were present from the earliest days of the Commission's work. The decision was to provide a progress report to the EB on January 26th 2008 and hopefully a final document to the WHA in May of that same year.

The final journey

The efforts to negotiate the strategy and plan of action continued during the IGWG2 resumed session in April. Much was brought to consensus and there were only a few areas left bracketed. Needless to say, the bracketed areas (indicating that agreement had not been reached) involved the age-old issue of IPR and access to medicines. On May 3rd, 2008 IGWG2 concluded without complete resolution of all action items, however much was in fact negotiated to a consensus on the part of all Member States. The document still required further negotiation in specific areas and that would transpire during the up-coming 2008 WHA.

Finally on May 24th, 2008 Resolution 61.21 reached the floor of the World Health Assembly as the document entitled "Global strategy and plan of action on public health, innovation, and intellectual property."[35] Though the diplomatic process was long and arduous the Member States agreed to a final resolution. However, in examining all the drafts it became clear that all the truly controversial issues regarding IPR and access to medicines had either been deleted or tempered down in the final document.

Lessons to be Learned

There were many important lessons that were learned from the IGWG process. As has been said many times, creativity is a messy process. An international negotiation is surely creative in all efforts to reach consensus. Certain key lessons were learned and are worth highlighting:

1) When working on controversial technical issues have a team of experts that has an in-depth knowledge about previously negotiated documents.

2) Maintain a focus on the overall objective and try not to get side-tracked by personal agendas, be it those of individuals, organisations, or governments.

3) Try to keep the real issues on the table and not temper them down simply to get consensus. If one chooses to do this then the document may end up lacking the strength needed to achieve the value-added change. It may not be easy, or even possible, to achieve but it is worth trying.

4) Public health negotiations are often about everything *but* public health. As such one must bring in the expertise from other domains

including, international treaty law, finance ministries, trade delegations, foreign affairs, international security, and any other areas that
are linked to the issues at hand.

5) As passionate as public health experts may be about the need to
improve global health, the reality is that, at the present time, public
health takes a backseat to other priorities set forth by Member States,
including commerce and finance. Hopefully, this will not always be
the case.

6) There often are big elephants in the room and sometimes it's important to just name them.

7) International agreements require significant patience. Delivering a
consensus may require negotiations that have a gestation period of 18
months; much like that of an elephant. Delivery of something really
good may be noisy but if done well it should be able to stand on its
own feet once it arrives.

Conclusion

Negotiating the contentious subject of how intellectual property and innovation are tied to public health occurred over several years. In fact, the
decision to develop the Commission started in May of 2003 and the final
agreement (with amendments) regarding both the Strategy and the Plan of
Action did not get signed until May 22nd 2009 as Resolution 62.16 at the
62nd WHA.[36]

The expenditure of time, money, human resources, emotional, and
intellectual horsepower invested in this process was tremendous. The
WHO's lack of authoritative power to assure the implementation of
the action items leads one to question the staying power of the adopted resolution. When looking at the plan of action, the time frame is 2008-2015
and the stakeholders for the majority of the elements and sub-elements are a
combination of governments, international organisations, non-governmental
organisations, and academia.

The final document is a work outcome of the diplomatic process of
reaching agreement amongst 193 Member States. However, the true test
of whether the IGWG process was a success is not in the words that are
on the paper, the resolutions in the binders, or the manuscripts on a shelf,

but in the improvement in the lives of people in the most impoverished nations on the Earth. Global health diplomacy cannot be an exercise in the artful craft of international resolutions in the absence of practical applications to the words that are inked in the six official languages of the World Health Organization. Only time will tell.

References

1. Estimating the Cost of New Drug Development: Is it Really $802 Million, Christopher Adams and Van Brantner, Health Affairs, 25 no. 2 (2006) 420–428.
2. Doha WTO Ministerial Declaration: 2001, http://www.wto.org/english/ thew-to_e/minist_e/min01_e/mindecl_e.htm.
3. World Health Assembly, Resolution 49.14 (1996).
4. World Health Assembly, Resolution 53.14 (2000).
5. World Health Assembly, Resolution 56.27 (2003).
6. World Health Assembly, Resolution 59.24 (2006).
7. World Health Assembly, Resolution 60.30 (2007).
8. World Health Assembly, Resolution 61.21 (2008).
9. World Health Assembly, Resolution 62.16 (2009).
10. World Health Assembly, Resolution 56.27 (2003).
11. Public Health: Innovation and intellectual Property Rights. Report of the Commission on Intellectual Property Rights, Innovation and Public Health, World Health Organization, c. 2006.
12. Trade-Related Aspects of Intellectual Property Rights, World Trade Organization, 1994: http://www.wto.org/english/tratop_e/trips_e/t_agm0_ e.htm.
13. Unhealthy Profits, by German Velasquez http://mondediplo.com/2003/07/ 10velasquez.
14. http://www.who.int/phi/en/.
15. Member State Submissions to the IGWG Document, A/PHI/IGWG/1/5.
16. Frequently Asked Questions about TRIPS http://www.wto.org/english/ tratop_e/trips_e/tripfq_e.htm.
17. Draft Global Strategy and Plan of Action on Public Health, Innovation and Intellectual Property — Report by the Secretariat, World Health Organization A/PHI/IGWG/1/6.

18. Declaration on the TRIPs agreement and public health. DOHA WTO Ministerial 2001 WT/MIN(01)Dec/2 Article 4.

19. Ministerial Declaration: DOHA WTO Ministerial 2001 WT/MIN/(01)Dec/1 Article 17.

20. The Role of Prizes in Stimulating R&D: Comment to WHO IGWG, Knowledge Ecology International, http://www.who.int/phi/public_hearings/second/contributions_section2/Section2_JamesLove-KEI_prizes.pdf.

21. Comments on IGWG Draft Global Strategy, International Federation of Pharmaceutical Manufacturers & Association, http://www.who.int/phi/public_hearings/second/contributions_section1/Section1_HarveyBale2_IFPMA_Full_Contribution.pdf.

22. A/PHI/IGWG/1/.

23. WTO: http://www.wto.org/english/tratop_e/trips_e/implem_para6_e.htm.

24. A/PHI/IGWG1/6.

25. Influenza Virus Samples, International Law, and Global Health Diplomacy, by David Fidler, in Emerging Infectious Diseases, Vol. 14. No. 1 January 2008, pp. 88–94.

26. World Health Organization, Executive Board, 120th Session: EB 120/INF.DOC./1 (January 2007).

27. Address to the Sixtieth World Health Assembly by Director-General Margaret Chan, May 2007: http://www.who.int/dg/speeches/2007/150507/en/index.html.

28. World Health Assembly, Resolution 60.30 (2007).

29. Personal notations from attendance at meeting.

30. Personal notation on comment by Mr. David Hohman, Health Attaché, US Mission in Geneva.

31. A/PHI/IGWG/2/2.

32. Report on Developments since the first session of the Intergovernmental Working Group on Public Health, Innovation and Intellectual Property, A/PHI/IGWG/2/3.

33. Ottawa Americas Regional IGWG: October 22-23, 2007: http://www.who.int/phi/public_hearings/second/regional_consultations/RC_AMRO.pdf.

34. International Centre for Trade and Sustainable Development — Tackling the Research Gap on Neglected Diseases, Vol. 11, No. 7 (November 2007) http://ictsd.org/i/news/bridges/3170/.

35. World Health Assembly, Resolution 61.21 (2008).

36. World Health Assembly, Resolution 62.16 (2009).

13

Taking the Fight Beyond Official Negotiations: Stakeholders Mobilise Against Counterfeit Drugs

James N. Class[i]

Abstract

Counterfeit medicines pose a serious global health risk as they can lead to treatment failure, including new resistance to medications, and even death. The problem is mired in politics, economics, trade, organised crime, public health, medicine, and power. This case study demonstrates how leadership has developed from the periphery in fighting this global health problem, rather than through the diplomatic arena. Diplomats confront counterfeit medicines through the World Health Organization, particularly through its "IMPACT" initiative, but have been slow in achieving results. Drawing on the experience of the Partnership for Safe Medicines, a federation of membership associations, results are being

[i] James N. Class, PhD, former Associate Vice President, International Affairs, Pharmaceutical Research and Manufacturers of America (PhRMA) (Washington, DC., USA) and former Executive Director (2005–2007), Partnership for Safe Medicines (PSM) (Vienna, VA, USA). This case study does not necessarily reflect the policy positions of PhRMA or the PSM. I would like to thank Bryan Liang, Tom Kubic, and Marv Shepherd for their comments.

achieved using unconventional approaches carried out by committed stakeholders from a variety of fields, such as industry, regulatory bodies, law enforcement, professional association, and patient groups.

The Problem

The counterfeiting of medicines is growing as a global problem with profound impacts on patients around the world. One can judge the importance of the problem by its prominent place of discussion at the May 2010 meeting of the World Health Assembly (WHA), the Executive Board of the World Health Organization (WHO). The WHO has worked on anti-counterfeiting issues for decades and most recently served as secretariat for the International Medical Products Anti-Counterfeiting Taskforce (IMPACT), a body formed in 2006 under the leadership of then WHO Assistant Director-General Howard Zucker, that was set up to centrally coordinate anti-counterfeiting activities worldwide. Though largely unfunded, the IMPACT has proven to be a controversial body, however, and concerns over its activities led to a resolution at the May 2010 WHA meeting that the WHA:

> "1. DECIDES to establish a time limited and results-oriented work-ing group on substandard/spurious/falsely-labelled/falsified/counterfeit medical products comprised of and open to all Member States."[1]

The working group's primary responsibility consists of producing a report by the May 2011 64th World Health Assembly. This report ostensibly will help clarify WHO's proper role in anti-counterfeiting.

A conventional way to approach the diplomatic issues surrounding anti-counterfeiting policies would entail looking at the negotiators at the WHA and those involved in or contesting the IMPACT. Such an approach, however, would overlook many important actors and activities. While analysis of the present situation might help clarify a path forward for good-faith negotiators, a more useful and practical approach involves examining the active stakeholders who are currently making a difference and carrying forward the fight against counterfeiting of medicines. These are not "diplomats" in the professional sense, but they certainly must handle complex negotiations and coordinate activities to maximise employment of scarce resources. These stakeholders are found in a variety of fields — industry, regulatory bodies, law enforcement, professional association, patient groups — and seem to be carrying on their activities and negotiations despite a lack of global leadership.

This case study analyses coordination challenges that these stakeholders face and what they are doing to succeed and demonstrate leadership. We provide a brief explanation of the problem of counterfeit drugs to identify barriers to action and highlight challenges and responses from the experience of the US-based Partnership for Safe Medicines (PSM). We then examine a number of groups that are making concrete efforts, negotiating amongst themselves, and producing results. Overall, we conclude that decentralised actors, not professional diplomats, are leading the way in negotiating common policy positions, showing commitment, and maximising the effectiveness of scarce resources.

Complexities of anti-counterfeiting policy issues

Drug counterfeiting is unquestionably an international issue, the complexity of which renders solutions extremely difficult. Even the definition of counterfeit drug lacks an international standard. Despite the diversity of definitions in national legislation, one ubiquitous feature is the concept of deception. Deception might relate to an intellectual property owner's trademark, but it is in no way limited to intellectual property rights (IPR) violations. Many IPR violations are patent-related and not related to counterfeiting at all (since no deception is involved). Or, as the International Federation of Pharmaceutical Manufacturers and Associations (IFPMA) put it, "Patents have nothing to do with counterfeiting and counterfeiting has nothing to do with patents."[2] Pharmaceutical supply chains are very complex and stretch from development of ingredients through manufacturing, distribution inside and outside of countries through clear and unclear distribution channels, to dispensing sites or pharmacies and ultimately to patients. Deception can take place at any point with the same possibility for physical harm to the patients who ultimately consume the medicine and financial harm to all the members of the supply chain and the governments who end up footing the bill through diminished tax

revenue or higher medical costs for the victimised patients. The advent of
Internet sales and virtual, unregulated distribution networks makes these
problems even more challenging. This extraordinary level of complexity
means that one stakeholder cannot be looked to for total responsibility —
or for total solutions. No technology will serve as a magic bullet; no individual corporate strategy, however robust, will solve the problem; and no
single government can wipe it out.

Hard data for the volume, financial value, and harm potential of counterfeit drugs also is woefully lacking, since one cannot measure the
deceivers' success. The best available data come from the Pharmaceutical
Security Institute (PSI), which uses an "incident" as the primary datum for
tracking. An incident can be as small as a Ziploc bag of pills ordered by a
customer off the Internet or as big as the results of a major raid involving
millions of pills and injectable medicines.[3] One might be able to rely on
law enforcement's estimation of the value of the incident, but it would be
almost impossible to quantify the harm potential of a large seizure. The
World Health Organization's 2010 counterfeit fact sheet quantified the
counterfeit drug problem only in broad terms:

> Counterfeiting is greatest in regions where regulatory and enforcement
> systems for medicines are weakest. In most industrialized countries with
> effective regulatory systems and market control (i.e. Australia, Canada,
> Japan, New Zealand, most of the European Union and the United States
> of America), incidence of counterfeit medicines is extremely low — less
> than 1% of market value according to the estimates of the countries con-
> cerned. But in many African countries, and in parts of Asia, Latin
> America, and countries in transition, a much higher percentage of the
> medicines on sale may be counterfeit.[4]

PSI data reveal other trends that should draw the attention of all health policy experts. First, counterfeit drugs are by no means limited to "lifestyle"
medicines, a derogatory term often used for medicines treating sexual dys-
function, hair loss, or weight loss. Since patients in many countries
purchase these types of medicines over the Internet to avoid interaction
with physicians, the "lifestyle drugs" can be associated with higher risk for
consumers. The fastest-increasing therapeutic categories of counterfeited

drugs from 2008–2009 were alimentary, anti-infective, and muscular-skeletal.[5] Second, incidents overall are increasing. In part, an increase in reported incidents bodes well for all stakeholders, because it means that more regulators and law enforcement officials are increasing anti-counterfeit activities with visible results. On the other hand, an expanded knowledge base indicates that the problem itself is much larger than previously had been believed. There is no sign that incidents will decrease. Analysis of cases from the US in recent years also indicates that drug counterfeiters are connected to organised crime and have used funds to support terrorist activities. Though these problems might not be "health" concerns, they are important to ordinary people, who seek security and a sense of protection. Political aspects of the problem and the players remove any negotiation from the sole domain of health professionals. Negotiations thus become even more complex and obstacle-ridden because security experts (to give one example) and health professionals do not necessarily speak the same professional language nor understand each others' perspectives, and their representatives are not necessarily experienced negotiators.

Furthermore, certain types of incidents should register significantly higher public safety concerns. Life-saving medicines are the object of drug counterfeiters. In the US, well-known cases involve erythropoietins (red-blood cell stimulating agents or EPOs); in Europe, drugs for prostate cancer and other diseases; in the developing world, anti-malarial drugs and a variety of other anti-infective drugs.[6] While the current situation should be cause enough for global attention and action, the prospect of new, untreatable forms of malaria should be inherently alarming.[7] Fortunately, some of the best examples of coordination on anti-counterfeiting have aimed at tackling the malaria drug problem and will be addressed below.

Barriers to effective centralised coordination mechanisms

Amongst the IMPACT, inter-governmental organisations, think tanks, patient and provider congresses, as well as the wide array of technology-related private sector conferences, hundreds of presentations are available on the problem of drug counterfeiting. A constant theme that recurs through these presentations is the need for coordination and negotiation amongst various types of groups and across countries. In principle, this requires a coordinating agent, such as the IMPACT (globally) or along the lines of the Partnership for Safe Medicines (nationally). Although widespread agreement seems to exist on the need for such entities, none are well funded or adequately staffed. Indeed, many factors cause organisational and coordination problems for anti-counterfeiting stakeholders.

Resources: Because of the diversity of the stakeholders needed for a solution, no one agency or entity emerges as the natural financier for anti-counterfeiting activities. Regulators can rightly assume that this is an industry problem. Industry can naturally assume that anything it does will taint the entire enterprise with assumed commercial motives. Even generic industry participation in any negotiation could be viewed as "big" generics trying to shut small local enterprises out of the market. Most patient and provider non-governmental organisations (NGOs) have expertise and robust networks but meagre project budgets. Government-based funding agencies must balance anti-counterfeiting with other initiatives that seem much more concrete, such as child immunization, emergency preparedness, and basic medical supplies. Furthermore, government grants often require the preparation of laborious grant proposals that volunteers in an NGO are unlikely to be able to write in their spare time.

Alignment: Conferences that employ the three-speaker panel format often do a good job of soliciting views, but very rarely challenge people to negotiate and achieve alignment. Everyone can and usually does agree that drug counterfeiting is an abominable problem, but people rarely engage in dialogue about agreeing on joint solutions and developing an action plan. Multilateral institutions are very un-useful for achieving alignment. When decisions are taken on a consensus basis, the lowest common denominator becomes the standard. Such an approach is not advisable on safety-related issues. Alignment should not be achieved at the cost of meaningful policy and action steps.

Commitment: Supposing that all relevant countries negotiated common preferred policy goals, coordinated legislation, and designated single points of contact, stakeholders could then start tackling the problem. Success however, would require much more. Success would require senior government officials to create inter-agency working groups; individual government agency directors to assign staff to this problem; industry associations to educate their members on concrete ways to assist; industry stakeholders to create education programs about their own products; NGOs to assign their working-groups to this issue with timelines and reports; scientists and others to have the resources to spend time and laboratory resources working on analytical characterisation of unknown materials. The people who implement policy need income and assurance that their efforts will be rewarded. Where appropriate, they need governing authorities to designate this issue as a priority and to be able to see benefits from their engagement. Commitment does not come from altruism across all groups. Commitment is tied inherently to the problem of coordination. You can coordinate only when you have on-going activities.

Achieving alignment on policy does not solve a problem; it merely enables the possibility for meaningful action. How these challenges can be tackled can be more clearly understood by looking at the experiences of a group that is dedicated to coordination of anti-counterfeiting activity.

The Partnership for Safe Medicines (PSM): An example of successful approaches to key challenges

The Partnership for Safe Medicines (PSM) was created in 2003 to raise public awareness of problems with counterfeit drugs and disseminate reliable information and alerts on counterfeit-related issues. During that year, disturbing information came to light in the US. The publication of the *Report of the Florida Grand Jury* detailed an economic underworld of diversion, counterfeiting, fraud, and abuse of Florida's drug supply chain.[8] Some of the most egregious abuses detailed in this report involved criminal networks purchasing HIV medicines on the street to sell back into "secondary" distribution networks. Reporting by investigative journalist Katherine Eban uncovered stories of highly-sensitive EPOs stored in Florida "gentlemens'" clubs and sold out of car trunks.[9] A case of counterfeit Lipitor (a drug used to control high cholesterol) spreading throughout the US into multiple states indicated that this problem was by no means confined to one state. Since these problems were so new and dramatic, many associations in the supply chain, professional provider associations, and patient groups thought there was urgent need for public education on the problem and joined the new association. The need was all the more pressing considering that many of the drugs mentioned in the report were certainly not "lifestyle" drugs or being purchased via the Internet.

The PSM's experience demonstrates how coordination challenges can be handled when resources are scarce. The PSM's activities were enabled largely because of the Board of Director's commitment and ability to support PSM activities with their time and occasional resources. The current Board was formed over dinner at the 1st Annual San Diego Health Policy Conference, hosted by Dr. Bryan Liang's Institute of Health Law Studies at California Western School of Law. In addition to Liang, the Board of Directors includes Marv Shepherd, a well-known researcher on drug supply issues and US consumers' importation habits from Mexico, and Tom Kubic, former Deputy Assistant Director of the Federal Bureau of Investigation and current CEO of the Pharmaceutical Security Institute (PSI), as well as myself. The Board Directors each have expertise in relevant areas: patient safety/medical, pharmacy, law enforcement, and international trade. Board members demonstrate commitment through funding their own travel for meetings, developing presentations and research proposals, writing opinion-editorials and media pieces, and through their outreach to expand Partnership activities. Further demonstrating their firm personal commitment, travel and PSM activity for the two Board members who are university professors requires that they negotiate permissions from Deans at their respective universities and means that they forego more lucrative research opportunities.

The PSM is best understood as a federation, a collection of member associations. Unlike trade federations however, the PSM is comprised of member associations from a variety of communities, primarily patient groups, pharmacy groups, pharmaceutical associations representing different actors in the supply chain, and some physician groups. The groups participate by developing educational materials in working-groups that are later approved by the Board and disseminated (see below).

Early in the PSM's existence the Board faced problems of alignment, but managed to achieve resolution by focusing on the goal to be achieved. The PSM wanted to raise public awareness about counterfeit medicines but realised that some products, which would not meet the criteria for counterfeit, might still pose significant safety risks for patients. Medical errors, medical devices, and the wider category of substandard drugs — both licit and illicit all added additional dimensions of safety which had the potential to fit within the scope of the PSM's public awareness-raising work. Mixing in all of these other issues however, would detract from the goal that the PSM had established as its focus. How to sort it all out? The Board went back to the WHO definition of "counterfeit drug" and decided to focus on the medicines where some kind of deception was involved because it considered that to be the greatest unaddressed threat to patients. The Board recognised however, that many drugs carry the same risks as counterfeit drugs even if they do not meet the strict criteria of "counterfeit." The Board addressed this by agreeing to focus on counterfeit and "contraband" drugs, per the definition of the National Association of Boards of Pharmacy in the US. For the purpose of this section, contraband includes: a Drug which is Counterfeit, stolen, Misbranded, obtained by fraud, purchased by a non-profit institution for its own use and placed in commerce in violation of the own use agreement for that Drug, or for which a Pedigree (if required) does not exist, or for which the Pedigree in existence has been forged, Counterfeited, falsely created, or contains any altered, false, or misrepresented information.[10]

Through these strategies, the PSM managed to maintain its focus on activities that were not undertaken by another NGO, which were certainly illegal, and which posed definite patient safety risks. Both commitment and flexibility played major roles in arriving at this resolution.

Problems with financial resources were encountered extremely early in the PSM's existence and persist to the present. The PSM survived for years with almost no funding, but that limitation actually prompted creativity to maximise resources. Success in this regard required a public affairs strategy leveraging low-cost resources.

Safe Meds Alert System: Undoubtedly, the Internet facilitates counterfeit and illicit drug sales. The Internet also can be a powerful tool against them. In 2005, the PSM converted the typical "email subscription" service into an alert system. Instead of lobbying the government, the PSM took government warnings and sent them to citizens. There were no copyright or liability issues because the government documents were in the public domain. The SafeMeds Alert System reflected the PSM's mission to raise awareness about counterfeit and contraband medicines. Medicines that are diverted from the legitimate supply chain, for instance, might not meet the legal threshold of "counterfeit," but there is no guarantee of their safety. Once the subscription service was set up, there was essentially zero cost to forward to the public by Internet alerts on counterfeit, diverted, stolen, or otherwise troublesome incidents. Recognising the fact that people do import drugs from other countries the PSM disseminated the Medicine and Healthcare products Regulatory Agency's (MHRA) alerts for the United Kingdom as well as alerts emanating from Asia. While WHO set up a "Rapid Alert System" for regulators to share information and to make progress on investigations, the PSM opened its system up completely to the public. Eventually the US Food and Drug Administration (FDA) signed a Memorandum of Understanding to add the PSM to its Counterfeit Alert Network.

Website Resources: In addition to government alerts and news links, the PSM built specific resources for the Safemedicines.org website. Developing new policy resources requires a great deal of negotiation, especially in an organisation with over 50 members, which the PSM had at the time. The PSM's educational material for patients — the SAFE-DRUG checklist — was largely adapted from the independent work of Bryan Liang. Marv Shepherd, from the University of Texas at Austin, oversaw development of the other key PSM resource: SAFE Sourcing. This guide was intended for small pharmacies to help them identify questionable shipments they might have received. Again, the PSM was able to draw on its expert resources — involving approximately a dozen PSM member associations between the two projects. Of no less importance and impact, the PSM also reached out to the FDA and the FDA's Office of Criminal Investigations for expert comment on the draft of the guide, in order to ensure that the PSM's recommendations would be helpful. It cost little to negotiate outcomes that met everyone's standards, but the members associations needed internal mandates to permit staff time for such an endeavour. As a result, the final version of Safe Sourcing was sent to WHO IMPACT for the Regulatory Working Group's activities on good distribution practices.

The News: The Internet also facilitates free global news monitoring. In 2004, the PSM started identifying key articles of interest to post on the website, but received feedback that no one had the time to read them. In response, the PSM started summarising the key articles of the week, providing links to original stories, and distributing the publication for free. Reader feedback underscored a general desire for basic facts such as which country, what happened, who did it, and what did the courts do? Although it did not require financial resources, this effort was labour-intensive and would have been impossible without a supportive employer.

The Conference Circuit: The PSM also leveraged the for-profit conference circuit to educate, network, and disseminate resources. The PSM regularly received invitations to conferences, the organisers of which would waive registration fees and sometimes pay travel costs. Although audiences often were industry members, these conferences did provide a means to expand media interest and to associate with policymakers and key stakeholders from the supply chain or patient and physician groups.

Overall, the PSM was unable to find access to large-scale financial resources in industry, the donor community, or government agencies, which would have enabled large-scale public awareness campaigns. Because of strong alignment and commitment from the Board level, the Executive Director's employer, and the member associations however, the PSM managed and continues to operate effectively notwithstanding significant resource constraints.

Leadership from the periphery

Despite the ubiquity of the challenges outlined above, the anti-counterfeiting movement is far stronger today than it was 2003. A May 2010 meeting of PSM staff with Indian government officials and civil society organisations could lead to the creation of an analogous group in India. Contacts also have been established in China, Thailand, and East Africa, and the first major Partnership for Safe Medicines conference is planned for September 2010 in Washington, D.C. In recent years the PSM has started translating materials into languages other than English and posting news around the world to appeal to broader audiences.

A similar group, the European Alliance for Access to Safe Medicines was launched in 2006 in London. The group actively raises awareness in the media about the dangers of illicit drug purchasing through the "counterfeiting superhighway" — the Internet.[11] The PSM has also made public its guide to starting a Partnership for stakeholders around the globe (see Annex I).

International stakeholders have leveraged strong working relationships and coordinated to produce tools for their members and patients. In May 2010, the World Health Professionals Alliance (WHPA) announced a campaign against drug counterfeiting called "Be Aware, Take Action." WHPA, which includes international member organisations representing physicians, nurses, pharmacists, physical therapists, and dentists, has coordinated activities for several years and issued press statements around IMPACT meetings. The "Be Aware, Take Action" campaign includes many new tools and information resources,[12] including:

- General Information
- Fact Sheets for health professionals, patients, and public health advocates on counterfeit medical products
- Communication with patients
- The Internet and counterfeit medical products
- You can help keep medical products safe
- Effective advocacy for change
- Campaign postcards
- Sample Reporting Form for health professionals
- Be Aware, Take Action poster
- A Medicines Checklist poster for hospital and clinic waiting rooms and pharmacies
- The WHPA Joint Statement of Counterfeiting of Medical Products

The WHPA materials are noteworthy for their emphasis on the joint efforts need by patients and health care professionals. These materials not only support members' professional practices, they also instruct on advocacy and arm people with facts. The WHPA's members have been active on the anti-counterfeiting issue for many years. The International Federation of Pharmacists was the first chair of the IMPACT working group on communications. The International Council of Nurses dedicated International Nurses Day 2005 to the problem. A sister association, the International Alliance of Patients' Organizations (IAPO), also has engaged in public repeatedly on counterfeit medicines, following its Board's decision to prioritise patient safety issues.[13] In 2010 the WHO issued a factsheet on counterfeit medicines (Annex II).

Regarding policy and legislation, the Council of Europe has exercised leadership in the development of the so-called "Medicrime Convention."[14] The Medicrime Convention follows on a number of other Council of Europe conventions and seeks to tackle counterfeit-related crime at the following levels:

- The manufacturing of counterfeit medical products;
- Supplying, offering to supply, and trafficking in counterfeit medical products;
- The falsification of documents linked to medical products;
- The unauthorised manufacturing or supplying of medicinal products and the marketing of medical devices that do not comply with conformity requirements.

The Medicrime Convention also handles the anti-counterfeit definition with general terms that pertain to the problem of deception: "the term "counterfeit" shall mean a false representation as regards identity and/or source."[15] The Convention document was developed in 2009 and will be available for signature and ratification by Council of Europe Members as of November 2010.[16]

National law enforcement authorities also have demonstrated that leadership can attract and inspire other their colleagues in other countries. The UK's Medicines and Healthcare Regulatory Products Agency (MHRA) deserves special mention. MHRA since 2006 has conducted an annual "Internet Day of Action," whereby it carries out raids and apprehends criminals connected to a variety of internet-based crimes involving medicines or medical devices. While the targets of the MHRA's actions were not all counterfeit cases, they all related to pharmaceutical crime. In the most recent example, MHRA investigated ten websites, seized fifteen computers, confiscated 147,000 tablets at just one postal centre, and made three arrests. Over time, MHRA's leadership has been rewarded with wider levels of participation. In 2008, MHRA christened the day "*International* Internet Day of Action" in coordination with eight countries and assistance from INTERPOL. In 2009, the total number of participating countries rose to 24, with support from INTERPOL, WHO, and IMPACT.[17]

Pharmaceutical manufacturers coordinate through the Pharmaceutical Security Institute (PSI) to support law enforcement investigations, including the Internet Days of Action. PSI staff help individual company investigators share key aspects of intelligence to build cases against pharmaceutical crime. Since any one investigation could lead to counterfeit products from a variety of companies, the PSI coordination role helps ensure that all the relevant industry resources target priority problems. It also provides strategic intelligence to law enforcement and regulators around the globe.

A *tour de force* case study of coordination and negotiation by law enforcement, scientists, multilateral organisations, and diplomats can be seen in efforts to investigate counterfeiting of anti-malarials in Southeast Asia. A team of researchers had identified and classified counterfeit forms of the anti-malarial medicine artesunate, including over a dozen[14] faked holographic security devices. Working with the WHO, scientists, pharmacists, and physicians joined with INTERPOL to seek a solution to the counterfeit artesunate plaguing Southeast Asia. After a variety of sophisticated forensic measures were used to find evidence that pointed toward a counterfeit source in Southeast China, the Secretary-General of INTERPOL intervened, requesting help from the Ministry of Public Security in China. Resulting actions led to several arrests and seizures of over half a million blister packs (individual units for a patient). While the results were significant, an article written by the authors underscored that such kinds of collaboration require serious investment and relationship building.[18]

Although coordination and negotiation across the globe proves increasingly difficult, these examples demonstrate that coordination within sectors is, in fact, thriving — even in the absence of central leadership. This limited examination of initiatives reveals major efforts and resources in public awareness, enforcement, and legislative activity. Results in the struggle against counterfeit drugs are coming from the action-oriented stakeholders who are taking the lead on their own initiative by banding together with like-minded allies.

Conclusion

Drug counterfeiting is a complex criminal activity, which requires a corresponding response by a wide variety of stakeholders and thus presents significant challenges for negotiation amongst those stakeholders. At the World Health Assembly, negotiations continue to proceed slowly, while official diplomats wrestle over definitional issues. The failure of negotiations at this level would preclude any hope for effective central coordination. Amongst diverse, decentralised health regulators, enforcement agencies, non-profit organisations, and other groups however, strong actions have started to catalyse momentum against drug counterfeiting. The PSM provides an example of how a small group can produce some significant benefits with limited resources. Other key initiatives in public awareness — raising, law enforcement, and legislative developments are bearing fruit by exercising pro-active leadership and recruiting partners as they go.

When she was Director-General of the Nigerian regulatory authority NAFDAC, Dr. Dora Akunyili used to tell the story of her fight against counterfeit drugs. She had no resources, but she had a car. So she would drive around to various local business councils and encourage them to join the fight and dedicate resources to it. She is now famous for tremendous successes and improved public awareness. She participated in the IMPACT and WHO meetings, but she did not wait for them. Nor are stakeholders waiting health diplomacy through the World Health Assembly to define a role for the WHO. Real progress on anti-counterfeiting has come from people with constrained resources but unlimited commitment. While the many initiatives are far from maturity, the high level of engagement clearly demonstrates that committed people are working through negotiations, developing action plans, and executing them. Whatever the fate of the IMPACT, one must hope that the anti-counterfeiting movement's commitment levels and willingness to coordinate will be stronger and more prosperous in the years to come.

Annex I

How to Start a Partnership for Safe Medicines

The Partnership for Safe Medicines is a coalition of more than 50 patient, physician, pharmacist, university, industry and other professional organizations committed to the safety of prescription drugs and protecting consumers against unapproved, counterfeit, substandard, mishandled or otherwise unsafe medicines.

Learn more about the dangers of contraband and counterfeit drugs at www.safemedicines.org or contact us at info@safemedicines.org.

1. Find Partners

Potential partners in the fight against counterfeit medicines include non-governmental organizations (NGOs), governmental departments and agencies, and for-profit companies who are committed to the safety of prescription drugs and protecting consumers from counterfeit drugs. Partners may come from universities, pharmacists and other healthcare professional organizations, as well as from the business and pharmaceutical sectors.

2. Designate a Main Contact

One of the partner organizations needs to take the lead and designate a staff person to serve as your partnership's executive direct and coordinate activities. This person can act as a spokesperson if needed, or you can recruit spokespersons from among the partners.

3. Collect Existing Information on Safe Medicines

Survey your partners to see if they have already created materials about counterfeit medicines, Internet safety problems or related issues. Put these in an electronic archive that you can use in step 4.

4. Create a Web site on Safe Medicines

You can use the Internet to create a Web site where you can post partners' existing materials (step 3), new materials created by your partnership, and news stories relevant to the Partners. If you want to use a page from safemedicines.org, contact the U.S. Partnership at info@safemedicines.org.

5. Join the SafeMeds Alert System

The SafeMeds Alert System is a free email service offered by the U.S. Partnership that sends official alerts from the FDA and other government agencies around the world to anyone—private citizens, public groups, corporations, healthcare practitioners, associations—when specific counterfeit drug incidents are detected. Individuals can enroll online at www.safemedicines.org or you can send a list of email addresses to info@safemedicines.org.

6. Expand the SafeMeds Alert System

Contact your local drug regulatory authority or relevant Health Ministry to see if it would participate in the SafeMeds Alert System. Ask it to send an email to U.S. Partnership at info@safemedicines.org when specific counterfeit drug incidents occur and the U.S. Partnership will forward them through the SafeMeds Alert System.

7. Start a Local Weekly News Update

Every week, the U.S. Partnership sends free weekly email that provides readers with a weekly roundup of what's happening around the world regarding counterfeit drugs, as well as the latest blog entry from the its experts. For an example of a current newsletter, contact the U.S. executive director at info@safemedicines.org.

8. Develop Educational Materials

Hold meetings with your partners to develop appropriate educational materials. You can use existing Partnership materials as templates: especially the "S.A.F.E. D.R.U.G." checklist for patients, the "L.E.A.D.E.R.'s Guide for Pharmacists" and the "Principles for Drug Safety" doctrine.

8100 Boone Blvd., Ste. 220
Vienna, VA 22182
USA

Phone: +1-866-300-1077
Fax: +1-703-848-0164
info@safemedicines.org
www.safemedicines.org

Annex II

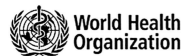

Fact sheet N°275
January 2010

Medicines: counterfeit medicines

Key facts

- Counterfeit medicines are medicines that are deliberately and fraudulently mislabelled with respect to identity and/or source.
- Use of counterfeit medicines can result in treatment failure or even death.
- Public confidence in health-delivery systems may be eroded following use and/or detection of counterfeit medicines.
- Both branded and generic products are subject to counterfeiting.
- All kinds of medicines have been counterfeited, from medicines for the treatment of life-threatening conditions to inexpensive generic versions of painkillers and antihistamines.
- Counterfeit medicines may include products with the correct ingredients or with the wrong ingredients, without active ingredients, with insufficient or too much active ingredient, or with fake packaging.

Counterfeit medicines are found everywhere in the world. They range from random mixtures of harmful toxic substances to inactive, ineffective preparations. Some contain a declared, active ingredient and look so similar to the genuine product that they deceive health professionals as well as patients. But in every case, the source of a counterfeit medicine is unknown and its content unreliable. Counterfeit medicines are always illegal. They can result in treatment failure or even death. Eliminating them is a considerable public health challenge.

Extent of the problem

Defining the extent of counterfeiting is difficult for a number of reasons.

The variety of information sources makes compiling statistics a difficult task. Sources of information include reports from national medicines regulatory authorities, enforcement agencies, pharmaceutical companies and nongovernmental organizations, as well as ad hoc studies on specific geographical areas or therapeutic groups.

The different methods used to produce reports and studies also make compiling and comparing statistics difficult.

Studies can only give snapshots of the immediate situation. Counterfeiters are extremely flexible in the methods they use to mimic products and prevent their detection. They can change these methods from day to day, so when the results of a study are released, they may already be outdated.

Finally, information about a case under legal investigation is sometimes only made public after the investigation has been concluded.

Counterfeiting is greatest in regions where regulatory and enforcement systems for medicines are weakest. In most industrialized countries with effective regulatory systems and market control (i.e. Australia, Canada, Japan, New Zealand, most of the European Union and the United States of America), incidence of counterfeit medicines is extremely low – less than 1% of market value according to the estimates of the countries concerned. But in many African countries, and in parts of Asia, Latin America, and countries in transition, a much higher percentage of the medicines on sale may be counterfeit.

Not only is there a huge variation between geographic regions in terms of incidence of counterfeit medicines, variation can also be significant within countries: for example, between urban and rural areas, and between cities.

All kinds of medicines have been counterfeited – branded and generic – ranging from medicines for the treatment of life-threatening conditions to inexpensive generic versions of painkillers and antihistamines (see table).

Table: Examples of counterfeit medicines

Counterfeit medicine	Country/Year	Report
Anti-diabetic traditional medicine (used to lower blood sugar)	China, 2009	Contained six times the normal dose of glibenclamide (two people died, nine people hospitalized)[1]
Metakelfin (antimalarial)	United Republic of Tanzania, 2009	Discovered in 40 pharmacies: lacked sufficient active ingredient[2]
Viagra & Cialis (for erectile dysfunction)	Thailand, 2008	Smuggled into Thailand from an unknown source in an unknown country[3]
Xenical (for fighting obesity)	United States of America, 2007	Contained no active ingredient and sold via Internet sites operated outside the USA[4]
Zyprexa (for treating bipolar disorder and schizophrenia)	United Kingdom, 2007	Detected in the legal supply chain: lacked sufficient active ingredient[5]
Lipitor (for lowering cholesterol)	United Kingdom, 2006	Detected in the legal supply chain: lacked sufficient active ingredient[6]

Internet sales

In over 50% of cases, medicines purchased over the Internet from illegal sites that conceal their physical address[7] have been found to be counterfeit.

Public health risks

Counterfeit medicines pose a public health risk because their content can be dangerous or they can lack active ingredients. Their use can result in treatment failure (and contribute to increased resistance in the case of antimalarials that contain insufficient active ingredient) or even death. Unlike substandard medicines where there are problems with the manufacturing process by a known manufacturer, counterfeit medicines are made by people with the intent to mislead.

The extreme difficulty in tracing the manufacturing and distribution channels of counterfeit medicines makes their circulation on markets difficult to stop. Even a single case of a counterfeit medicine is unacceptable since it indicates that the pharmaceutical supply system in which it was detected is vulnerable. Worse, it undermines the credibility of national health and enforcement authorities.

Contributory factors

Several factors contribute to the counterfeit medicine problem.

Paying for medicines can consume a significant proportion of individual or family income. Some people seek medicines that are sold more cheaply. These are often available from non-regulated outlets, where the incidence of counterfeit medicines is likely to be higher.

People might also purchase medicines from non-regulated outlets if, as is often the case in the rural areas of developing countries, medicines supplies at regular health facilities do not meet demand.

Counterfeiting medicines can be very lucrative. Since many countries have not yet enacted deterrent legislation, counterfeiters often do not fear prosecution.

The growth in international trade of pharmaceutical ingredients and medicines adds a further dimension of complexity to this issue. For example, trade through brokers and free trade zones where regulation is lax or absent (and medicines repackaged and relabelled to conceal country of origin) is increasing.

WHO response

Stringent regulatory control of medicines and enforcement by national medicines regulatory authorities contributes significantly to prevention and detection of counterfeit medicines. WHO provides direct country and regional support for strengthening medicines regulation.

To fight counterfeit medicines effectively, a range of stakeholders – not just health professionals – is needed. In 2006, WHO helped to create the International Medical Products Anti-Counterfeiting Taskforce, or IMPACT. The aim is to involve a range of stakeholders in collaborative efforts to protect people from buying and taking counterfeit medicines. To prevent the manufacture and distribution of counterfeit medicines, IMPACT's areas of focus are:

- legislative and regulatory infrastructure
- regulatory implementation
- enforcement
- technology
- communication.

1. Deadly counterfeit diabetes drug found outside China's Xinjiang, China View, 5 February 2009.

2. Tanzania Food and Drugs Authority

3. Center for Combating Counterfeit Drug, Thailand

4. US Food and Drug Administration

5. The Medicines and Healthcare products Regulatory Agency, United Kingdom

6. The Medicines and Healthcare products Regulatory Agency, United Kingdom

7. Some Internet pharmacies are legal operations, established to offer clients convenience and savings. They deliver medications from government-licensed facilities and sell only on the basis of a prescription.

For more information contact:

WHO Media centre
Telephone: +41 22 791 2222
E-mail: mediainquiries@who.int

References

1. 63rd World Health Assembly (2010) *Decisions and List of Resolutions. WHA 63(10)* http://apps.who.int/gb/ebwha/pdf_files/WHA63/A63_DIV3-en.pdf; all links accessed 26 June 2010.

2. IFPMA (2010) *The IFPMA Ten Principles on Counterfeit Medicines.* http://www.ifpma.org/documents/NR13800/IFPMA_Ten_Principles_on_Co unterfeit_Medicines_12May2010.pdf.

3. "An incident is a discrete event triggered by the discovery of counterfeit, illegally diverted or stolen pharmaceuticals. PSI considers an incident to be a unique occurrence. It must have adequate factual information such as a particular date, time, place and type of pharmaceutical product involved in order for it to be considered a unique incident". See PSI. *Counterfeit Situation: Definitions.* http://psi-inc.org/counterfeitSituation.cfm.

4. WHO (2010) *Medicines: Counterfeit Medicines. Fact Sheet No 275.* http://www.who.int/mediacentre/factsheets/fs275/en/index.html.

5. http://psi-inc.org/therapeuticCategories.cfm

6. See the research especially of Paul Newton, Newton P *et al.* Impact of poor-quality medicines in the 'developing' world. *Trends in Pharmacol Sci* (2010) 31 (3), 99–101; Newton, P *et al.* Counterfeit anti-infective medicines. *Lancet Inf Dis* (2006) 6, 602–613; Newton, P. *et al.* A collaborative epidemiological investigation into the criminal fake artesunate trade in South East Asia. *PLoS Medicine* (2008) 5 (2): e32.

7. Newton (2010) 100.

8. Supreme Court of the State of Florida (2003) *First Interim Report of the Seventeenth Statewide Grand Jury. Case No: SC02-2645.* http://www. turkewitzlaw.com/cases/pdf/GrandJuryFlorida303.pdf.

9. Eban K (2005) *Dangerous Doses*, Harcourt Books, Orlando, FL.

10. NABP (2009) *Model State Pharmacy Act and Model Rules of the National Association of Boards of Pharmacy*, Section 105(ee); (http://www.nabp.net/ publications/assets/2009%20Model%20Act.doc).

11. EAASM (2008) *The Counterfeiting Superhighway.* http://www.eaasm.eu/ Media_centre/News/The_Counterfeiting_Superhighway

12. WHPA. *WHPA Counterfeit Medical Products Campaign.* http://whpa.org/ counterfeit_campaign.htm

13. IAPO. *Counterfeit Medicines.* http://www.patientsorganizations.org/showarticle. pl?id=759&n=37200

14. CoE-Medicrime. *Introduction.* http://www.coe.int/t/DGHL/StandardSetting/ MediCrime/Default_en.asp

15. CoE. European Committee on Crime Problems. (2009) *Draft Council of Europe Convention on Counterfeiting of Medical Products and Similar Crimes Involving Threats to Public Health.* http://www.coe.int/t/dghl/stan-dardsetting/medicrime/CDPC%20_2009_15Fin%20E%20Draft%20Conven tion%2009%2011%2009CM.pdf Article 4j.

16. CoE (2010) *Fact Sheet: Counterfeit Medicines and Similar Crimes.* http://www.coe.int/t/dghl/standardsetting/medicrime/FactSheetE.pdf

17. MHRA (2009) *Press release: International Operation Combats the Online Supply of Counterfeit and Unlicensed Medicines.* http://www.mhra.gov.uk/ NewsCentre/Pressreleases/CON062909

18. Newton (2008).

14

Global Health Workforce Alliance: Negotiating for Access to Health Workers for All

Mubashar Sheikh[i] *and Muhammad Mahmood Afzal*[ii]

Abstract

Pressing health needs across the globe cannot be met without a well-trained, adequate, and available health workforce. Whilst the validity and importance of this fact is widely agreed upon, the practical realisation is amongst the greatest challenges for health diplomats today. This case study describes how The Global Health Workforce Alliance developed as an international leader and focal point for consolidated action on this complex and multi-dimensional critical global health problem. The Alliance works with a membership of over 300 diverse stakeholder groups, such as representatives of United Nations agencies, national governments, academia, civil society organisations, private corporations, philanthropic organisations, professional associations, hospitals, and trade unions. This story describes the importance of strategic leadership,

[i] Dr. Mubashar Sheikh is the Executive Director of the Global Health Workforce Alliance.
[ii] Dr. Muhammad Mahmood Afzal is a former staff member of the Global Health Workforce Alliance.

cross-ministry dialogue, effective timing, and capacity building in developing countries as amongst the key messages universally valid for diplomats working with different areas of focus.

The Problem

Health workers are the heart and soul of health care systems. The world is faced with a chronic shortage of health workers. After decades of neglect, dramatic shortages in the health workforce has been recognised as one of the most critical constraints faced by health sectors to achieving progress on reaching health and development goals, such as the Millennium Development Goals.

Even in the decade of exponential increases in donor funding for global health and despite a scaling up of disease-specific interventions, health services remained out of reach for those who need them most. As a result, millions of people throughout the world do not have access to skilled health care providers. The crisis is noticed particularly in provision of essential life-saving interventions such as childhood immunization, safe pregnancy and delivery services for mothers, and access to prevention and treatment for HIV/AIDS, malaria and tuberculosis, predominantly in poor countries and across Sub-Saharan Africa.

The significant shortage of health workers is also noticed in preparedness for and response to the global security threats posed by emerging and epidemic-prone diseases such as Severe Acute Respiratory Syndrome (SARS), avian flu, and hemorrhagic fevers, as well as the consequences of climate change and disasters like war, earthquake, and other mass emergencies.

In addition to a critical shortage of health workforce, health workers are also inequitably distributed throughout the world. With severe imbalances between developed and developing countries, this global workforce shortage is made even worse by imbalances within countries. In general, there is a lack of adequate staff in rural areas compared to cities. In developing countries, the priority disease programmes are competing for scarce human resources; whereas, in the developed countries, a rise in chronic health conditions among ageing populations and the overall ageing of countries' workforces has led to an ever-growing demand for health workers. The pull of higher salaries in industrialised countries and the push of poor working conditions at home drive thousands of health workers to jobs abroad each year. Yet developing countries face an escalating double burden of both infectious and non communicable diseases and are in need of massive scaling up of training programmes and retention interventions.

The Local and External Players and Their Roles

Global Health Workforce Alliance: evidence-based evolution

Over the years, more and more evidence has been revealed on the need for equitable access to health workers, if the international community is committed to the achievement of the Millennium Development Goals (MDGs) in the developing countries.

Acknowledging the issue with its multi-dimensional causes and outcomes, the global stakeholders initiated a process for assessing the situation and building the evidence needed to negotiate and design appropriate solutions to address this momentous challenge. In this context, the Joint Learning Initiative (JLI), implemented by JSI Research & Training Institute Inc.[iii] and coordinated by the Global Equity Initiative at Harvard University, was launched in 2002, bringing together over 100 health professionals and experts from academia, countries, and international agencies to examine the problems in Human Resources for Health (HRH) in greater depth with the view toward improving overall equity in global health. This initiative was funded by the Rockefeller Foundation and others donors.

The JLI created seven working groups to analyse current trends in human resources availability and shortages, holding consultations in countries, developing regional best practices, and creating a strategy report on global human resources for health. The aim of the report was to inform, influence, and make an impact on government policymakers, donors, and human resources for health managers.

[iii] JSI Research & Training Institute, Inc. is non-profit affiliate of John Snow, Inc. Both are public health research and consulting firms dedicated to improving the health of individuals and communities throughout the world.

The groundbreaking report of the JLI, "Human Resources for Health — overcoming crisis," released in 2004, changed the history of debates and discussion on the topic and succeeded in highlighting the crisis. The report indicated that:

> ...mirroring today's global health crisis, we face a global crisis of the health workforce. There are not enough health workers, they do not have the right skills and support networks, they are overstretched and over-stressed, and often they are not in the right place...Three major things went wrong: investment was replaced by neglect, the market for health workers went global, and — worst of all — the HIV/AIDS epidemic added horrendous new burdens on precisely those health systems least able to cope.[1]

Providing strong evidence with precision about challenges, the JLI report called for immediate global action to harness the power of health workers for global health equity and development. Failure of such action will result in "stark failures to achieve the MDGs, epidemics spiralling out of control, and the unnecessary loss of many lives" and perhaps most importantly, the report stated "at stake is nothing less than the course of global health and development in the 21st century."

The JLI report was followed by a range of key policy discussions and negotiations that took place to drive the initiative forward. In February 2005, the Oslo Consultation brought together key global stakeholders to achieve consensus around a "common global platform of action." During this consultation, the decision was taken to create a new global partnership–the Alliance–to address the health workforce crisis. To kick start the Alliance, a special technical working group was formed.

During the winter of 2005–2006, work started on the Strategic Plan of what would become the Global Health Workforce Alliance (hereafter referred to as the Alliance or the GHWA). The Working Group met in January 2006 to put final touches on the Strategic Plan and to gear up for the launch of the Alliance later in the year. In Lusaka, in April 2006, a sub-regional meeting on HRH was held, convened by the Working Group, just prior to the launch of the World Health Report 2006, which has served as the scientific basis for the Alliance's work ever since.

Meanwhile during 2004–2005, three High Level Forum meetings on health-related MDGs were held in Geneva, Abuja, and Paris. Outcomes of these three meetings identified the HRH challenges and endorsed a plan of action called "Working Together" in a global alliance.[2]

During the World Health Day campaign celebrated around the world on 6 April 2006, the World Health Organization (WHO) informed the global community about the most critical findings revealed in its World Health Report 2006, indicating a serious shortage of health workers — 4,250,000 health workers, at least 2,360,000 health service providers including doctors, nurses, and midwives, and 1,890,000 management support workers urgently needed to fill the gap, with 1.5 million needed for Africa alone. The report stated that at least 1.3 billion people worldwide lack access to the most basic healthcare services, often because there is no health worker. The shortage is global, but the burden is greatest in countries overwhelmed by poverty and disease. Across the world, 57 countries have been identified as having "critical shortages"–36 of these are in Africa. Shortages are most severe in sub-Saharan Africa, which has 11% of the world's population and 24% of the global burden of disease, but only 3% of the world's health workers.[3]

Launching the report, WHO set out a 10-year plan to address the crisis, calling for national leadership to urgently formulate and implement country strategies for the health workforce. WHO also called for more international support and investment in the training and support of health workers. The report recommended that of all new donor funds for health, 50% should be dedicated to strengthening health systems, of which 50% should be dedicated specifically to training, retaining, and sustaining the health workforce.

WHO facilitated the process for establishment of this global level Alliance with the appreciation of new facts all over the world and an understanding that a number of players are involved or can be engaged in the health workforce-related processes, whereas a single organisation cannot offer solutions to this global and multi-dimensional crisis thus necessitating a common platform or alliance of key players where all can contribute to addressing this global challenge.

With this backdrop, the Global Health Workforce Alliance (GHWA) was officially launched on 25 May 2006, after a rational negotiation and decision in the 59th World Health Assembly in Geneva. Its core mission was fixed as to become an unprecedented global focal point — the 'joint platform' for consolidated action on the health workforce crisis — bringing together multiple stakeholders to work collaboratively to increase and improve desperately needed human resources for health, to scale up access to key services, and to strengthen health systems performance, both public and private. It was designed to be the global advocating voice on the issue, to draw together the major stakeholders and players from all sectors — governments, civil society, international and regional institutions, professional associations, academia, and the private sector, and to work to combine the key components of the issue — health, but also labour, management, governance, finance, education, research, data collection, and planning. The mandate was, and still is, broad, the challenges great, but the commitment level is high.[4]

Former WHO Director-General Dr. Jong-Wook Lee appointed Dr. Francis Omaswa as Special Advisor to the Director-General on HRH and assigned him the task of setting up the Alliance. Later, he was appointed as Executive Director of the Alliance. The Director-General also appointed Dr. Lincoln Chen, one of the JLI's co-chairs, as his Special Envoy on HRH. The new Alliance was to become a JLI successor initiative to work in parallel with WHO's development of the World Health Report 2006 "Working Together for Health" focusing on HRH challenges.

The GHWA relations with WHO, its governance, and the secretariat

The Global Health Workforce Alliance and WHO have a special relationship established through a Memorandum of Understanding (MOU) negotiated during the evolutionary process of the Alliance. Negotiating and establishing the MOU with the host organization — WHO — took at least five months during the initial phase of the Alliance due to diverse challenges. The main challenges were related to the Alliance's governance

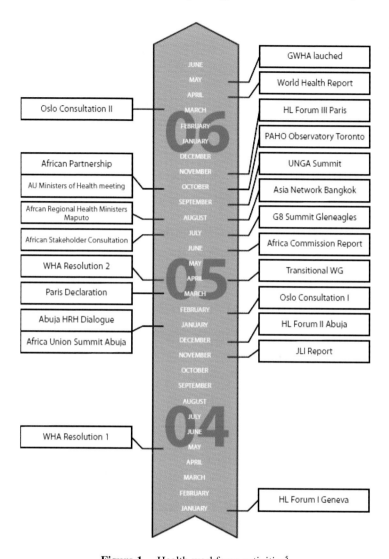

Figure 1.   Health workforce activities[5]

system, its functions and roles, its links with WHO and other partners, and the required supporting mechanisms. An intense negotiation and dialogue process assisted in bringing a consensus about key aspects, including the Alliance's governance, management systems, roles, and relations with WHO.

Based upon this MOU, the GHWA works independently and not as a part of WHO. For administrative and legal purposes, the Alliance Secretariat is housed within the headquarters of the WHO in Geneva, Switzerland; however, WHO does not fund, nor does it control the Alliance's operations. While maintaining the independence of its functions, the GHWA Secretariat follows the management and financial procedures as well as regulations and guidelines of WHO, whereas WHO facilitates the Alliance's functions through its regular supporting mechanisms.

Importantly, the GHWA is governed by a Board. The Board of the Global Health Workforce Alliance is composed of a selection of the key stakeholders in human resources for health, as well as its funding partners. WHO, being a founding member and partner of the Alliance, has a permanent seat on the Board of the Alliance, as are professional associations, non-governmental organisations (NGOs), and other constituencies including donor governments. Board meetings occur twice a year. Along with overseeing the work of the GHWA, the Board also sets its policies and strategic directions. The Board was joined by 18 member organisations by the end of 2007 and it now has 20 members.[6]

The GHWA Secretariat[7] is led by an Executive Director who is an official staff member of the WHO, but who reports to the Board of the Alliance and leads the Secretariat to implement the Alliance's work plan as determined by the Board. Dr. Francis Omaswa, the first Executive Director of the Alliance, was followed in 2008 by Dr. Mubashar Sheikh who was re-assigned from his position as WHO Representative in the Islamic Republic of Iran. The GHWA Secretariat staff members either are recruited through WHO procedures or seconded by the Alliance partners. Initially there were only two staff members in the Alliance Secretariat; currently that number has increased to 17 staff members.

The GHWA also has close technical relations with WHO, as WHO strategic objectives and core functions are linked with the health workforce. The Department of Human Resources for Health at WHO's headquarters in Geneva, related departments of six WHO regional offices, as well as WHO country offices all collaborate closely with the Alliance on many joint activities, and with the stakeholders in the countries, regions, and at the global level.

Working together for health workforce

The Global Health Workforce Alliance has a broad base of members[iv] and partners[v] that work on a common platform to address the health workforce challenges. This network of members and partners is growing consistently with time. The list of members and partners include academic and research institutions, foundations, national governments, non-governmental and civil society organisations, private corporations, professional associations, United Nations agencies, hospital networks, unions, and many more throughout the world, in all regions.

The initial partners of the Alliance included the Bill & Melinda Gates Foundation, the Canadian International Development Agency, the European Commission, the Global Alliance for Vaccines and Immunization, the Global Equity Initiative at Harvard University, the International Council of Nurses, the New Partnership for Africa's Development, the Norwegian Agency for Development Cooperation, the Ministry of Public Health of Thailand, Physicians for Human Rights, the World Bank, and WHO. The Government of Norway donated US$3.5 million towards the Alliance's operations during its first year. Seed money for its start-up also was donated by the governments of Canada, Ireland, and Sweden. Later on, partnerships expanded and while some have a funding relationship with the Alliance, others have been central in the Task Forces and Working Groups, e.g. Realizing Rights, Duke University, and Physicians for Human Rights. WHO is, of course, a significant partner. The GHWA donors have included the Bill & Melinda Gates Foundation, Canadian International Development Agency (CIDA), European Union (EU), French Development Agency, Deutsche Gesellschaft für Technische Zusammenarbeit, Germany (GTZ), Irish Aid, NORAD/Ministry of Foreign Affairs Norway, Department for International Development of the United Kingdom (DFID), and the United Sates Agency for International Development (USAID). The regional networks like the Asia-Pacific Action Alliance on Human Resources for Health (AAAH) and the African Platform are also significant collaborators.

[iv] Members are the organisations that joined the Alliance through an application process.
[v] Partners provide funding and other support and collaborate with the Alliance members and the Secretariat.

Membership to the GHWA requires a commitment to resolving the health workforce crisis and the development of human resources for health, in accordance with the Alliance's guiding principles, strategic framework, and internationally-agreed guidance. To become a member of the Global Health Workforce Alliance, the interested organisation fills in and submits the on-line application form or sends through email. An organisation seeking membership with the Alliance should: be active in the area of human resources for health, or a closely related field; endorse the values and general principles of the Alliance, as reflected in its strategic plan; represent an institution, agency, or government active in the Alliance's priority areas; and be actively supporting the attainment of the Kampala Declaration and the Agenda for Global Action on HRH.

The Alliance's membership base has expanded exponentially over a relatively short period of time. As of July 2010, the Alliance had 248 members including: 80 academic and research institutions, one financial institution, 13 foundations, 15 national governments, 66 non-governmental and civil society organisations, 22 private corporations, 18 professional associations, seven United Nations agencies, and 26 members of other categories such as hospitals, networks, and trade unions.[8]

The GHWA vision and mission

The Global Health Workforce Alliance, being a global partnership, highlights the crisis of human resources for health and keeps it on the global agenda, convenes members, partners, and countries to work together to find solutions, advocates for their effective implementation and facilitate the sharing of knowledge and best practices on health workforce issues.

This purpose of the Alliance is in line with its vision that "all people everywhere will have access to a skilled, motivated and supported health worker, within a robust health system" and mission "to advocate and catalyse global and country actions to resolve the human resources for health crisis, to support the achievement of the health-related millennium development goals and health for all."[9]

First global forum on HRH and international commitments

In March 2008, the Alliance convened the First Global Forum on Human Resources for Health with the theme "Time is now: Action on the Health workforce."[10] The Forum was held in Kampala, Uganda. The aims of the Forum were to build consensus on how to accelerate human resources for health (HRH) action at the global and country levels; strengthen implementation capacity for HRH action at these levels; and develop alliances to work as a global network on HRH. The Forum was attended by some 1500 participants from Africa, the Americas, Asia, Europe, and the Middle East. Participants included government ministers, international HRH experts, health professionals, researchers, and policy-makers, who shared current research, best practices, and promising innovations for scaling up the health workforce.

The Forum culminated in the adoption of the Kampala Declaration and the Agenda for Global Action.[11] These two documents serve as a framework to guide the development of HRH over the next decade. Strategies are provided to overcome health workforce challenges and to translate into action the many commitments that have been made all over the world to resolve the health workforce crisis. Though global in scope, the Agenda for Global Action relies on individual countries to design their own national policies based on local circumstances.

The Agenda for Action presents the main steps needed to be taken by countries, the international community, civil society, and health workers to ensure determined, coordinated and evidence-based action to address and solve the crisis of health worker shortages. Six fundamental and inter-connected strategies are outlined in The Agenda for Action:

1. Building coherent national and global leadership
2. Scaling up education and training
3. Managing pressures of the international health workforce market and its impact on migration
4. Retaining an effective, responsive and equitably distributed health workforce

5. Securing additional and more productive investment in the health workforce
6. Ensuring capacity for an informed response based on evidence and joint learning

The Alliance was tasked to monitor the implementation of the Declaration and Agenda for Global Action, and to report back on their status at the second Global Forum on Human Resources for Health, scheduled to be held in January 2011 in Bangkok, Thailand.

Following the first Forum, a host of positive endorsements were made. Dr. Mubashar Sheikh joined as Executive Director of the Alliance and streamlined its programmes and policy actions according to outcomes of the Global Forum. There was a welcomed increase of high level commitments on HRH at the G8 Summits in 2008 and 2009. At these two summits pledges were made by governments to address the critical shortages of health workers across the world as a fundamental component for progress in health — also noting the work of GHWA and its partners, as well as the Kampala Declaration and Agenda for Global Action. Specific donor commitments were made by Japan, Norway, the United Kingdom, and the United States, all of whom pledged specific funds in 2008 for training new health workers in Africa.

At the UN High Level Meeting on the MDGs in September 2008, resolving the health workforce crisis was underlined as central to the achievement of the health-related targets. A new task force on Innovative Financing for Health was launched, the mandate of which includes finding solutions for funding over one million additional health workers by 2015. Significant commitments also were made by the Clinton Global Initiative, the GAVI Alliance, the Global Fund for HIV/AIDS, Tuberculosis and Malaria, and the Gates Foundation. The African Union adopted the Africa Health Strategy: 2007–2015, which places addressing the health workforce crisis at the centre of the action plan.

During July 2009, the G8 Summit at L'Aquila, Italy acknowledged the health workforce issue and the active role played by the Global Health Workforce Alliance in the G8 Leaders Declaration: *Responsible leadership for a sustainable future.*[12] At that summit, the G8 Leaders also endorsed the Health Experts Group report "Promoting Global Health," which highlighted the necessity of addressing the scarcity of health workers in developing countries and acknowledged the role of health systems strengthening in ensuring universal access to health services and in attaining the Millennium Development Goals.

Collaborating with countries and regional bodies

Aiming for impact in countries where health workers are still working and living under constraints has been one of the Alliance's key objectives. As stated in the World Health Report 2006, 57 countries are suffering from an acute shortage of health workforce. The Alliance's Board decided that country action should start in a set of eight "fast-track" countries, all in the group of the 57 most critical. These eight countries (called "pathfinder countries") included: Angola, Benin, Cameroon, Ethiopia, Haiti, Sudan, Vietnam, and Zambia. The Alliance provided catalytic funding to address the most critical concerns.

Given the complexity and richness of the human resources for health issues in countries, where many sectors outside the portfolio of the Ministries of Health, such as institutions in education, labour, and finance have decision-making roles on key issues, the Alliance aimed to convene all partners to identify common challenges and to find joint solutions. Many of the "pathfinder countries" have capitalised on this initial approach by employing full-time HRH focal points, mainly within the Ministry of Health, to facilitate the creation of the Multi-sector Country teams (MCT). By 2010, virtually all "pathfinder countries" have developed national HRH plans — an important indicator of progress in improving health workforce situations in priority countries. In addition, the GHWA also provided catalytic support to countries such as Djibouti, Pakistan, Somalia, South Sudan, and Zambia for dealing with the HRH crisis and carrying out specific projects.

The Alliance worked in partnership with ministries of health, WHO headquarters, and WHO regional and country offices to support the development of a series of HRH country profiles with the aim of accelerating the availability of synthesized and accurate information. The target is to complete HRH profiles in most of the crisis countries by the end of 2010. In addition, the Alliance also supported proposals from 18 African States to develop comprehensive, costed HRH plans while strengthening their HRH information systems and establishing HRH observatories. By the end of 2009, 14 countries tabled progress reports and all aimed to finalise their HRH plans by 2010.[13]

Community health workers represent a largely untapped potential solution to help alleviate the global HRH crisis. In 2009, the Alliance, with support from the United States Agency for International Development, conducted a global systematic review and eight in-depth country case studies in sub-Saharan Africa (Ethiopia, Mozambique, Uganda), South-East Asia (Bangladesh, Pakistan, Thailand) and Latin America (Brazil, Haiti). The study focused on maternal and child health, HIV/AIDS, tuberculosis and malaria, and also covered mental health and non-communicable diseases. This exercise identified and shared best practices that could be adapted to crisis and priority country contexts to assist attainment of the Millennium Development Goals. It also shared evidence with policymakers and informed them of how to expand the cadre of community health workers in resource-strapped settings.

In an effort to further expand political and policy buy-in in affected regions, the Alliance worked to support regional bodies in further promoting HRH issues. For Africa, the Alliance has supported the foundations of the African Platform on Human Resources for Health (AP-HRH). In Asia, the Asia-Pacific Action Alliance for Human Resources for Health (AAAH) was created with assistance from the Alliance. In the Americas, the Alliance's main partner is the Pan American Health Organization (PAHO), which is the WHO's regional arm for Latin America and the Caribbean. PAHO's dynamism and expertise in health workforce issues specific to that region are tremendous assets. Joint plans also are being implemented in the HRH crisis countries of the Eastern Mediterranean Region, with more focus on developing and implementing national plans in addressing the health workforce needs.

Addressing key issues through task forces and working groups

GHWA launched several initiatives to tackle specific HRH related issues and challenges whose nature warranted a global, multi-stakeholder approach.

In order to deliver on its core objectives, the Alliance has embarked on addressing specific workforce challenges by establishing mission-oriented, time bound international Task Forces and Working Groups[14] to address specific areas that impact on human resources for health. The Alliance has so far commissioned six Task Forces, on the following themes: Financing, Migration, Private Sector, Scaling up Education and Training, Tools and Guidelines, and Universal Access to HIV treatment.

The work of the Task Forces and Working Groups is guided by terms of reference and budgeted work plans, approved by the Board of GHWA. The purpose of the work of the Task Forces and Working Groups is to produce evidence that will impact on and accelerate action on improving the workforce.

The Task Force on Tools and Guidelines has developed a framework and indicators to assist policy makers in planning, assessing, managing, and monitoring the health workforce in countries. The Human Resources for Health Action Framework (HAF) is one of the group's main products. It seeks to compile the guidelines, tools, knowledge, and best practices on health workforce planning into a single, user-friendly, web-based tool.[15]

The Task Force on Scaling Up Education and Training was set up in March 2007 with the aim of finding evidence of previous scale-up initiatives around the world and how best to replicate these examples on a larger scale. It responds specifically to the 2006 World Health Assembly Resolution 59.23, where Member States urged particular attention to the issue of rapidly increasing the quantity and quality of health personnel. The Task Force concluded its work in mid 2008 and its report "Scaling up Saving Lives" was launched at the 61st World Health Assembly in May 2008. Accompanying the report is a series of country case studies, commissioned as part of the Task Force's work. The country case studies are from Bangladesh, Ethiopia, Ghana, Malawi, and Pakistan. These case studies describe successful scale up models which are central in bringing about improvements in the health status of their populations.[16]

The Health Worker Migration Policy Initiative[17] was launched during the World Health Assembly in May 2007, to identify and recommend solutions to what drives migration — the "push" factor, which means health workers want to leave their countries of origin (usually low-income countries), and the "pull" factor, which is observed in some rich countries whose health care workforces are not sufficient and where working conditions are better. The Initiative released recommendations to the WHO's Director-General with regard to an international Code of Practice on ethical recruitment of health personnel, which was presented to the World Health Assembly in 2009 for consideration and finally adopted at the same forum in 2010.

Financing human resources represent the largest single cost element in providing health services in developing countries. To improve the effectiveness of financing policies for HRH in developing countries, the Alliance established a Task Force on Financing in January 2008. It now completed its work and has coordinated the development of Resource Requirements Tool (RRT) and related technical papers, along with training of consultants and national personnel in Liberia, Ethiopia, the Philippines, Uganda, Peru, and Ghana on the use of the RRT.

The Task Force on the Private Sector, established in 2008 to identify additional and innovative sources of health workers from the non-State sector, undertook an assessment in three countries: Kenya, Mali, and Zambia — for the development of a health workforce incubator — a pilot model that offers technical capability, access to business expertise, and private and public financing. It also helps identify and develop partnerships with local affiliates, technical partners, and potential investors. Under this initiative, the Alliance supported the expansion of a distance learning initiative, which accelerates the certification of nurses in Kenya for deployment into other sub-Saharan countries.

The technical working group on "Access to HIV/AIDS Prevention, Treatment, Care and Support" was established in recognition of the fact that health worker shortages are a major obstacle to universal access to HIV/AIDS-related services. This technical working group was launched in March 2008 to review new and innovative strategies for scaling up, and to synthesise existing evidence and concrete experiences in order to identify approaches needed to respond to the HRH requirements for expanding HIV/AIDS-related services in a country. A number of country-based case studies have led to a set of recommendations on how different stakeholders can assist countries to reach universal access targets for HIV/AIDS prevention, treatment, care, and support.

Reliable data and evidence are the backbone of effective policy building in countries. Despite the view that rigorous statistics are scarce, diverse sources of information can be potentially used to produce relevant information, even in low-income countries. The Health Workforce Information Reference Group (HIRG) was created to address the challenges in improving HRH information. The ultimate goal is to establish and bolster country health workforce monitoring systems to support policy, planning, and research. The HIRG has developed the basis for a 2010–2011 biennium action plan to develop and implement a global strategy to promote standardised approaches to monitoring health workforce development; build institutional and individual capacities for HRH data collection, analysis, presentation, sharing, synthesis and use; and to mobilise technical and financial support for countries to monitor their health workforce.

GHWA also established a Reference Group, composed of academic institutions, global alliances, non-governmental organisations, professional associations, private sector entities, and country partners, to integrate their work that would accelerate country HRH action. Its first meeting was held in December 2009 in Geneva. The meeting recommended that the Reference Group will act as a think tank, and recommend innovative approaches with respect to knowledge brokering. The aim is to achieve the coordinated, cost-effective, efficient, and sustainable use of HRH-related products, tools, and methodologies at country level.

Other key initiatives of the GHWA

The Alliance also started communication and information exchange amongst stakeholders groups. The Health Workforce Advocacy Initiative (HWAI)[18] is dedicated to one of the Alliance's core functions, namely to keep human resources for health at the top of the agenda at the country, regional, and international level. HWAI is a civil society-led network affiliated with the Global Health Workforce Alliance. The initiative engages in evidence-based advocacy with the goal of enabling everyone to access skilled, motivated, and supported health workers who are part of well-functioning health systems. Towards this end, HWAI has launched a Campaign on Sustained and Adequate Health Workforce Financing to mobilise the considerable new resources required from wealthy countries and developing country governments, as well as to ensure that macroeconomic policies are consistent with health and other development financing needs. Along with the focus on adequate funding for health workforce and related health system strengthening, HWAI promotes the development of human rights-based health workforce strategies that are designed to achieve the Millennium Development Goals, universal access to HIV/AIDS treatment, prevention, care, and support by 2010, and other health goals and obligations. Working primarily through issue-focused teams that are open to anyone to join, HWAI is building a broader network of civil society, health workers, and anyone else interested in international health workforce advocacy.

The Alliance is also supporting the initiative of Positive Practice Environments (PPE) Campaign.[19] It is a worldwide campaign to generate public awareness and political will to introduce and maintain improved working conditions and environments within health systems. This is a country and facility-centred initiative focusing on all health care settings. The campaign aims to improve the quality of health services by raising awareness, identifying good practice, and developing tools for managers and health professionals in the field. Working collaboratively, the campaign has been initiated by the International Council of Nurses, The International Pharmaceutical Federation, the World Dental Federation, The World Medical Association, the International Hospital Federation, and the World Confederation for Physical Therapy, with the support of the Alliance.

The Alliance expanded the number of spokespersons to include new categories of representatives who could speak out on behalf of health workforce issues. It secured Princess Haya Bint Al Hussein of Dubai as Special Advocate. The Alliance also selected four other high-profile individuals as its champions. These new champions included in 2009 are: Professor Sheila Tlou, former Health Minister, Botswana; Lord Nigel Crisp, former Chief Executive of the National Health Service, United Kingdom; Professor Keizo Takemi, former State Secretary for Foreign Affairs of Japan; and Dr. Marc Danzon, former Regional Director of the WHO Regional Office for Europe.

The Alliance also supported the WHO-led E-Portuguese initiative in Angola, Brazil, Cape Verde, Guinea-Bissau, Mozambique, Portugal, Sao Tome and Principe, and Timor Leste to promote and strengthen collaboration among Portuguese-speaking countries. It contributes to the training and capacity building of the health workforce in these countries while enabling governments to have their own technical and scientific portal with a local directory of health events, health sites, and health legislation. These countries have developed their own national health libraries and strengthened HRH capacity by using information and communication technology (ICT) tools such as distance learning platforms and they have strengthened collaboration with other strategic initiatives, such as the Evidence-Informed Policy Network (EVIPNet), a WHO-hosted site that encourages policy makers to use evidence to improve health systems planning.

Challenges Faced and the Outcomes

Challenges

The health workforce related challenges are complex and multidimensional. The Alliance has actually used some of these challenges as a comparative advantage, in particular using them to provide a sound basis for the strategies, plans, and actions of the Alliance. Such challenges include the following:

1. The prevailing serious shortage of skilled health workers is most apparent and most critical in poor and developing countries. The effects of this shortage of manpower are further exacerbated by an inadequate and inequitable distribution of health workers where they do exist, and the complexity of diverse needs various regions and countries. This shortage of health workers in poor and underdeveloped countries is made even worse by their limited capacity, particularly their technical and institutional capacities.
2. These newly emerging health needs are overstretching the already over-burdened health sectors. Rising scales of global health issues and the emergence of new health problems further complicate the situation and require new skills among existing health staff. Coupled with this, disasters, wars, and conflicts create not only demand for specialised skills among existing health workers, but also make the security situation in work settings unsafe. These conditions contribute significantly to an increase in the brain drain of health workers to more secure and rich countries.

3. Resource limitation has been recognised as a key constraint in developing and poor countries. The available resources mostly are tagged with donors' objectives and agendas. The situation of resource constraints is particularly worsening in this era of economic crisis where countries have many other pressing needs influencing their priorities.
4. Regional and national interests are diverse, mostly determined according to their health care needs, political motives, and political agendas. Market forces also play an important role in this context. Many rich countries are benefiting from the health workforce migrated from poor countries but in most cases have failed to provide a justifiable level of financial, material, and technical support to the "losing" counties as a compensation for their lost resources.
5. Working environments and the practice of safety standards in different countries and institutions are usually a neglected area. At the same time, the implementation of quality standards and related regulations are also erratic in many settings whilst there is a need for their uniform application and practice.
6. Regional and cross border cooperation usually is not up to mark. This results in deficient collaboration amongst regional players and neighbouring countries, and inadequate regional policies and plans associated with variable practice of standards for training and education of a health workforce.
7. Along with increased trends of the double burden of disease of communicable and non-communicable diseases, ageing populations and a steep increase in chronic diseases worldwide are placing new demands on health workforces that are already inadequate, themselves ageing, and whose numbers are stagnating.
8. Poor governance and lack of transparency, particularly in the poor and underdeveloped countries, are mostly associated with pitiable health system planning and management, as well as an absence of implementation and monitoring systems. Redressing these challenges requires a great degree of top-level political commitment together with policy actions.

The outcomes

Together with its partners, the GHWA is striving to address complex challenges related to the health workforce crisis. The Alliance has maintained its dedication to the six interconnected strategies of the global Agenda for Action, while continuing to work in line with the guiding principles outlined in the "Moving Forward from Kampala" framework. Sticking to these broader lines of commitment in a dynamic global environment means remaining receptive to emerging issues. In a crowded environment of competing priorities, wider goals such as the MDGs, addressing the social determinants of health and renewed Primary Health Care (PHC), and the global crises in food, fuel, finance, and climate change, it is important to stay abreast of, and to respond to, emerging challenges to global HRH work. Furthermore, as the Alliance grows and its reach from the global arena into closer regional and national ties is extended and strengthened, re-confirming its position as a convener and player at all levels will be achieved through its work and actions.

At the global level, the Alliance has stayed abreast of the developments regarding the WHO process of developing a Code of Practice for the International Recruitment of Health Personnel. Along with the initiative of the Alliance's Health Worker Migration Policy Initiative, two consecutive World Health Assemblies have issued resolutions: WHA57.19[20] urging WHO and Members States for policy actions pertaining to "International migration of health personnel," and WHA 58.17[21] asking to intensify efforts on the resolution on "International migration of health personnel" and to strengthen WHO's programme on human resources for health by allocating to it adequate resources, in particular financial and human resources. The Alliance, its partners, and the Board have actively engaged in WHO discussions and negotiations, including civil society motions at the WHO's 126th Executive Board session in January 2010. The draft Code of Practice was discussed and negotiated at the 63rd WHA in May 2010.

In order to support countries in streamlining their coordination and management in addressing human resources for health challenges, the Alliance has started a series of consultations and negotiations with countries, based on a guidance document "Country Coordination and Facilitation," (CCF) with accompanying country assessment, tracking, and policy planning tools. The CCF is a coordinating process that builds on existing country mechanisms, promoted by the Alliance along the directions set out in the Kampala Declaration, but not owned or implemented by GHWA. It is the national leadership to decide on the use of the CCF as a framework for action. Seventeen countries are at various stages of developing their own costed

HRH plans utilising CCF mechanisms. GHWA members and partners in countries can support and facilitate such comprehensive, cross-sectoral dialogue in countries by integrating the CCF into their own approaches as stakeholders in health system support.

At the global level, the Alliance has gradually established important networks that were possible through negotiation and dialogue with the concerned stakeholders and interested parties. It also built bridges with other health-related partnerships in an effort to raise awareness of HRH which is one of the main bottlenecks that these partnerships face in fulfilling their mandates. GHWA has participated in discussions on the Global Fund's role in health systems; it is a member of the Health Systems Strengthening committee of the GAVI Alliance; it is a member of the Health Metrics Network steering committee; and it has commissioned joint work with the Alliance for Health Policy and Systems Research. The GHWA is sharing the HRH related information through its website as well as regular emailing of bulletins and other types of communication.

Lessons to be Learned

Working in multiple dimensions and arenas while addressing the health workforce-related challenges, GHWA has come across a number of lessons that need special consideration at all times. Some of these are described below.

1. Pressing health needs across the globe cannot be met without a well-trained, adequate, and available health workforce, and the health workers shortage has been a major impediment to making progress on meeting the health-related Millennium Development Goals.
2. Critical shortage of essentially required health workforce desperately indicates the urgent need to incorporate HRH in developmental strategies and plans. In particular, investment in health workforces needs to be enhanced based upon the local requirements and future projections.
3. Improving the national and local capacities can be significantly instrumental in achieving their health workforce-related targets and goals. Along with building institutional capacities, the under developed countries should also be provided with health workforce-related

development models and technical materials for their own adaptation and implementation.

4. Countries with critical shortages of health workforce should develop national plans incorporating a more efficient use of the existing health workforce and measures like improving governance and management systems with robust policies like task shifting — some simple health care tasks assigned to highly skilled personnel can be delegated to less skilled workers.

5. Sudden catastrophic events like natural disasters can quickly overwhelm local and national health systems already suffering from staff shortages or a lack of funds. Comprehensive preparedness plans in a country for a workforce response to outbreaks and emergencies should include plans for how health workers will collaborate with staff in the military, transport, and education sectors to maximise the efficiency of scarce human resources.

6. Conflicts and wars often cause severe and long-lasting damage to the health workforce in a country. Qualified personnel may be killed or forced to abandon their jobs. In protracted conflicts, a number of trends generally emerge, such as civilian workers flee from health centres and hospitals in dangerous areas, and those in safer areas become overstaffed; management systems collapse; working environments deteriorate; and professional values are eroded. In conflicts, health workers re-assigned to areas in need require protection and support. In this context, international donors and other major actors need to take measures to protect existing health worker networks.

7. Civil society and the private sector can play pivotal roles in health workforce development and retention. Their roles should be duly recognised, promoted, and streamlined to compensate the limitation of public sector resources and capacities. Better strategies to more actively engaging the communities and patients in their own health care have proven their worth in improving the quality of care and health outcomes.

Protection and fairer treatment of health workers in line with the international standards need due focus as workers face difficult and often dangerous working conditions, and receive poor salaries and incentives in many developing countries. With this, encouragement of women to enter the health profession can help in addressing the health workforce crisis. The specific requirements of women should be accommodated through flexible work arrangements and leadership career tracks adapted to family life.

8. Orientation and induction courses along with in-service training and development programmes can help in staff retention. Career incentives to health workers as a means of encouraging service in rural and disadvantaged areas would help counteract the tendency of health workers to cluster around cities.

9. Domestic cross-sector leadership is essential, together with well-tailored collaboration with partners in developing evidence-based knowledge and tools, enabling policies for collaboration through education and training, finance, information, management, and retention. Health sector plans and programmes, linked to donor instruments and collaborative frameworks for public and private service providers and professional bodies, exist in many countries in varying degrees of functionality.

10. The human resources for health challenges must be understood as a critical element of the efforts to strengthen health systems by all actors in development. Ministries of Health, Finance, Labour, and Education are key actors for diagnosing the constraints and finding the right solutions in human resources for health, along with regulatory bodies, public service commissions, professional associations, civil society, and other private and public actors around the health workforce market.

11. Measures as salary top ups, training of special cadres, and varied incentive systems for retention and results need to be assessed in a broader framework than the health sector alone, including with partners in the world of work and the impact of these measures on both the public and the private domain.

12. Research should be promoted to build an updated evidence base on health workforces, particularly for needs assessments, future projections, and identifying local and national level potentials, since an evidence base can provide a sound basis for policy and planning development, as well as monitoring of goals and objectives.

Conclusion

The Alliance has established itself as a global leader in health workforce advocacy, convening, and knowledge-brokering, advocating for health workforce issues, and directly supporting the countries and partners. Keeping in view the extent of the health workforce needs in various countries and regions, and viewing the complexity of the related issues, the GHWA is working through global, regional, and national entities and partners to quantify the problems, mobilise the partnerships, generate resources, build local capacities, and implement need-based health workforce developmental programmes. The Alliance is privileged by a special relationship with the WHO. In rolling out its various programmes of work, and through its Country Coordination and Facilitation (CCF) mechanism, it is also increasingly recognised at global, regional, national, and local levels.

Since the First Forum, a growing body of evidence and experience from countries has become available that underline the basic principles of the Kampala Declaration and Agenda for Global Action, specifically — that sustainable solutions to close the gaps in access to skilled health workers need to be found on country-by-country basis.

Carrying forward the Agenda for Global Action and the Kampala Declaration, the Second Global Forum on Human Resources for Health (the Forum) is being convened by the Global Health Workforce Alliance, the Prince Mahidol Award Conference, the World Health Organization, the Japan International Cooperation Agency, with additional support by many other agencies, especially the Rockefeller Foundation, the China Medical Board, and the World Bank. The Forum will be held in Bangkok, Thailand from 25–29 January, 2011. The principal theme of the Forum is "reviewing progress, renewing commitments to health workers towards MDGs and beyond." The Forum will build upon the successes achieved in Kampala and will provide a platform to review progress made in fulfilling the commitments outlined in the Kampala Declaration and the Agenda for Global Action. It will be an opportunity to further galvanize and accelerate the global movement on HRH towards achieving the Millennium Development Goals and Universal Health Coverage. The Second Global Forum on HRH will also honour successful country case stories and individual health workers with prestigious HRH awards. This is the first time that such recognition will be conferred to health sector human resource efforts.

Whilst these are a central focus of the Alliance's work in the build-up to the Second Forum, the Alliance and particularly its Secretariat responded to the success of Kampala in elaborating "Moving Forward from Kampala," which lays out the Alliance's programme of work for 2009–2011 according to five broad areas of activity:

1. Facilitating country actions
2. Continuing advocacy
3. Brokering knowledge
4. Promoting synergy amongst partners
5. Monitoring the effectiveness of interventions

The Global Health Workforce Alliance will continue to build upon its achievements. Its foundations are firmly set in the Kampala Declaration and the Agenda for Global Action, and guided by the workplan detailed in "Moving Forward from Kampala."[22] Looking beyond 2011, in striving to think more globally and act more locally, new issues and challenges will arise on the road to achieving the Alliance's vision.

References

1. The Joint Learning Initiative, Harvard University Press (2004) "Overcoming the Crisis: Report of the Joint Learning Initiative", and http://www.healthgap.org/camp/hcw_docs/JLi_Human_Resources_for_Health.pdf, accessed on 10 March 2010.
2. High-level Forum on Health MDGs, accessed from http://www.hlfhealth-mdgs.org/, accessed on 12 July 2010.
3. World Health Report 2006 "Working together for health", accessed from http://www.who.int/whr/2006/en/index.html, on 12 July 2010.
4. GHWA website: History of the Alliance: accessed from http://www.who.int/workforcealliance/about/history/en/index.html, on 12 July 2010.
5. Global Health Workforce Alliance: Strategic Plan (2006); accessed from http://www.who.int/workforcealliance/GHWA_STRATEGIC%20PLAN_ENGLISH_WEB.pdf, on 10 March 2010.

6. GHWA website: Alliance Board: accessed from http://www.who.int/ workforcealliance/about/governance/board/en/index.html on 12 July 2010.

7. GHWA website: Alliance Secretariat: accessed from http://www.who. int/workforcealliance/about/governance/secretariat/en/index.html, on 12 July 2010.

8. GHWA website: Members and Partners: accessed from http://www.who.int/ workforcealliance/members_partners/en/, on 12 July 2010.

9. GHWA website: Alliance vision and mission: accessed from http://www.who. int/workforcealliance/about/vision_mission/en/index.html, on 12 July 2010.

10. GHWA website: First Global Forum on Human resources for Health, 2-7 March 2008, Kampala, Uganda: accessed from http://www.who.int/ workforcealliance/forum/2008/en/index.html, on 12 July 2010.

11. GHWA (2008) The Kampala Declaration and Agenda for Global Action, accessed from ttp://www.who.int/workforcealliance/knowledge/resources/ kampala_declaration/en/index.html, on 12 July 2010.

12. http://www.g8italia2009.it/static/G8_Allegato/G8_Declaration_08_07_ 09_final,0.pdf (para 121).

13. GHWA (2009) Catalyst for Change report, 19_6_10_HQ_AR_Final Final for distribution, accessed on 12 Aug 2010.

14. GHWA website: Task Forces and Working Groups: accessed from http:// www.who.int/workforcealliance/about/taskforces/en/index.html, on 12 July 2010.

15. GHWA website: Working Group on Tools and Guidelines: accessed from http://www.who.int/workforcealliance/about/taskforces/tools_guidelines/en/ index.html, on 12 July 2010.

16. GHWA website: Task Force on Education and Training: accessed from http://www.who.int/workforcealliance/about/taskforces/education_training/ en/, on 12 July 2010.

17. GHWA website: Task force on Migration — health Workers migration Policy Initiative: accessed from http://www.who.int/workforcealliance/about/ taskforces/migration/en/index.html, on 12 July 2010.

18. GHWA website: Health Workforce Advocacy Initiative: accessed from http://www.who.int/workforcealliance/about/initiatives/hwai/en/index.html, on 12 July 2010.

19. GHWA website: Positive Practice environments Campaign: accessed from http://www.who.int/workforcealliance/about/initiatives/ppe/en/index.html, on 12 July 2010.

20. WHA57.19 International migration of health personnel: a challenge for health systems in developing countries: accessed from http://apps.who.int/gb/ebwha/pdf_files/WHA57/A57_R19-en.pdf, on 12 July 2010.

21. WHA58.17 International migration of health personnel: a challenge for health systems in developing countries: accessed from http://apps.who.int/gb/ebwha/pdf_files/WHA58/WHA58_17-en.pdf, on 12 July 2010.

22. GHWA: Moving Forward from Kampala (2009): accessed from http://www.who.int/workforcealliance/knowledge/resources/moving_forward/en/index.html, on 12 July 2010.

15

The US President's Emergency Plan for AIDS Relief: Negotiating a Recreation in Global Health and Development

Mark Dybul[i]

Abstract

Against the emergency of the HIV/AIDS pandemic, U.S. President George W. Bush launched the USD15 billion President's Emergency Plan for AIDS Relief (PEPFAR) — the largest international health initiative in history targeting a single disease, and a milestone for public diplomacy. This case study tells the story of the complex, and not always uncontroversial, process of bringing a wide variety of stakeholders to work together on the same agenda. PEPFAR's success led to a new U.S. government approach in international development and global health. It catalysed a paradigm shift from paternalism to action by empowered citizens through partnership. PEPFAR created collaboration amongst U.S. government departments, foreign governments, civil society, and other stakeholders active in the fight against HIV/AIDS. These efforts also have resulted in better relations between nations.

---

[i] The Hon. Mark Dybul is currently a Distinguished Scholar and Co-Director of the Global Health Center of the O'Neill Institute for National and International Health Law, Georgetown University and the inaugural Global Health Fellow of the George W. Bush Institute. He was the US Global AIDS Coordinator from 2006 to 2009.

The Problem

In 2003, it was estimated that 42 million people were living with HIV, more than 20 million had died, 3 million were dying and 5 million were becoming infected each year and there were 12 million AIDS orphans. HIV was called the Black Plague of the modern era. Two-thirds of the disease was concentrated in Sub-Saharan Africa. Yet the global response was anemic. Despite significant expressions of concern, less than $4 billion per year was dedicated to combating the pandemic. By contrast, in the US nearly $16 billion was being spent annually for one million HIV positive people and 40,000 new infections per year.

Against that backdrop, President George W. Bush launched the $15 billion US President's Emergency Plan for AIDS Relief (PEPFAR), the largest international health initiative in history for a single disease, designed to support national scale-up of integrated prevention, treatment and care programs with specific targets in countries with half the disease in the world. The Journal *Lancet* called PEPFAR "the largest and most successful bilateral HIV/AIDS programme in the world,"[1] the news magazine television show *60 Minutes* hailed it as "monumental,"[2] President Obama has praised the initiative and President Bush for his efforts; and Secretary of State Hilary Clinton described it as the "one of our countries' most notable successes in development."[3] The strong bipartisan Congressional support that was required to initiate and maintain PEPFAR was reflected by the provision of $18.8 billion for 2004 to 2008 and a legislative renewal at the previously unimaginable level of $39 billion for HIV/AIDS for the following 5 years. Perhaps most important, African Heads of State, First Ladies, Ministers of Health, and local leaders from every sector have pointed to PEPFAR as a great life saving measure that helped to usher in a new era in development that put them in charge and moved from paternalism to partnership.

But such laudatory statements were not always forthcoming. Following the initial round of positive reactions to the announcement, concerns began to surface. As the US Government process moved from a Presidential announcement to the passage of enacting legislation, difficult and controversial issues emerged. In many ways, the early problems were a direct manifestation of the policy process that led to the creation of PEPFAR. President Bush had decided that there was a global emergency that required a rapid response. He also decided that a new way of doing business was needed — that the solution was not just to "write a bigger check." In 2002, President Bush led an historic agreement on a new approach to development — the Monterrey Consensus. Reduced to its essence, the Communiqué, adopted by Heads of State from high-, low- and middle-income countries in Monterrey, Mexico, shifted development to a partnership framework based in the need for countries to "own" development efforts in their country, including strategic leadership and economic growth as the ultimate engine of true development. Country ownership requires good governance, a results-based approach and all sectors, including non-governmental and private sectors, being engaged and acknowledging economic growth as the ultimate engine of sustainable development. These foundational elements were the core of Bush's approach to development and were a prerequisite for his more than doubling of resources, including a six-fold increase for Africa[4] and served as the animating principles for his key international development initiatives — the Millennium Challenge Corporation, the President's Malaria Initiative, the African and International Education Initiatives, the Women's Empowerment and Justice Initiative and, the largest, PEPFAR.

On the day that President Bush announced his International Prevention of Mother and Child HIV Initiative (Mother and Child Initiative), a $500 million effort to reduce the transmission of the virus from mothers to children by half in 12 countries and the Caribbean, he instructed then Deputy Chief of Staff, Josh Bolten, to "think big." That direction was quickly relayed to the small team that was to develop the implementation plan that the President adopted and which served as the basis for the enacting legislation and the operationalisation of the programme.

The normal US Government policy process would have been an interagency negotiation that can be extremely lengthy and tends to go from bold ideas to the least common denominator to satisfy the many stakeholders involved. Such a process is useful and sound for routine business to ensure all viewpoints and options are explored. But it is not well suited to an emergency situation. And one of the three main activities of the initiative alongside prevention and care was treatment. PEPFAR was the first global effort to squarely acknowledge the public health requirement to integrate prevention with treatment and care and that arguing in favour of one over the other was deadly. With 5 million people receiving antiretroviral therapy in low- and middle-income countries today,[5] it is difficult to remember that in 2003 there was little support for it. Leaders in international organisations and the US Government thought treatment was not possible and some even claimed it was wrong to do anything but prevention. Such forces colluded to preclude a treatment goal for HIV among the Millennium Development Goals. Resolving such a contentious issue through the inter-agency process would have been time-consuming and there was no guarantee of ultimate success or support. At the direction of the President, that process was to be by-passed to ensure an urgent response to the global crisis. The development of the plan and the plan itself were kept secret amongst a very small group of advisors and was not made public until the State of the Union Address (SOTU) in January 2003. The SOTU is the most important policy address for the President and sets the priorities for the coming year.

While keeping PEPFAR secret had the advantage of rapid and bold action including a treatment component, there were downsides. While US Presidents have significant authority and power, the separation of powers in the governing structure gives Congress the power of the purse. President Bush calling for $15 billion for a focused programme on HIV was only a starting point — Congress and the many constituency groups with influence and their own priorities related to HIV and to development more broadly would need to support the programme and agree to resource allocations. Although the President is the head of the Executive Branch, the bureaucracy has long-established processes to slow, undermine, and even prevent the implementation of Presidential directives. Cabinet Secretaries, members of Congress, and key leaders in the Executive Branch were informed of the President's decision and the content of the SOTU the day before or morning of the speech. Very few advocates and members of key HIV and development constituencies knew about the initiative until they heard it in the SOTU. It is the nature of human beings and bureaucracies to resist ideas and programmes unless they were engaged in their creation. While there were initial laudatory comments from many sectors, grumbling, discontent, and doubt followed shortly thereafter.

Perhaps of greatest concern was the fact that although PEPFAR was to encompass all US Government activities in global HIV, the vast majority of new resources were to be concentrated in 14 "focus countries" in Africa and Latin America which were home to half the disease burden in the world (of note, Vietnam was added following Congressional direction that a country in another region be selected). The governments of those countries were notified within 48 hours of the announcement. Because of the President's leadership in creating the Monterrey Consensus with its foundational principle of country ownership and his strong personal belief in the need to move from paternalism to partnership in development, an announcement that money would be dedicated and prevention, treatment, and care goals would be set by the US for 14 countries was not without difficulties. Compounding the problem was that certain countries already had strong national leadership and programmes and certain Heads of State were not interested in large HIV programmes.

The fundamental problem was how to harness all of the positive energy engendered by President Bush's personal commitment to the largest international health initiative for a single disease in history while attenuating the less positive reaction to a surprise announcement and secret plan that was developed without the input of stakeholders who would be essential to its success. The diplomatic challenge was to get everyone under the same tent.

The Local and External Players and Their Roles

President George W. Bush

President Bush's role in PEPFAR cannot be overstated. Quite simply, PEPFAR would not exist without him, and the global response to HIV would be a slim shadow of what it is today. From the creation through its implementation and legislative renewal, he was the driving force. There have been published hypotheses as to why he acted, who was whispering in his ear, the geopolitics involved, etc. They are inaccurate and have been proffered by people without access to him or the people who were engaged in the process. He is a voracious reader and knew about global HIV without technocrats or advocates providing information — although he has acknowledged that Condi Rice, the top national security advisor to then-Governor and Presidential candidate Bush, pressed engagement in

Africa during the 2000 campaign. He did it because he felt deeply that it was the right thing to do. In nearly every public or private comment about PEPFAR and the many other development initiatives he pursued while doubling resources, he quoted from the Bible: "to whom much is given, much is required." The reason PEPFAR succeeded was because of the personal and direct interest and engagement of President Bush. It is also important to note that First Lady Laura Bush played key roles shining a light on PEPFAR in the US, on her trips that took her to many countries around the world and as a strong supporter within the White House.

The Bush administration

The President was ably supported by members of the White House under the direct supervision of then Deputy Chief of Staff Josh Bolten. Josh was the high-level "angel" of President Bush's efforts on HIV in his different Administration incarnations including Director of the Office of Management and Budget and Chief of Staff. A small team from the White House (Gary Edson, Jay Lefkowtiz, Margaret Spellings, Robin Cleveland, Kristen Silverberg and, later, Joseph O'Neill) and Dr. Anthony Fauci from the National Institutes of Health (NIH) and I, then at NIH, worked to develop the plan that became the basis for the SOTU announcement, the enacting legislation, and the implementation of the programme.

In 2003, President Bush nominated, and Congress later confirmed Ambassador Randall Tobias as the first US Global AIDS Coordinator (the Coordinator). He is a thoughtful and wise man who brought gravitas to the programme due to his long and distinguished career in the private sector. I served Ambassador Tobias as Deputy Chief Medical Officer, Assistant Coordinator, and Deputy Coordinator before becoming Acting Coordinator and, ultimately, Coordinator when Ambassador Tobias became Administrator of USAID and the first Director of US Foreign Assistance to work to integrate the entire US development portfolio.

One of the important aspects of PEPFAR was to bring the various US Departments and Agencies together under a unified funding source and strategic vision. The Coordinator reported to the Secretary of State by law. For the first time, the Department of State became the major player in HIV with the engagement of the top political leadership as well as the Ambassadors in each of the 14 focus country. However, the role of the State Department was in setting strategic direction and directing resources. Secretary Powell and Secretary Rice were strong supporters of PEPFAR. Implementation was the domain of organisations that had on-going HIV programmes and, in many cases, staff on the ground. The largest actors were the US Agency for International Development (USAID), the Department of Health and Human Services (HHS) and its operating divisions — most notably the Center for Disease Control and Prevention (CDC), however the Health Resources and Services Administration (HRSA) and the National Institutes of Health (NIH) were also engaged (Secretary Thompson led several important delegations to Africa and his successor, Secretary Leavitt, was engaged and supportive). In addition, the Department of Defense and the Peace Corps were involved. Because of the personal commitment and engagement of the President, the highest political level in each organisation paid attention to PEPFAR.

The Congress of the United States

As noted above, the separation of powers in the United States gives the power of the purse to the Congress. The Congress has two main legislative functions: to authorise the use of resources and the appropriation and oversight of the use of those resources. Authorising legislation generally covers a resource envelope for several years, while appropriations is an annual activity following the submission of a budget request by the President to Congress. The principal Congressional Committees with oversight over authorisation and appropriations for PEPFAR have a long history of bipartisanship and that set the tone for significant support from both parties and overwhelming majorities to adopt the authorising and re-authorising legislation and annual appropriations that exceeded the $15 billion total that was originally proposed. The bipartisan support was maintained regardless of which party was in power. In November of 2006, the President's Party lost control of both chambers, yet resource commitment remained strong and the 2008 re-authorisation passed under their watch. After initial difficulties due to the surprise announcement, PEPFAR enjoyed strong bipartisan support, the importance of which cannot be overstated. There were many important leaders in Congress from both sides of the aisle who supported PEPFAR and they had some of the most talented and thoughtful staff in Washington, DC.

Civil society

Once President Bush made the decision to pursue a massive effort on global HIV and announced it in his SOTU, the support from various elements of civil society became important for the passage of both authorisations and the annual budgets. There was an effective coalition of traditional non-governmental organisations and HIV advocates that tend to the more liberal end of the political spectrum, faith-based organisations with a wide range of political views but strong engagement of a number of more conservative groups, and the corporate sector. The broad spectrum of advocacy for PEPFAR promoted the strong bipartisan support for the programme. However, as with any loose coalition that tries to find common ground among various perspectives, the PEPFAR coalition was fragile and disagreements about a few policy issues were difficult to manage. Very conservative and very liberal groups, which likely constituted no more than ten per cent of individuals and organisations, occasionally tried to divide the moderate majority. But civil society generally held together and supported the package of tradeoffs and compromises for both authorising laws and annual appropriations legislation. The organisations and individuals are too numerous to mention.

National governments and local civil society

The final partner is the most important partner — the people of the countries in which PEPFAR served. One key strategic decision in the design of PEPFAR was to support national scale-up of prevention, treatment, and care. While pilot projects can be managed from the US or Europe, widespread services requires local leadership and the involvement of all sectors of a country's society. Because of President Bush's personal commitment to PEPFAR and his insistence that it lead an effort to move from paternalism to partnership in development, Heads of State were engaged. It was known that when there was a meeting with Bush, part of the agenda would be PEPFAR, other Presidential initiatives, and development in general. In certain countries, the Heads of State were already engaged. President Mojae in Botswana had begun a significant effort with his national budget and support from the Gates Foundation and the Merck company. Ministers of Health and their staff led the national strategic processes and in nearly all countries were fully involved and committed. In certain countries, the public sector was the main provider of health care as well as the leader in planning. In other countries, non-government implementers were the dominant implementers. For example, the World Health Organization (WHO) estimates that 30 to 70 per cent of health care in Sub-Saharan Africa is provided by faith-based organizations.[6] In several countries, local groups that had begun as support groups for the dying became significant health service providers for the living. Although nascent in many places, local advocacy groups became very active over time.

Challenges Faced and the Outcomes

One of the greatest challenges in the development and implementation of PEPFAR was to build support for a programme that was developed in secret and to bring a wide variety of stakeholders and actors to work together with the same agenda to achieve the same goals.

The Executive Branch of the United States government

When President Bush took office, the US Government's commitment was approximately $500 million. President Bush was clear that the solution was not simply "to write a bigger" check, but that part of the solution had to be to change the culture and structure of the US Government. When PEPFAR began, six US Government Departments and Agencies were active in global HIV. USAID had long-standing programmes and staff throughout the world with national and regional programmes and controlled more than 60 per cent of the resources. The Global AIDS Program (GAP) of CDC was active with staff in 25 countries with a few regional offices and an annual budget of approximately $150 million. The Department of Defense dedicated a little under $10 million per year to work with militaries, which are heavily affected by HIV. Peace Corps volunteers in endemic areas were trained in basic HIV facts and prevention education. The Department of Labor had a small programme with staff in a handful of countries dedicated to workplace issues, generally in partnership with the International Labour Organization of the United Nations. The Department of State nominally oversaw all activities of the US Government in-country and in a few places had public education programmes. In Africa, several Ambassadors used resources from their limited "Ambassador's Fund" for HIV projects.

Prior to PEPFAR, each organisation functioned independently. There was no common strategic framework for the deployment of staff or resources. It was not uncommon for staff from different agencies working in the same country, sometimes in the same area of the country, on the same intervention not to know each other. To ensure the autonomy of the agencies, the US Ambassador was rarely informed about the specifics of what they were doing or funding levels. The culture was that each organisation was responsible to their headquarters and to the Congressional Committee with oversight for their funding. The headquarters culture was often more insular than the field. It was at the central level that turf protection was at its peak, often driven by competition for resources and the natural tendency of human beings to want to be in charge. A deeper problem with competition for resources was that the US development culture was driven largely by the dollars dedicated, not to results achieved.

Organisational structure followed culture — planning and reporting were kept internal to the organisation and its Congressional funders. It was not, and still is not, uncommon for agencies to work with Congress to circumvent the President's budget request or policy direction. In some sense, the HIV activities of the US Government were as closely guarded a secret as the process that created PEPFAR. None of this was unique to global HIV or development. But obviously, such an arrangement did not allow for strategic allocation of resources, caused duplication and inefficiency, and was a poor use of US taxpayer dollars.

Perhaps more troubling, the host government had little idea of what the US Government was doing in their country, or how much money was being committed. International and local partners also were in the dark. While there would be collaboration and cooperation with the national and local government and international partners on specific projects or even each organisation's overall approach, there was no clear picture of the totality of US Government engagement on HIV within the US Government or with any of its partners. In such a setting, it was difficult for the national governments to develop comprehensive strategic plans. In other words, country ownership was effectively impossible.

The environment naturally set bureaucratic wheels in motion to stop, slow, or redirect a plan that was developed in secret by a small team, launched by the President without input from stakeholders and with very short advanced notice to even top political leadership. Presidential Initiatives are not uncommon — at the time PEPFAR was announced, USAID was managing more than a dozen of them. Many programmes have been launched only to languish in a system that knows that it need only throw up enough roadblocks to get through one or at most two Presidential terms of four years, and that with competing priorities and many initiatives, the President and White House staff cannot stay on top of all of them. An opening salvo was fired when a key member of one of the larger implementing agencies publicly referred to PEPFAR as "half baked."

The outcome: changing organisational culture and structure

Results-based financing

Perhaps the most lasting legacy of President Bush in development is the shift from a culture dominated by resources promised to results achieved. From today's perspective with the persistent mantra of results-based financing, it is difficult to recall that PEPFAR was heavily criticised for setting numeric targets. Development was too complex for concrete, short-term results. While a results-base was a core principle of the Monterrey Consensus, it had not yet become engrained in the culture of development.

President Bush insisted that PEPFAR set aggressive but achievable targets, and that intermediary benchmarks be set to assess progress. From those targets, a budget would be determined. He would not write a bigger check and then try to figure out what to do with the money. The goals the President set were to support treatment for 2 million people (half the estimated persons requiring treatment in the Focus Countries), the prevention of 7 million new infections (a 60 per cent reduction in projected new infections in the Focus Countries), and care for 10 million HIV-positive persons and the orphans left behind. The treatment and care targets were to be reached in 5 years, the prevention goal in seven years, based on available forecasts for results with dollars committed and the fact that evaluations of infections averted cannot be accurately done more than every few years in each country. The targets were ordered not to indicate prioritisation, but to provide a tool for public diplomacy and create an internal culture of results orientation — "2-7–10" rolls off the tongue with greater ease than "7-10-2" or "10-7-2." Focusing on saving and lifting up lives was not only important for the historic re-direction of the purpose of development, it was important for the day-to-day management of the culture of US Government organisations. The vast majority of personnel in the Departments and Agencies of the US Government engaged in global HIV, and in fact in development, are amongst the most talented, caring, dedicated, and decent human beings one will ever come across. They give much of themselves, sometimes even their lives, to serve others. They did not commit to traveling to distant lands removed from family and friends to fight for control of budgets. Focusing on 2-7-10 elevated the purpose of the programme to save and lift up lives — which is why they signed up. The goals provided a sense of being part of something much bigger than institutional loyalty. PEPFAR became the opportunity to fulfill the life ambition of service for those fortunate to be engaged. That sense of service, and of seeing results reported twice per year, provided a powerful incentive to overcome the initial territorial resistance to the programme.

But it is human nature that the early energy engendered by a new life saving programme will wane as the machinery of government inexorably takes over. A lasting effect of the culture of results is creating a new competition between implementing agencies. Competition for resources was tied to competition for results: whichever organisation was achieving more would be far more likely to secure a greater piece of the resource pie. That shift in culture, like the global shift the Monterrey Consensus began and PEPFAR did much to advance, is likely to be a lasting legacy.

Finally, 2-7-10 was an important tool of public diplomacy. It told host countries that PEPFAR was serious about making the money work and it told Congress that the resources they committed would be put to good use, and reinforced the notion of a high return on investment.

Presidential engagement

To re-set organisational culture and build a structure that would ensure results required the direct and personal engagement of President Bush and, through him, his inner circle at the White House. The President's team was aware of the agency resistance that would be fueled by a surprise announcement that did not include their input. Several key steps were taken to ensure that a strong message was delivered that PEPFAR was not just another Presidential Initiative. The first step was dedicating several paragraphs in the SOTU, the most important policy speech a President delivers. Every word in each Address is parsed and reconsidered. However, not all new programmes announced in the SOTU come to fruition — and the bureaucracy knows that. To reinforce the importance of PEPFAR, the President called together leaders in government and the development community to the White House Complex to deliver a separate speech on PEPFAR several days after the SOTU. Weekly inter-agency meetings were convened by the White House to begin the planning process even before Congressional action on authorisation or appropriations. When Congress was slower to act than was desired, President Bush held an event in the East Room of the White House to encourage swift action with the leaders of the key Congressional Committees from each chamber, and a large representation from civil society who could put pressure on them. The President signed the legislation two months later.

The role of Coordinator was at the level of an Assistant Secretary of State. Presidents hold formal events or press conferences to announce the nomination of Cabinet members. The announcement of Assistant Secretaries, and even Deputy and Under Secretaries, is usually relegated to a release of all new nominations that day. However, President Bush held a press conference in the meeting room adjacent to the Oval Office to introduce Randall Tobias as his nominee to become the first US Global AIDS Coordinator. In 2004, the President held the first ever World AIDS Day event at the White House, dedicated almost entirely to global HIV. Regardless of the demands of his schedule, he and Mrs. Bush commemorated every World AIDS Day with an event at the White House, or even traveling to meet with the "foot soldiers of compassion" implementing programmes. In 2007, the White House broke with long-standing tradition not to adorn the White House with the various ribbons that mark causes and draped a massive red ribbon — symbolizing solidarity in the fight against HIV- on the North Portico — a practice that has continued in the Obama Administration. The President mentioned PEPFAR in speeches related to foreign affairs with great regularity — often going off script to provide greater emphasis to his knowledge of and support for the programme. Importantly, with the assent of the Secretary of State, it was well known within the system that the Coordinator had direct access to the most senior members of the White House and, effectively, reported to the President.

The many actions of the President were done with great intent by him and his staff and had the desired effect, sending a clear message of the personal commitment and engagement of the President that reverberated from the political leadership of Departments and agencies to staff in the field and provided the foundation for significant changes in culture and structure. In effect, the President and his Administration were engaged in public diplomacy directed at the Executive Branch of the United States Government.

New money controlled by the coordinator

There is no doubt that the infusion of significant new resources was essential for achieving the prevention, treatment, and care targets, but also to open the way for cultural and structural change. It is very difficult to move a bureaucracy if there is no incentive beyond pleasing the President. Fifteen billion dollars — 10 of it new money — would allow the career development and health officials and their political leadership to fulfill their desire to make a significant difference in the world. Simply dividing the money among the US Government organisations implementing global HIV programmes to achieve targets would not have fixed the fundamental duplication and inefficiencies inherent in the existing fragmented approach. During the planning process, the White House members of the small planning team decided on the need for one person to provide strategic direction with control of resources to guarantee that direction was followed. The Coordinator was to develop a unified approach to the use of resources squarely focused on achieving the targets.

To ensure that the Coordinator had the necessary leverage and power to succeed, Congress codified into law that the President would appoint, and the Senate would confirm, a Global AIDS Coordinator with the rank of Ambassador who would report directly to the Secretary of State. The magnitude of budgetary control cannot be overstated. A Coordinator that does not control the allocation of resources has little ability to effect change.

Following the well-established pattern by the White House staff to use public diplomacy directed at the US Government, the President chose to sign the authorising legislation at a ceremony held at the Department of State, sending a clear signal that the center of gravity for PEPFAR would be there. Soon after Ambassador Tobias was confirmed by the Senate, President Bush convened a meeting in the Oval Office with Secretaries Powell and Thompson and Administrator Natsios of USAID, gave Tobias the seat of honour despite his lower rank and made clear his instructions that their staff were to follow his lead. The message was received. From that day forward, there was no question about who was in charge.

Inter-agency ownership

While control over resources was an essential starting point in the organisational structure, overreaching can be counterproductive. It was important to establish a strong inter-agency approach both at headquarters and in the field, to create an effective division of labour between organisations and between staff in headquarters and stationed abroad. To draw the best out of each person and agency, all parties needed to have a sense of ownership. PEPFAR was fortunate to follow the Mother and Child Initiative, which struggled through the development of inter-agency processes and the balance between headquarters and the field that were continued and expanded. An essential component of the structural reforms of both Initiatives was to listen to concerns of staff and to continually change as lessons were learned. The Institute of Medicine called PEPFAR a "learning organization" in its Congressionally required review of the programme.[7]

A weekly headquarters meeting of inter-agency Principals chaired by the Coordinator was quickly created to review major policy and strategy issues.

Although final decisions rested with the Coordinator, there was an openness to all viewpoints and collegial debate. The group, however, was dominated by political appointees. It was quickly determined that a similar meeting of the top career staff from each implementing agency was required to create buy-in and ownership throughout the organisations and to ensure continuity when political leadership changed. A weekly Deputy Principals meeting was established to precede the Principals meeting to work through implementation issues and to develop agenda items and recommendations for the Principals. Inter-agency Core Teams were established for groups of two to three focus countries to interact with the field, including communicating and clarifying strategic and policy direction, securing technical support, and serving as an advocate at headquarters. Inter-agency technical teams, eventually for 15 technical areas, were created to further promote programmatic cohesion, integrity, and consistency, and to integrate the agencies at all levels.

The inter-agency structure at headquarters was to be reflected in each focus country, and later in an expanding universe of countries with significant resources. Regular inter-agency meetings were established in each country and inter-agency technical groups were also created. Co-location of at least USAID and CDC was strongly encouraged — in some countries they were several hours removed by car due to traffic.

Key role of the US Ambassador

A lesson learned from the experience of the Mother and Child Initiative was that someone in a position of authority including the power of the purse had to be responsible for inter-agency coordination in the field. As the President's representative and an official of the Department of State, the US Ambassador/Chief of Mission was a natural choice. However, as noted above, historically agencies were not always forthcoming with the Ambassador regarding their activities or budget levels. To overcome that obstacle and empower the Ambassador, the funding structure was designed to require the Chief of Mission to approve the annual Country Operations Plan (COP) in each focus country before it was submitted to headquarters for review. In fact, the COP had to be submitted *by* the Ambassador. The COP included an overall strategy for US engagement including an explanation of how US resources supported the national strategy and leveraged other resources available in that country, annual and five-year targets for key indicators, resources and staff for each agency, and a list of partners with funding level and targets related to 2-7-10 for each partner. The COP was then submitted to the Coordinator for review by inter-agency technical and policy teams and presented by the Deputy Principals for final decisions by the Coordinator. The COP was a key innovation to ensure a unified strategy and inter-agency coordination both at headquarters and in the field. Because the Ambassador had to approve and submit the COP, and therefore was responsible for its content and results, they became very engaged.

To encourage the active participation of the Chief of Mission, successive Secretaries, Deputy Secretaries and Undersecretaries for Political Affairs reinforced the responsibility of the Ambassador to make PEPFAR a success, including through formal cables to the field. In a few cases, the Assistant Secretary of State for Africa telephoned a recalcitrant Ambassador. The availability of significant new resources and, for the first time, the ability to actively engage with the agencies in how they were used and to resolve disputes, certainly contributed to the interest of the Chief of Mission in PEPFAR.

To further encourage the participation of Ambassadors and foreign service officers, basic HIV education became, for the first time, part of the curriculum of the Foreign Service Academy and became, for the first time, part of the formal training for out-going Ambassadors. The new Ambassadors to the focus countries had routine meetings with the Coordinator before being posted or when back in Washington, D.C. for consultations and the Coordinator spoke at each annual meeting of Chiefs of Mission from Africa. There was also an annual PEPFAR meeting to review major policy, strategy, and implementation issues and the Ambassadors were featured on panels. Finally, a monthly phone call between the Coordinator and the Ambassadors in the focus countries was held for about one year before that became unnecessary.

Despite all of the structural changes that were made to promote inter-agency coordination, it became clear that much depended on the inclination of individuals and over time, as the novelty of the programme waned, inter-agency turf battles increased. One of the insights of PEPFAR was that an effective response to global HIV required all agencies, with their different strengths and expertise, to engage with a division of labour that would maximise efficiencies. However, over time the agencies began to replicate each other, for example USAID began hiring many more technical experts while CDC was growing its procurement staff. This growing inefficiency led to a significant increase in staff that seemed to have duplicative functions. In response, the "Staffing for Results" initiative was launched. The concept was that there should be one organisational chart for US Government personnel engaged in PEPFAR that identified the roles that were needed to get the job done. Ambassadors were directed to work with their coordinator and agencies to develop such an organisational chart, and then populate it with existing staff or hire those needed irrespective of home agency. For example, a working group on prevention should have an expert manager who was engaged in all prevention programmes regardless of which agency was implementing the programme. There was significant resistance to this approach among certain agencies, but certain Ambassadors implemented it with great success.

The active engagement of Ambassadors had an important corollary benefit — significant public relations for the US. Most Ambassadors in the focus countries incorporated HIV, the host country's response and PEPFAR into nearly every public appearance or speech they made. That effort reached from Heads of State to the village level. Often when traveling, I was asked to "thank President Bush" or "thank the American people for caring about us." After the head of a remote, rural clinic in Africa referred to PEPFAR several times, I asked him "What does PEPFAR mean?" His answer was remarkable: "PEPFAR means the American people care about us." It is not a surprise that 8 of 10 countries with the highest favourability rating of the US were in Africa in 2008.[8] The HIV resources were frequently the largest investment by the American people in a country. As one Ambassador said, that gave him a regular entry point to the Head of State and senior government officials and a seat at tables otherwise not available to him. During PEPFAR reauthorisation, Ambassador Mark Green from Tanzania sent a powerful letter to members of Congress extolling the significant public diplomacy and public relations benefits of PEPFAR. That letter was read and referred to in many Congressional speeches and hearings. The fact that Ambassador Green was a former Congressman who served on the House Foreign Affairs Committee during the initial PEPFAR authorising legislation added significant weight to his perspective.

Balancing headquarters and the field

A chronic problem in any global bureaucracy, in the public or private sector, is balancing the roles of headquarters and the field. PEPFAR's goal to support national scale-up of HIV prevention, treatment, and care services required nearly all of the work to be managed and done in-country. Based on the Mother and Child Initiative, the headquarters was to provide strategy and policy direction and the field was to implement. We understood that staff from Washington or Atlanta (where the CDC is based) could not and should not attempt to micromanage programmes on the ground. As Ambassador Tobias liked to say, "the what would be determined centrally and the how would be determined in the field." Three months before the first appropriation of resources by Congress, each Focus Country was asked to send two representatives to Washington, D.C. for a two-week meeting to develop a detailed implementation strategy and to draft the first centrally issued Requests for Application (RFA) for funding under PEPFAR. There were regular calls with staff remaining in-country, including a concluding "all hands" call with Ambassador Tobias. The interest was overwhelming and it created a sense of ownership and buy-in from the field staff that was essential. More than any single action, that early meeting with the field created the culture and structure for a balance between headquarters and the field.

While central RFAs were issued in the first year to move money rapidly, field-driven implementation required field-driven RFAs to ensure that the programmes that were funded would achieve the goals. This was a bit of a revolution: central funding reduced administrative burden and the need for procurement officers and legal advisors in-country. We believed the investment would have a high return by limiting large international partners with broad grant agreements that were not designed with a focus on the needs of individual countries. Although the five-year goals for each country were determined in advance, the annual goals were determined by the country team, with each country establishing a different pace depending on partners on the ground and existing capacity. In certain countries, for example Nigeria, there was a two-year period when low targets were expected as capacity was developed. In contrast, Uganda targeted meeting its five-year goal in a few years.

Congress and civil society

While initial public reactions by members of Congress to the announcement of PEPFAR in the SOTU were very positive, behind the scenes there was a mixed picture. Both sides of the aisle were discontent that such a major initiative was developed without their knowledge or consultation. Republicans who chaired development committees were a bit confused and perhaps disgruntled that they had recently been asked to shepherd legislation to create and finance the Millennium Challenge Corporation and to secure resources for the President's pledge of $200 million to the Global Fund for AIDS, Tuberculosis and Malaria (the Global Fund) — the first pledge from any country — and would now have to pivot to garnering support for PEPFAR. Congressional pique was heightened when senior members of the Administration proposed that broad authorising legislation consisting of a few pages be quickly adopted. The Congressional leadership responded by making it clear that a regular legislative process would be followed.

Reactions in civil society mirrored those in Congress. There was strong support for a significant increase in resources but there was concern about the details and disappointment that there had not been widespread consultations for such a momentous decision. Certain groups that strongly supported a multilateral strategy through the Global Fund expressed consternation about the heavy tilt towards the bilateral programme. Congress and civil society intended to make their imprint on PEPFAR as it moved from an announced Presidential initiative to the authorisation and appropriations processes.

The outcome: balance and compromise

There is no such thing as a perfect piece of legislation. Competing interests must be resolved and, in the US system, a small number of Congressional members can slow or stop the process. Although 99 per cent of the proposed law had strong bipartisan support, the enacting legislation of 2003 had several controversial issues regarding a requirement that 33 per cent of prevention funds (or 7 per cent of the overall budget) be dedicated to "abstinence until marriage" and a requirement that those receiving funds have a "policy opposing prostitution and sex trafficking." Both amendments were passed in the House Committee along Party lines and survived in the final legislation. When the House bill was taken up by the Senate, several important Republican members supported modifying disputed sections. Because both chambers must pass identical language before a piece of legislation can be sent to the President, any changes would have resulted in substantial delays in final passage. It would mean that the law would have to go to a Conference so the Senate and House versions could be reconciled and that version would have to be passed without amendments by each chamber before being sent to the President. Many bills have died in Conference.

There was an important public diplomacy reason to quickly adopt the law enacting PEPFAR. President Bush was determined to take a freshly minted PEPFAR authorisation of $15 billion over 5 years to the G8 to press global leaders to commit $30 billion. At the time it was estimated that $45 billion was needed for a comprehensive response and the President was hopeful that if the US committed the first third, the world would respond accordingly. Perhaps the greatest miscalculation of PEPFAR was the belief that others shared the same strong commitment to turning the tide on the modern day Black Plague. With the time pressure of the G8, the Senate passed the legislation without amendment, allowing it to go to the President's desk for signature.

The abstinence language led to the loss of support among some Democrats and segments of civil society. While the prostitution issue had its objectors, it remained part of the re-authorisation legislation of 2008 that was supported by all but one Democrat in the entire Congress (and that "no" vote was not related to the prostitution clause). Others recognised that opposing such a massive humanitarian effort because of disagreement on one issue was not tenable. It is interesting to consider what the world would look like today had the largest international health initiative in history for a single disease never happened because of 12 words.

One reason a few issues were not able to stop the PEPFAR enacting legislation was the recognition that there could be administrative methods to implement the legal requirements. The law stipulated that the

Coordinator should define "abstinence until marriage." In a Report to Congress in June of 2004, abstinence until marriage was defined to include programmes to promote a single sexual partnership — what was known as the "B" of the ABC approach (Abstinence, Be faithful, and Correct and consistent condom use) that was pioneered in Africa and was part of every African national AIDS strategy. In real terms, "abstinence until marriage" in particular would include programmes to promote gender equality and reduce trans-generational sex. In the calculations to report on the funding requirement, country teams were directed to pro-rate the "AB" components of comprehensive ABC programmes as appropriate and justifiable. Because the requirement was for all countries combined, not each individual country, guidance instructed countries to craft a prevention programme relevant to their epidemic. For example, in Vietnam where intravenous drug use and commercial sex work were fueling the epidemic, the country team was instructed to focus on condom distribution and methadone substitution therapy. If PEPFAR did not coin the term "combination prevention," it was the earliest adopter and largest implementer of that strategy.

Other contentious issues were managed in the annual budget cycles. After a year of competition between the Global Fund and the bilateral programme for resources, the Administration did not actively fight increased resources for the Global Fund and a significant element of civil society shifted to support "full funding" for *both* the bilateral programme and the Global Fund. Congress responded favourably.

In 2008, nearly all of the contentious issues embedded in PEPFAR had been resolved and the programme enjoyed widespread support in Congress and civil society. The re-authorisation process had its share of controversies and compromises. Of note, in the Senate, then Senator Biden sponsored the legislation with Senator Lugar and then Senators Obama and Clinton were co-sponsors. A good, if not perfect, law was passed with large bipartisan majorities in a Congress controlled by the Democratic Party and signed by a Republican President in a very upbeat ceremony in the East Room of the White House with a large presence by members from both sides of the aisle on the stage and a large crowd of supporters from a broad spectrum of public health, political, and policy perspectives.

National government and local civil society

Shifting from paternalism to partnership and building country ownership was a key objective of President Bush's strategy for development that was embraced by PEPFAR. However, bureaucratic tendencies developed over decades were difficult to overcome. A concerted effort to change culture and structure was again needed, and evolved over time.

To begin to change the culture of paternalism, President Bush addressed it head on in nearly every major speech on development in his last few years in office. He convened a major White House Summit on a "New Era in Development" to press the issue of country ownership and the principles of the Monterrey Consensus. In his two trips to Africa , he emphasised that the country was "in charge" and the US was there to support the government and people to implement their national strategy and to achieve their goals. Mrs. Bush made trips to 12 focus countries, half on her own, delivering a similar message with a special emphasis on the role of women in changing society. The Coordinator visited focus countries with great regularity, building on the need to create partnerships — often referring to the US Government as the "junior partner" in the relationship with the national government and local civil society.

As always, structure must follow culture. US development, like nearly all bilateral and multilateral development for decades, has not focused on partnership and country ownership. The COP was a key structural element in simply providing local authorities for the first time with comprehensive information about US financial commitments and programmatic efforts in their country — essential data to develop a national strategy. The COP also required the inter-agency team to delineate efforts to support the national strategy and to leverage and align with other resources available, in particular through the Global Fund. Guidance issued by the Coordinator required consultation with the national and local governments and civil society to create the COP, including an explanation of the process and local agreement before the COP would be approved, and encourage innovative approaches. In Nigeria, the Ambassador created a PEPFAR steering committee chaired by the Minister of Health and him. In Uganda, a PEPFAR advisory group, chaired by a former Prime Minister, was formed. Most focus countries held large partner meetings to define priorities for the COP.

When the Coordinator transferred resources to the implementing agencies, the Memorandum of Understanding required that all grants issued to international implementers include language with benchmarks on transferring management and programmatic efforts to local organisations — governments or non-governmental organisations — with increases in resources dependent on meeting the targets.

Despite radical structural changes, there was insufficient progress. When President Bush called for the re-authorisation of PEPFAR, he insisted on Partnership Compacts.[9] The Compacts were to outline five-year programmatic, policy and financial commitments between the US Government and the government of each of 33 countries. Guidance instructed country teams to take a broad view and work with all sectors, including non-government-, faith- and community-based organisations and the private sector to design a strategy that placed the response to HIV within health services and systems and the broader development picture. The Congress endorsed the President's approach in the new authorising legislation. Although the State Department lawyers insisted that the word "compact" be changed to "framework," Partnership Frameworks are a cornerstone of the Obama Administration's approach to PEPFAR.

Lessons to be Learned

Recreating development

To recreate development, a new vision and philosophy was needed. The vision was codified in the Monterrey Consensus and then the Paris Declaration and Accra Accord and required a fundamental shift from paternalism to partnership and a focus on results-based financing, good governance, and the engagement of all sectors, not just governments. President Bush insisted that PEPFAR be a direct manifestation of the vision for a new era in development, not just an expansion of the approaches of the past. In many ways, PEPFAR played a lead role in the renaissance in development.

Changing a bureaucracy

New ideas that are not well executed are just dreams. Implementing PEPFAR required a fundamental change to the culture and structure of the

US development bureaucracy. That change required a clear purpose and vision, an extraordinary level of commitment and personal involvement of President Bush, significant new resources, inter-agency engagement at all levels, the use of public diplomacy directed at the bureaucracy, and constant evaluation and re-creation based on lessons learned.

The lessons learned from PEPFAR are applicable to any bold and revolutionary effort in bilateral and multilateral development — and, in fact, any significant and fundamental change in well-established systems.

Conclusion

Transformation of the organisational culture and structure of the US Government and its relationship to partner countries was key to the success of PEPFAR and to overcoming the initial resistance to a major Presidential Initiative. The changes that were made allowed the aggressive targets to be achieved early and on-budget. In simple terms, millions of lives were saved and lifted up. These achievements laid the foundation for widespread changes in US development under President Bush, such as creation of the President's Malaria Initiative and the first Director of Foreign Assistance to develop one strategic, integrated approach with a focus on partnership and results. The Global Health Initiative of the Obama Administration is a fluid extension and evolution of the work that began with President Bush's Mother and Child Initiative and PEPFAR. There have also been domestic implications for the US — the new Obama National HIV/AIDS Strategy[10] was developed based on the PEPFAR accountability model. PEPFAR has saved and lifted up millions of lives and provided a new window into the heart of Americans. Beyond that, the lasting legacies include significant contributions to a shift in the global culture of development from a culture of money committed to a culture of results-based financing and a shattering of the myth that low- and middle-income countries were not capable of providing complicated, comprehensive, health services as part of a broad movement from paternalism to partnership. As President Bush said when he launched PEPFAR, "Seldom has history offered an opportunity to do so much for so many." Those words proved to be true beyond any expectation or imagination.

References

1. Appointment of PEPFAR head should be merit based (2009) [editorial]. *Lancet*, 373: 354. doi:10.1016/s0140-6736(09)60112-4.
2. http://www.cbsnews.com/stories/2010/04/04/60minutes/main6362203.shtml
3. http://www.foreignpolicy.com/articles/2010/01/06/hillary_clinton_on_development_in_the_21st_century
4. http://www.foreignaffairs.com/articles/66464/princeton-n-lyman-and-stephen-b-wittels/no-good-deed-goes-unpunished
5. http://www.who.int/hiv/en/
6. http://www.who.int/mediacentre/news/notes/2007/np05/en/index.html
7. http://www.iom.edu/Reports/2007/PEPFAR-Implementation-Progress-and-Promise.aspx
8. http://www.gallup.com/poll/106306/us-leadership-approval-highest-subsaharan-africa.aspx
9. http://georgewbush-whitehouse.archives.gov/news/releases/2007/05/20070530-5.html
10. http://www.whitehouse.gov/sites/default/files/uploads/NHAS.pdf

16

Negotiating ARV Prices with Pharmaceutical Companies and the South African Government: A Civil Society/Legal Approach

Christopher J. Colvin[i] and Mark Heywood[ii]

Abstract

Amidst the complex political dynamics of post-apartheid South Africa and the HIV/AIDS epidemic, a case for intellectual property rights violation before a national court led to a turning point in South African civil society's efforts to secure affordable treatment for people with HIV/AIDS. A complicated negotiation process took place between the Government of South Africa and the claimant, the Pharmaceutical Manufacturers' Association (PMA) — representing 40 global pharmaceutical companies. The Treatment Action Campaign (TAC), a key civil society actor, mobilised to achieve more equitable access to

[i] Christopher J. Colvin is a researcher at the School of Public Health, University of Cape Town.

[ii] Mark Heywood is the Executive Director of SECTION27, incorporating the AIDS Law Project in Johannesburg, South Africa. He is also an executive member of the Treatment Action Campaign. More information about the work of SECTION27 and TAC can be found at www.section27.org.za and www.tac.org.za

HIV/AIDS treatment services. TAC applied innovative approaches including legal and political activism to build alliances on the local and global level, ensure timely support from a wide range of players, and maintain public pressure on the PMA and the Government of South Africa.

The Problem

This case study in global health diplomacy examines the potential for a combination of civil society-led activism and litigation to promote and protect the right to health. It describes the intervention of South Africa's Treatment Action Campaign (TAC) and its partner the AIDS Law Project (ALP) in a court case between the South African government and the Pharmaceutical Manufacturers' Association (PMA) over the state's plans to improve access to healthcare through the regulation of drug pricing and measures to increase competition. The ALP and TAC's interventions — both inside and outside the courtroom — were arguably central in the eventual decision of the PMA to unconditionally withdraw its legal challenge to the state's limited restrictions of its use of its intellectual property rights.[iii]

Health care inequities and amendments to the medicines and related substances control act

In 1994, multi-party, non-racial elections in South Africa brought to an end nearly 50 years of apartheid rule and another 300 years of colonial oppression before that. This long history of marginalisation and oppression of the majority of South Africa's population by a small, white "settler" minority resulted in a wide-ranging and persisting set of social and political challenges including deep suspicion and separation across racial lines, mistrust

---

[iii] Much of the material for this case study has been adapted from Mark Heywood's (2001) article entitled "Debunking 'Conglomo-talk': A case study of the *amicus curiae* as an instrument for advocacy, investigation and mobilisation."[1]

of the government, high levels of poverty, and deepening forms of social and economic inequality. The new post-apartheid government inherited these challenges and despite its many efforts, nearly 20 years on, the consequences of apartheid's race-based policies of discrimination continue to permeate the lives of South Africans.

These enduring inequities are visible in any number of areas but it is perhaps in health and healthcare that the contrasts are most stark. We know that the health of a population is shaped by a wide number of broad "determinants" of health including education, employment, legal and political rights, social relationships and capital, clean water and air, decent infrastructure, and protection of the environment.[2] Apartheid policies systematically privileged white South Africans in all of these domains and the dramatic health disparities between white South Africans and South Africans of the other "population groups" bear testimony to the profound impact of discrimination and inequality on health.

The public and private health systems in South Africa also reflect these inequities. Roughly 80% of the South African population, most of them poor and working class, makes use of the public health system though only 40% of the country's health expenditure is spent in the public system. The private sector, on the other hand, spends 60% of the health expenditure on treating the remaining 20% of the population, mostly middle and upper class. In addition, the apartheid government's privileging of high-tech medicine and medical specialisation resulted in both a neglect of "primary health care approaches" as well as a rapidly increasing rate of medical inflation in both the public and private sectors. Though post-apartheid governments have tried to re-orient the public system towards the primary health care approach (which emphasises prevention and early intervention), it has struggled to rein in escalating costs in both the public and private sectors. These escalating costs are one of the main drivers behind the deepening inequalities in the health of the South African population overall. They are also making responding to the crisis of HIV and AIDS in the country even more difficult. In a country of roughly 50 million people, about 5.7 million or 11.4% of the population are infected with HIV and about 1.7 million of these need access to anti-retroviral treatment.[3]

As one way of addressing its growing inability to provide access to healthcare for the majority of the population, the South African government decided in 1997 to amend the 1965 Medicines and Related Substances Control Act (hereafter "the Act") to allow for greater control over the pricing of drugs used in the public and private health systems. By gaining more control over the prices of essential drugs, it was hoped that medical costs in both the public and private sector could be brought down.

These amendments centred around three mechanisms for negotiating and reducing drug pricing: parallel importation, generic substitution, and setting up a state pricing committee. Parallel importation involves the importation of brand name drugs from other countries where they are being sold by the same company at a lower price. For example, if a brand name drug is sold in Thailand for half the price of that same drug in South Africa, the South African government could import this drug from Thailand and use it in South Africa despite the fact that the owner of the patent on the drug had not agreed to its sale at this lower price in South Africa.

Generic substitution involves policies that either incentivise or require the substitution of generics when available for all prescriptions for name-brand medications. Patients and healthcare providers usually have the right to "opt-out" of generic substitutions but the default would be to fill prescriptions for branded medications with legally available generics when possible. The pricing committee anticipated in the amendments to the Act would have had the power to directly set "exit prices" (the final prices paid by retailers or consumers) and dispensing fees for all medications.

All three of these mechanisms represent a limitation to one degree or another of the patent rights of pharmaceutical manufacturers. Patent rights however, like all rights, can only be protected and promoted in the context of other competing rights and obligations. The Trade Related Aspects of Intellectual Property Rights (or "TRIPS") agreement is the principle vehicle for the protection and negotiation of intellectual property rights in the context of trade. TRIPS makes provisions for these types of limitations to intellectual property rights under specific conditions.

Lawsuit between PMA and the South African government and TAC's *amicus curiae* brief

Though these kinds of limitations to patent rights were standard practice in a number of developed countries and were compliant with the regulations in the TRIPS agreement, the Pharmaceutical Manufacturers' Association decided that these amendments to the Act were a significant threat to its business in South Africa. The PMA was also concerned that other countries in the developing world might follow South Africa's lead and put in place stronger limitations on patent rights for medications. Their concern was significant enough that in early 1998, the PMA launched a court action in the Pretoria High Court, accusing the South African government of violating its own Constitutional protections to private property in the amendments (Case 4183/98).

Though the South African government defended itself against the PMA's court action, its capacity to respond to the PMA's legal briefs was limited and progress was slow. This suited the drug companies since delays in the legal process meant the continued suspension of the amendments to the Act. It was only in late 2000 that a court date was quietly set down for the trial to begin in March 2001.

In the period between early 1998 and early 2001 however, there were a number of important political shifts and developments in the country.[4] Thabo Mbeki became State President in 1999. Early in his administration, he discovered and began promoting critics of mainstream AIDS research that questioned the science behind HIV virology and were suspicious of the political and economic interests behind the search for an effective treatment for AIDS. Some of the critics Mbeki promoted even questioned the existence of AIDS and/or the link between HIV and AIDS. This "denialist" position would come to occupy the attention of AIDS activists for the rest of Mbeki's administration.[5]

At the beginning of Mbeki's term however, the powers of these denialist views on HIV and AIDS were not yet clear. Conflicts between AIDS activists and global pharmaceutical companies around the pricing of important AIDS-related medications however, had catalysed a growing social movement in the country around affordable access to AIDS drugs. The Treatment Action Campaign (TAC) emerged in this time period as the key organisation fighting for access to free treatment in the public sector and more affordable treatment in the private sector. By the time the court date was set for the PMA's suit in early 2001, TAC had already launched a number of high profile protests and actions including the unauthorised importation from Thailand of a generic version of an important anti-fungal drug for treating opportunistic infections that was affordable in Thailand but unaffordable in South Africa because it was still under patent to Pfizer.

When news eventually got to TAC that a court date for the PMA suit had been set, TAC decided to try to join the lawsuit. Working with the AIDS Law Project, a non-governmental organisation (NGO) that specialises in HIV law and promoting the rights of people living with HIV, the TAC applied to be a "friend of the court" and sought permission from the government and the PMA to file an *amicus curiae* brief in support of the government's amendments to the law. Its objective was first to contrast the PMA's defence of its intellectual property rights with a legal argument about the state's positive duties to reasonably regulate the price of medicines: a right the Constitutional Court later affirmed in the New Clicks case stating "The right to health care services includes the right of access to medicines that are affordable. The state has an obligation to promote access to medicines that are affordable."[6] It also aimed to bring international attention to bear on the court proceedings and generate momentum in a legal process that had been already stalled for several years. TAC could have tried to join the court action as a full party to the suit, but were warned that this might lead to significant delays in the process. An *amicus curiae* brief had the advantage of allowing TAC to present information and legal argument to the court — and bring increased public and media scrutiny to the proceedings — without going through this longer process.

At the same time that it decided to pursue a legal strategy supporting the government's case against the drug companies, TAC also set into motion plans for a parallel process of social and political mobilisation at both the local and international levels. This political activism outside the courts was intended to closely support and drive the legal process that was taking place inside the courts.

Key Points

- Inequity in access to health care in South Africa was a growing concern after the end of apartheid and the government put in place mechanisms and amended laws for negotiating and reducing drug prices as one response to the problem.
- The Pharmaceutical Manufacturers' Association (PMA) contested the constitutionality of these mechanisms in the South African courts on the grounds that they violated the intellectual property rights of drug manufacturers.
- The South African government's defence of this court action was joined in an *amicus curiae* brief by the Treatment Action Campaign (TAC), a social movement campaigning for free access to anti-retroviral (ARVs) and other essential medicines in the public sector health system.

The Local and External Players and Their Roles

This section outlines both the central players in the legal process — PMA, the South African government, and TAC — as well as the other actors who played important roles at different steps outside the courtroom. It was in this parallel process that we can see the true breadth of the important roleplayers in TAC's and the government's defence against the PMA.

The pharmaceutical companies, the SA government, and TAC

The Pharmaceutical Manufacturers' Association, at the time, represented 40 global pharmaceutical companies including Merck, Pfizer, Glaxo-Wellcome, Bayer, and Bristol-Meyers. The PMA was publicly supported in its case against South Africa however, not only by the multinational drug companies it represented but also by the US government, the European Union, and PhRMA (the Pharmaceutical Research and Manufacturers of America). This support came in the form of both diplomatic and economic pressure as will be described below.

In 1999, the South African government was still very much a government in transition. The Department of Health had spent several years after the end of apartheid just trying to integrate and rationalise a bloated and fragmented public health system. The HIV/AIDS crisis was of increasing concern though the coming scale of the epidemic was not yet widely known or accepted and the government's response to the epidemic in the first five years after apartheid was weak and uncoordinated. During the first year of the PMA's suit, the Presidency of the South African government switched from Nelson Mandela to Thabo Mbeki. Though Mbeki's denialist stance on HIV/AIDS would come to dominate the politics of HIV and define TAC's agenda throughout most of the next 10 years, in 1999 and 2000, affordability was still the dominant reason given by the state for not providing anti-retrovirals (ARVs) in the public sector. As a result, movements like TAC were focusing more during this period on the global pharmaceutical industry and the struggle to reduce prices for these medications.

Despite its focus at the time on the drug companies and the question of pricing however, the relationship between TAC and the South African government wasn't easy. There were, in particular, difficult relations between TAC and the Office of the Presidency but TAC's relationships to the Department of Health at different levels were also difficult. These tensions were the result of TAC's strategy of focusing its activism not only on the drug companies themselves but also on the duties of the South African state to make essential medicines available to the poor. Its argument was that the South African state had a legal duty to protect and promote the right to health for its citizens. If medicines essential for the health of the population were unaffordable, then it was the government's responsibility, they argued, to use its power and resources to bring those prices down.

TAC's internal and external allies

One of the keys to TAC's success in the PMA case came from the support from a broad range of allies they were able to draw on both inside and outside the courtroom. The Congress of South African Trade Unions (COSATU) was one of TAC's principle internal political allies during the case. COSATU is the largest federation of trade unions in South Africa and a member of the important "tripartite alliance" of political players between itself, the ruling African National Congress, and the South African Communist Party. COSATU's support for TAC was crucial both for the political weight it could bring to bear within the tripartite alliance as well as for the number of supporters COSATU could mobilise for TAC's mass actions.

TAC also drew on a number of prominent activist and development organisations during the case including Medicins sans Frontieres (MSF, also known as Doctors Without Borders), Oxfam, Action for Southern Africa in the UK, and the Health-GAP coalition in the US. These partners played a number of important roles. AIDS activists from an earlier generation of activism in the US came to South Africa to bring TAC members up to speed on technical development in AIDS treatments and help them strategise politically. MSF and Oxfam helped to organise international pressure through petitions and large demonstrations.

Individuals at research and academic institutions also played an important role inside and outside the courtroom. Along with US AIDS activists, they contributed to the initial education of TAC members on the scientific issues at stake in HIV and AIDS treatment. They also proved invaluable during the legal process itself when TAC needed to make arguments and present evidence based on research it did not have the capacity to conduct rapidly.

Finally, the local and global media were instrumental in enabling public pressure on the PMA within South Africa and abroad. TAC cultivated close relationships with media outlets and provided journalists with a steady stream of both compelling stories about the human impacts of exorbitant drug pricing as well as detailed scientific and legal responses to the PMA challenge.

Key Points

- The original players in the lawsuit — PMA and the South African government — were joined by TAC who filed a brief in support of the government's defence of the amendments.
- TAC's strategy of combining legal action with social mobilisation and protest meant that a number of other players, including political allies, activist organisations, medical experts and the media, both local and global, were crucial to the success of the process.

Challenges Faced and the Outcome

The actual series of events between TAC's decision to join the PMA case and the eventual decision by the PMA to drop it were fairly rapid. Shamir[7] has called it the "slow rise and fast fall of the PMA case." The period of the "slow rise" of the case was mostly driven by the PMA who mounted a three-pronged attack on the South African government. Firstly, the legal action itself consumed considerable time and resources from the government and there were frequent requests from their side for postponements in the proceedings. Secondly, the PMA mounted economic pressure on South Africa by having PhRMA and its associated drug companies lobby for South Africa's inclusion on a "watch list" of global violators of intellectual property rights and a range of sanctions and warnings from the US government followed. Finally, the US government and the European Union mounted diplomatic pressure on the South African government, warning them of the potentially far-reaching political and economic consequences of the amendments to the Act (see ref. 7 for more detail).

Though South Africa's inclusion on this watch list was later reversed under pressure from international AIDS activists and President Clinton's issuance of an executive order recognising the rights of African countries to pass TRIPS-compliant legislation without interference from the US, this didn't really change the course of the PMA's legal case in South Africa. By the end of 2000, the two parties were finally ready to go to court and the court date was set down in November for March 2001.

TAC, which was at that time aware of the PMA's case but not directly involved, learned of the anticipated court date on 11 Jaunary. The "rapid fall" of the PMA's case began with TAC's decision to join the legal action as a "friend of the court" and present its own evidence and argument against the PMA's position. The table below summarises some of the key elements inside and outside the courtroom.

A quick glance at the table reveals some of the broad outlines of the encounter between TAC, the government and the PMA. The legal process centred around 1) TAC's application to join the suit, 2) a series of affidavits exchanged between TAC and the PMA after the Court's

Month	Day(s)	The Battle in the Courts	The Battle for Public Opinion
January	15 & 16	TAC's National Executive Committee meets and decided to file an *amicus curiae* brief	TAC holds a press conference and calls for "Global Day of Action" on 5 March, first day of court case.
	26	TAC delivers letter to SA government and PMA seeking admission as an *amicus curiae*	
February	6 & 14	Replies to TAC from government (positive) and PMA (negative)	
	16	TAC files its Founding Affidavit and Notice of Motion	
	18		TAC-led march of 1000 people to Parliament in Cape Town; TAC produces "AIDS profiteer poster" against GlaxoSmithKline CEO
	22	Answering Affidavit from PMA	
March	1	TAC's Replying Affidavit to PMA	TAC, MSF, Oxfam, COSATU International Press Conference
	4		TAC and COSATU night vigil in Pretoria
	5	Argument begins in the Pretoria High Court	Global Day of Action in 30 cities worldwide led by 250 organisations. 5000 people march from Pretoria High Court to US Embassy with broad national and international media attention
	6	TAC is admitted as amicus and PMA is told to reply to TAC's Founding Affidavit; case is postponed to 18 April	COSATU pickets outside court European union issues resolution calling for PMA to withdraw

(Continued)

(Continued)

Month	Day(s)	The Battle in the Courts	The Battle for Public Opinion
	28	PMA files Answering Affidavit	
April	10	TAC and SA government file eplying Affidavits	Pickets held outside the court and strong presence of TAC
	17	TAC's Heads of Argument are filed with the court	supporters in the courtroom. MSF delivers 250,000 name
	18	Court case resumes and is soon adjourned at PMA's request	petition to PMA TAC, MSF, and Oxfam hold international press conference
	19	PMA withdraws its case unconditionally	to celebrate. South African government holds a separate press conference and doesn't mention TAC's involvement

*adapted from Appendices 1 and 2 in Heywood (1)

decision to accept TAC's "friend of the court" brief, and 3) PMA's withdrawal before argument could really begin. The advocacy process outside the courtroom closely paralleled the legal process with carefully timed and large-scale actions including marches, vigils, petitions, pickets, and press conferences at both national and international levels.

The details of the legal arguments put forward in this case have been summarised by Heywood[1,8,9] and Shamir.[7] Instead of reviewing these in detail, this section highlights some of the key challenges in the legal and political process faced by TAC and the strategies it developed in response.

One of TAC's first challenges was that the court case brought by the PMA centred on fairly narrow Constitutional questions on the infringement of intellectual property rights and on the delegation of what they asserted were overly broad and overly vague powers to the Health Minister to dictate drug policy and pricing. The South African government's response to these arguments were equally narrow and focused primarily on the question of the delegation of powers to the Minister. TAC attempted to introduce a new legal argument that the limitation of property rights was justifiable in the context of a number of other Constitutionally protected rights that would be promoted through the amendments, including the right to access to health services, to life, to dignity, and to equality.

Although the amendments themselves were not specific to AIDS-related medications and only gave the government the abstract power to regulate pricing, import, and licensing policies, TAC's focusing of the Court's attention on the AIDS epidemic in South Africa provided a powerful and concrete example of how the provisions outlined in the amendments could be enacted in such a way that balanced the right to property with, in this case, more compelling obligations by the government to respond to a national public health emergency. That is, the Court and the "court of public opinion" had an easy time recognising how the AIDS crisis in South Africa, which was threatening to turn into a catastrophe, could be considered a grave enough threat to the public good to limit the property rights of patent holders.

Another strategy TAC used to garner support both inside and outside the courtroom was to attach appendices to its affidavits containing the dramatic testimony of a number of people living with or affected by HIV/AIDS as well as three doctors treating AIDS patients. These were included as part of its legal argument around the severity of the AIDS epidemic and the reasonableness of limited abrogations of property rights in response to overwhelming public need. These testimonies became an official part of the Court record however, and helped to sway opinion both with the judge and with those outside the courtroom.

TAC was also able to bait the PMA into including some valuable appendices to their own affidavits. TAC argued, for example, that the drug companies' right to profit from their inventions was not unduly limited in these cases since the companies had already more than made back their costs for research and development of AIDS drugs. They didn't have evidence of these costs however, since the drug companies refused to release this information. In their response to

TAC, the companies in fact released valuable information about the internal costs and revenues for certain drugs. Similarly, in responding to TAC's emphasis on the high cost of AIDS drugs in its brief, the PMA argued that this argument was null and void given the fact that the drug companies had recently offered the South African government steep discounts on these drugs and their affordability was therefore not such a pressing concern. This argument had little bearing on the case but the South African government had never revealed these offers and had long maintained that affordability was still their key concern. Having this internal data on drug development costs and pricing structures, and negotiations helped TAC immensely both in the case with the PMA and in its subsequent activism against the government.

Another important challenge faced by TAC was the complexity of the legal, economic, and scientific arguments around drug development, distribution, and pricing, and around the pharmacology of AIDS-related drugs. This information was vital both for the lawyers who were preparing TAC's affidavits as well as for the broader public and organisations allied to TAC who struggled to understand many of the technical details of the case.

TAC addressed these challenged in two ways. First, it set about educating its own members and those of key allies in politics and the media about AIDS medicines and the technicalities of the court case. It held workshops with overseas activists to educate its own members. It met with political leaders in COSATU during their all-night vigils to workshop the political and legal issues at stake. It made all of the court papers from the PMA, the government, and themselves readily accessible on their website as soon as they were available. And it was very responsive to media requests for further information and clarification on the issues.

Second, TAC recruited the help of a number of national and international experts in the drafting of its affidavits for the case. When TAC was officially accepted in its *amicus* role, there was a great deal of research needed on a wide range of issues including health economics, drug pricing, and interactions of the public and private sectors; on the real costs and real profits of drug development and distribution; and on the standards of practice for generic substitutions and medicine price control in other countries. TAC managed to secure supporting affidavits on all of these issues by recruiting a wide number of experts including health system personnel (local and foreign), national and international professors of health economics, pharmacology, and law, and even groups of students from Yale University and the University of Minnesota.

In the end, the PMA quickly dropped its suit after only a couple of days of court hearings and entered into a negotiated settlement with the South African government that merely required that the government "consult" pharmaceutical companies before introducing drug pricing controls. This was a great public relations victory for TAC and the government and it was largely the result of growing international attention to the cause of people with HIV/AIDS in South Africa and other developing countries struggling to manage the costs of addressing the epidemic. If the PMA had not withdrawn its case, it might have suffered an even greater setback in the form of a negative judgement from the court which would have more firmly established a precedent for the limitation of property rights in the context of rights to health. Nonetheless, their withdrawal provided momentum for a growing movement globally to assert the rights of developing countries to limit in certain cases the trade rights of rich northern countries and companies in the interests of their own public good.

Unfortunately for TAC and the millions of people in South Africa with HIV/AIDS, the South African government had other plans. At its press conference after the victory, it did not even mention TAC's involvement and proceeded to announce that despite the victory over the drug companies, it would not be exploring pricing controls for ARVs since providing ARVs in the public sector was not government policy. This statement marked an important shift in the government's explanations for its refusal to provide ARVs — a move from arguments about affordability to a politics of AIDS denialism that would occupy TAC for the next seven years.

Key Points

- TAC was opposed by the PMA in its application to join as a friend of the court.
- TAC used its role as a friend of the court to introduce new legal argument and a wide range of evidence into the proceedings.
- TAC used a multi-pronged strategy both inside and outside the court and drew on multiple resources to develop its legal submissions while also building alliances to maintain public pressure on the PMA.
- In the end, the PMA withdrew its legal challenge unconditionally, leaving the government free to implement the new amendments.
- The government however, chose not to make use of its new powers to reduce the cost of ARVs.

Lessons to be Learned

A number of lessons about the potential role of civil society in global health diplomacy can be gleaned from this case study.

The first lesson is about the importance of combining legal activism with political mobilisation in these kinds of efforts. Though TAC's court action was independent of its political activism and represented a novel legal strategy in protecting human rights, the two processes reinforced each other in a number of important ways described above.

The second lesson, closely connected to the first, is that these kinds of actions often require the input from a wide range of actors including the media, other activist organisations, key political allies, academic experts, and health system personnel. Despite its outsized influence in South African health activism, TAC was not at the time a large or well-resourced organisation. Throughout its activism, it has depended on its ability to mobilise affected communities, supported by a diverse array of actors who can provide critical input, resources, and support at the right time.

The third lesson is about the possibility and importance of shifting legal and political debates around intellectual property rights to concerns around social and economic rights, the right to health, and the positive duty of governments to protect and promote these. Though there is a growing recognition of these rights as a platform for legal and political activism in health and in many other areas, in 2001, this was still a fairly new and untested approach.

The fourth lesson concerns the importance of using the AIDS crisis in South Africa as a rallying point and concrete focus for its campaign. At the time there were over three million people infected with HIV in South Africa. Most are poor and not able to afford medicines, therefore making them dependent on the public health system. The amendments to the Medicines Control Act that were attacked by the PMA were not specific to HIV/AIDS. But legal battles over abstract constitutional principles and international trade agreements will always run the risk of failing to galvanize sufficient public and political response. TAC's framing of the AIDS "emergency" in South Africa not only offered a compelling case study for the Court in terms of the question of justifying the limitation of property rights — it also made possible the broad and strong public and political support TAC was able to organise in a very short time. This lesson can and should be translated into other health challenges beyond HIV/AIDS. The challenge here is one of how to make the respective crises in health "real" and real in a way that can be heard both by the courts of public opinion and by the equally important judicial courts of law.

The final lesson for this case study centres around the importance of educating those involved in negotiations around health issues about the technical legal, scientific, economic, and social issues involved. TAC did this in some conventional ways — by educating themselves about the issues, and mobilising expert opinion for their affidavits. It also did this in some more unusual ways — feeding journalists with extensive information and references, workshopping the details with their political allies, and perhaps most importantly, putting an emphasis on educating their own membership beyond just the leadership. In fact, one of TAC's principle longer-term strategies has been to develop the "treatment literacy" of its ordinary members. Their argument is that better understanding the science of HIV/AIDS disease and treatment will not only improve the ability of individuals to take care of themselves, it will also make it more possible for them to advocate on their own behalf for the social and economic rights afforded to them in the Constitution. This focus on patient empowerment and improving their ability to access justice (without always having to go through expert intermediaries) is one of the cornerstone's of TAC's activism.

Key Points

- The combination of legal action and political activism was critical to TAC's success.
- The involvement of a wide range of players who could mobilise critical resources and support at strategic times was another key factor in its success.
- It is important — and effective — to introduce a "human rights approach" to social and economic rights in the negotiation of health issues.
- Using the specific case of HIV/AIDS as a way to mobilise various players and to frame the broader court action around drug pricing and generics was an effective strategy.
- TAC's focus on the education and scientific literacy of its members, the Court, and the broader public is an important component of levelling the playing field in global health negotiations.

Conclusion

TAC's victory over the PMA in 2001 was still an early part of the organisation's efforts to secure access to affordable treatment for HIV/AIDS. After the lawsuit was withdrawn, the political challenges for TAC changed as President Thabo Mbeki's and his Health Minister's denialism around AIDS took shape and the scale of the epidemic became clearer to the broader public.

TAC continued to develop and refine its strategy of pairing legal and political activism and turned its attention to putting pressure not only on the drug companies but on the state as well. In 2002, for example, it won a groundbreaking case against the South African government in the Constitutional Court which led to the government being ordered to provide anti-retroviral medicines to pregnant women with HIV. In 2003 it forced the government to announce a treatment plan that by 2010 had led to over one million people receiving ARV medicines. However, it also diversified its legal strategies beyond litigation and threats of litigation against these parties to also include complaints to regulatory bodies like the Competition Commission, providing advice and assistance to the government on how to purchase cheaper medicines through its procurement policies, and through placing pressure on the Medicines Control Council to register ARVs expeditiously and to prohibit the marketing of fake medicines. Though these activities are not all staged in a court of law, they are central to the effective translation of law into practice through the development and application of appropriate policies and regulations.

As TAC's legal and political strategies evolved, many of the same lessons still held. Their emphasis on scientific literacy within poor communities, their rich engagement with the media and academic experts, and their connection of "technical" health issues to the broader principles of social and economic rights continue to be hallmarks of an effective strategy for participating in health negotiations at both the national and international levels.

Their success wasn't, of course, pre-ordained and their strategies don't necessarily always translate easily. Respect for the rule of law and the independence of the judiciary in South Africa could be seen as one of the necessary conditions for TAC's numerous legal victories in the last 10 years. Judicial branches of government in many other countries are not so insulated from political pressure. And a human rights approach obviously will only have teeth in those countries that have afforded significant human rights protections in their Constitutions. Particularly important is the fact that South Africa has a specific clause in its Bill of Rights which relates to the right to health. Section 27 grants "everyone" a right of "access to health care services, including reproductive health care" and says that the state must take "reasonable legislative and other measures, within its available resources, to progressively realise the right." This is an important legal foundation and instruction to the state, on which much of TAC's work is founded.

Similarly, the publicity that "AIDS in Africa" has been able to elicit, because of AIDS activism, is hard to match by other health challenges that appear as if they are not as compelling. Health activism on these issues has not been as successful as that which developed around AIDS, and yet often these other diseases cause as much illness and death. This is the most immediate challenge faced today. TAC was able to prompt an international outcry about the behaviour of the drug companies and link this to efforts to raise awareness about the character of this epidemic and the impact it is having in Africa in particular. Diseases like malaria, TB, infant and maternal mortality have, thus far, struggled to capture the imagination of the public in the same way.

There is also the question of TAC's strategic relationship with the state. Though the media attention around TAC typically portrays it as a sworn enemy of the South African government (at least during the period of official denialism), it has always in fact tried to maintain a delicate balance between challenging the state in court and in public whilst at the same time partnering with the state — and government officials working in the health system in particular. These partnerships include support for and participation in bodies like the South African National AIDS Council (SANAC), the development of health systems strengthening and HIV prevention interventions, and legal actions like the one described here where TAC stood with the state to challenge the practices of multinational drug corporations.

In the end, it is the flexibility and variety of the ALP and TAC's approaches to health activism and negotiation — and the diversity of its network of supporters — that have proven to be key elements of its successes.

Key Points

- TAC's emphasis on scientific literacy, media, and academic engagement, and the relevance of social and economic rights in health activism have continued to be key success factors in its work.
- There are some important limitations and necessary conditions to the success described in this case study including the presence of an independent judiciary and a cause around which global opinion can be quickly mobilised.
- TAC has maintained a shifting relationship to the state and the public health system that allows it to both strongly challenge the state while also participating with government in strengthening the health system in other ways.
- The flexibility and variety in TAC's approaches to health activism and its diverse network of supporters are key elements of its success.

References

1. Heywood M. (2001) Debunking 'Conglomo-talk': A case study of the *amicus curiae* as an instrument for advocacy, investigation and mobilisation. *Law, Democracy and Development*, 5 (2) 133–162.
2. Commission on the Social Determinants of Health (2008). Closing the Gap in a Generation: Health Equity through Action on the Social Determinants of Health. World Health Organization, Geneva.
3. Republic of South Africa (2010) Country Progress Report on the Declaration of Commitment on HIV/AIDS: 2010 Report. Department of Health, Pretoria, South Africa.
4. Gray A, Matsebula T, Blaauw D, Schneider H, Gilson, L (2001) Analysis of the Drug Policy Process in South Africa, 1989–2000. Center for Health Policy University of the Witwatersrand, Johannesburg, South Africa.
5. Kalichman S. (2009) *Denying AIDS: Conspiracy Theories, Pseudoscience and Human Tragedy.* Springer, New York.

6. Constitutional Court of South Africa (2006) *Minister of Health & Another v New Clicks* South Africa *(Pty) Ltd & Others* 2006 (2) SA 311 (CC) at 253. (Paragraph 514).
7. Shamir, R. (2005) Corporate responsibility and the South African drug wars: Outline of a new frontier for cause lawyers. In: Sarat A and Scheingold SA (eds), *The World Cause Lawyers Make: Structure and Agency in Legal Practice*, pp. 37–62. Stanford University Press, Stanford.
8. Heywood, M. Drug Access (2004) Patents and Global Health" 'chaffed and waxed sufficient' in Global Health and Governance HIV/AIDS, Third World Quarterly Series, Palgrave Macmillan.
9. Heywood, M., Loff, B. (2002) Patents on Drugs: manufacturing Scarcity or Advancing Health. *Journal of Law, Medicine and Ethics*, 30 (4).

17

Negotiating Health Reform in Kyrgyzstan: Government Management of Donors and Stakeholders

Judyth L. Twigg[i]

Abstract

In a turbulent political context, the Manas ten-year programme for health care reform in the Kyrgyz Republic was introduced to re-build an essentially non functioning health care system and redress inequities in access to basic health services. This case study describes how the reform process oriented the system toward preventive and primary health care in stark contrast to the former Soviet style tertiary care based system. Along with the health-related achievements and universal access to basic health services, the story conveys a broader message for effective government-led sector development with the assistance of an array of external donors and key stakeholders on the national level. Central in the process have been coherence,

---

[i] Professor of Government and Public Affairs, Virginia Commonwealth University. This case study is based on the author's "Project Performance Assessment Report (PPAR): Kyrgyz Republic Health Sector Reform Project and Second Health Sector Reform Project," Sector Evaluation Division, Independent Evaluation Group, The World Bank, June 30, 2008.

commitment, country-ownership, strategic planning, inter-ministerial cooperation, consistent donor support, stable mechanisms to steer "harmonisation," and timely capacity building.

The Problem

The system of health care governing the Soviet Union since the 1950s was riddled with inefficiencies and weaknesses. The Kyrgyz Republic was part of this system before the Soviet collapse, inheriting it into the 1990s. The system was fragmented into four levels of government administration — republican (national), oblast (regional), city, and rayon (district) — that served overlapping populations.[1] It performed well in terms of guaranteeing access to health care and promoting a relatively equitable distribution of health resources, but it was structurally inefficient, with heavy reliance on inpatient and tertiary hospital-based care. The system was structured to deliver hospital-based *treatment* rather than primary health care with a focus on prevention. The emphasis on costly inpatient care was evidenced in the large numbers of hospital beds and physicians and high use rates compared to western industrialised countries.[2] As a result, there was virtually no diagnostic capacity and equipment at lower, less costly levels of the system. Instead of treating patients at these lower levels, patients were typically referred upwards for treatment at the tertiary, more highly specialised level.

The system of health financing perpetuated these inefficiencies. Budgeting norms based on physical capacity (numbers of beds or numbers of doctors) encouraged overstaffing, provision of more beds than dictated by medical need, and utilisation of inpatient services at levels higher than medically necessary. More inpatient services were used than what would normally be needed under a system based on a primary health care approach oriented toward prevention rather than advanced-stage and lengthy treatment. Combined with a rigidly enforced 18-line budgeting system used to pay medical care providers (hospitals and polyclinics), there were no incentives for primary care providers to use cost-effective ambulatory treatment protocols or to perform a "gate-keeping" function of screening inappropriate referrals. Reliance on capacity-based budgeting promoted inefficiency and waste. The impact of these inefficiencies was exacerbated by low levels of total (government plus private) health care spending: US$156.00 per capita in 1990 (using purchasing power parities), declining to US$37.00 in 1993.[2] In the context of these declining levels of budget spending on health care, a rise in informal health payments during the immediate post-Soviet period led to a rapid transition from universal, free-of-charge access to health services to a *de facto* fee-for-service system. With GNP per capita (in current dollars) around US$400.00 during the early 1990s, the population could scarcely afford high out-of-pocket payments. Corruption was also rampant, as was the case throughout the health sectors of all the post-Soviet countries.

Health indicators were poor as the Kyrgyz Republic emerged from the Soviet Union, with the country facing the double challenge throughout the 1990s of controlling high rates of communicable and non-communicable diseases simultaneously. In addition to high rates of childhood mortality due to infectious diseases, the Kyrgyz Republic also had very high rates of adult mortality largely due to cardio-vascular disease, cancer, and injuries.[3] In the early 1990s, there were significant increases in the incidence of highly infectious diseases such as tuberculosis (TB) and sexually transmitted infections (STIs).

The Local and External Players and Their Roles: Negotiating with and Managing Donors

In response to these challenges, the Kyrgyz government initiated a series of measures aimed at improving the performance of the health sector. From 1994 through 1996, the government worked together with the World Health Organization's Regional Office for Europe (WHO/EURO), the United Nations Development Programme (UNDP), and TICA, the Turkish development agency, financed by a US$300,000 UNDP grant, to create a ten-year (1996–2005) health system reform programme known as the Manas programme (named after a famous Kyrgyz leader, about whom the 1000-year-old national epic poem "Manas" was written). Formally adopted by the government in 1996, the programme defined four broad goals: health gain, equity, efficiency, and effective and high quality health care. Its programme elements were focused on (i) improving the health of the population and access to care; (ii) reducing disparities in health; (iii) guaranteeing the population's access to existing health services; (iv) improving the effectiveness and quality of care provided by the health system; and (v) increasing the responsibility of citizens for their own health, while protecting patients' rights.

The Manas programme also established specific objectives to be achieved during the first several years of implementation, the late 1990s, particularly related to a focus on re-orienting the health care system towards primary health care and away from specialised hospital care. This shift was to be supported by a re-allocation of the government's health resources, accompanied by a reduction in the number of hospital beds and the closure of some hospitals. The goal was to improve the quality of care at all levels, updating and standardising clinical practices for examination and treatment and protocols for referral to inpatient care. In addition, new management models were to be developed for hospitals as a basis for greater managerial autonomy in the future, supported by new management structures and information systems.

The World Bank implemented two consecutive Health Reform Projects that were explicitly designed to support key elements of the Manas Programme. The design of the first project (which ran from 1996–2002) took place at the same time that the government was crafting Manas, and therefore the two emerged deliberately in parallel, with the Bank-financed project forming the backbone of Manas programme implementation. Although the WHO and the Bank worked hand in hand with the government during project preparation, ultimately the lead was taken by the government. Indeed, the government's Manas strategy itself contained an unusually high level of feasibility analysis and implementation details, and the Bank-sponsored project was derived squarely and logically from the detailed set of government priorities. As a result, the Ministry of Health (MOH) claimed strong ownership of the project and of the reforms, with the project based not on WHO opinion or Bank opinion, but on government opinion. Also in 1994, the United States Agency for International Development (USAID) began to support an initial health reform pilot project in one of the country's regions (Issyk-Kul) through its ZdravReform programme. USAID's work was closely aligned with the development of the Manas programme, and many of the specific measures implemented in Issyk-Kul became a part of the Manas strategy. As this array of donors became involved in the Kyrgyz health sector beginning in 1994–1996, the Manas programme was the umbrella for all the international and bilateral organisations working in the health sector in the country.

There exists a wide range of opinion on the explanation for the emergence of strong and sustained government commitment to progressive health care reform, including the existence of a small but committed group of "champions" of reform — in this case, all currently-serving government officials in the health sector — who were responsible for the creation of the Manas programme. Some stakeholders attribute the commitment to reform to the Kyrgyz nomadic culture, rendering the country naturally more open to new ideas than its neighbours. Others cite the extreme poverty in the country during the immediate post-Soviet period, claiming that the country had no choice but to adopt strategies to use its scarce resources more efficiently. The unique presence of several strong Kyrgyz "policy entrepreneurs" who were able to negotiate and collaborate effectively with donors was clearly a major factor.

Health care sector reform in the Kyrgyz Republic has benefited from the continuity of donor personnel in place. USAID and WHO kept the same personnel on the ground for well over a decade, from the mid-1990s through the mid 2000s, and in some cases even longer, and there has been similar longevity among many key World Bank personnel. Over time, a productive division of labour has developed, where each donor — at the initiative and prodding of the Kyrgyz "champions" who launched the Manas strategy — has successfully carved out its own "niche" of comparative advantage in the health sector reform effort. This continuity has contributed to a remarkably strong sense of familiarity and teamwork within the donor community, and between the donor community and the government. While it is widely acknowledged that the World Bank has served as the convener and leader of donor efforts in the Kyrgyz health sector, the Kyrgyz government has effectively managed and coordinated donor interventions throughout the reform process.

From the outset, it was envisaged that the Manas programme would be implemented through a sector-wide approach (SWAp), defined as a comprehensive approach to sector development. The SWAp in the Kyrgyz health sector context was defined as having four core elements:

- a government-led process to define the vision for the health sector in the form of an explicit health sector strategy with clear goals, priority interventions, and costs;
- a medium-term budget framework (MTBF) to programme annual spending with mechanisms to ensure that annual budgets will correspond to the MTBF, and that budgetary execution matches agreed commitments;
- a joint sector performance monitoring and evaluation system integrated with the monitoring and evaluation framework of the MTBF as well as of the National Poverty Reduction Strategy; and
- a formalised government-led aid coordination mechanism, with the MOH responsible for overall coordination of international partners' contributions to the programme and for setting up a system of regular meetings, forums for discussion and negotiations, and joint review meetings.

In addition, donor funding (with the notable exception of USAID) is pooled, with external contributions not ring-fenced but instead intermingled with government funds supporting the health sector strategy. Three mechanisms continue to govern the process of donor coordination supporting the Kyrgyz health sector: twice-yearly Health Summits, one in May and one in September, intended to review progress and develop Programmes of Work for successive years; memoranda of support and understanding, the latter among the joint financiers and the government, specifying issues of special relevance to the pooled funds (these issues of special relevance include institutional arrangements, fiduciary arrangements and capacity building requirements, assessment and monitoring provisions, disbursement arrangements, information-sharing and conflict resolution expectations, and arrangements for adding new partners during implementation); and joint supervision arrangements, including regular joint supervision missions and coordination of policy dialogue.

Overall policy oversight and project steering is now the responsibility of an Inter-ministerial Coordination Committee (IMCC), chaired by the

Minister of Health. The IMCC focuses on the coordination of activities and harmonisation across ministries and sectors, and the Health Policy Council serves as the forum for implementation coordination. Within the Health Policy Council, two sub-committees have been formed: an internal Reform Implementation Coordinating Committee (RICC) for internal MOH coordination, and an external health sector RICC for external dialogue and coordination. The MOH and its Department of Strategic Planning and Reform Implementation hold responsibility for programme management and day-to-day implementation, with a 64-person staff tasked explicitly to implementation of health reform. The IMCC and the Minister of Health ensure that this system does not become overly bureaucratic, with coordination and communication flowing smoothly across departments and agencies.

Over time, the Ministry of Health has both sustained ownership of the health reform programme and acquired increasing capacity to make the "right" policy and investment choices. MOH staff receive special training at a WHO-run Health Management Institute so that they know how to programme resources coming from various donors. The training helps to enable financial specialists in the MOH to work side by side with technical specialists who are actually implementing programmes. The MOH as a whole has learned to take into account the entire resource envelope in the sector: what are the resources available, where to get those resources, who the major players are, and what the priorities are. Similarly, early in the reform programme, the MOH exhibited the traditional reluctance to spend money on technical assistance and training; more recently, however, the MOH has realised that budgets should be programmed based not on what the MOH wants to buy, but based on what objectives the MOH wants to achieve — and the MOH is spending around 15% of its procurement budget on technical assistance. Rather than deciding the correct approach in this and other cases on behalf of the government, the donors' role has transitioned to one of continuous engagement, dialogue, and persuasion, with the expectation — fulfilled in this case — that the government will eventually mature to make the "right" decision. The MOH is not a passive beneficiary of external aid.

Over the course of the Manas programme, the MOH and Ministry of Finance (MOF) have come to realise that their goal is not simply to satisfy donors, but also to satisfy broad development objectives. Capacity is being pushed down, from the ministerial/deputy ministerial level to the department heads and below. As this process develops, the prospects for sustainability no longer lie in the hands of just a few champions, but instead in personnel and institutional capacity across the MOH. The MOH and MOF now work collaboratively, and they co-chair the biannual Health Summits, while donors have transitioned from a supervisory to an advisory role. This "push-down" of capacity also applies to the center-region relationship. Whereas the MOH early in the reform process would instruct the regions on reform measures in a top-down manner, now it increasingly transmits objectives to work teams at the oblast and rayon levels, offering only broad guidance as the work teams figure out how to meet those objectives.

Outputs, Challenges, and Outcomes: negotiating domestic resistance to reform

Outputs

Reform activities included establishing the basis of an effective health insurance system that pools resources within a single purchaser, with a newly-established Mandatory Health Insurance Fund (MHIF) as the purchaser. The MHIF is separate from the providers of health services, and reimbursement of providers in some regions is based on capitation at the outpatient level and on case-based payments in hospitals. A modern Management Information System was established to connect purchasers and providers, and to track health indicators. The MHIF became the sole purchasing agency for health care services at the regional (oblast) level, combining state budget resources and health insurance premiums. These pooled funds are then distributed to outpatient facilities on a capitation basis and to hospitals on a case-based payment model. The case-based payment system introduced the concept of output-oriented payment to the health system.[4] The single payer reforms were pilot tested in two oblasts (Issyk-Kul and Chui, with USAID supporting the pilot in the former) in 2001, and then systematically rolled out to the rest of the country, adding two additional oblasts each year, until the entire health financing system operated on the single-payer model in 2004. The perceived effectiveness of the reforms was so strong that two regions scheduled to implement them in 2004 requested permission to do so a year earlier. In 2006, the oblast purchasing pools were further centralised into one national purchasing pool. The latter shift provided the opportunity for cross-national subsidy of poorer regions and expanded the risk pool to the national level.

Equally important, the foundation was laid for comprehensive restructuring of the primary care sector through the establishment of new primary care group practices (Family Group Practices, or FGPs). These were established in all regions. These FGPs are independent health care facilities, accessed by free choice of the population and an open enrollment process, subject to reimbursement based on financial incentives for quality and cost-effectiveness of care. In accord with international best practices, family physicians were trained to treat adults, pregnant women, and children.

Another key element of the reforms was the development of the State Guaranteed Benefits Package (SGBP). Created by government decree in February of 2002, the SGBP explicitly defined entitlements to health care coverage, including the following:[1,3]

- free primary care, with co-payments for some laboratory and diagnostic tests;
- hospital care provided for a flat fee co-payment, payable upon admission; this co-pay varies with insurance status, exemption status (designed to protect populations with high expected usage of health care), case type, and whether or not the patient has a written referral from a primary health care physician, with explicit attention to ensuring that the exemption policy protects those too poor to afford the co-payments; and
- an Additional Outpatient Drug Benefit to subsidise the price of medicines provided on an outpatient basis for the management of primary care sensitive conditions like anemia, ulcers, pneumonia, and hypertension, in order to reduce unnecessary hospitalisations.

A small handful of key Kyrgyz players, including an eventual Minister of Health and an eventual General Director of the MHIF, were instrumental throughout the implementation of reform. They initiated the creation of the Manas strategy, brought donors into the conversation and coordinated donor activities, sustained the intellectual and political energy driving the reforms, and steered the reforms through sometimes turbulent political waters. They served as archetypal "champions" of reform. Despite difficult challenges to the overall reform programme, including the almost-constant risk of non-availability of funds, these champions managed to keep health sector reform high on the political agenda and successfully defended against political attack.

Challenges

From the outset, resistance to rationalisation of the health sector was anticipated from medical professionals and auxiliary staff fearing job loss (particularly in the large tertiary facilities in the capital, Bishkek), and also from users in catchment areas of facilities being closed. It was recognised that consultations would be necessary with various constituencies such as doctors, other medical staff, users in urban and rural areas, MOH staff, Parliament, and others, to develop support for rationalisation, design a compensation package, identify re-training opportunities, disseminate information on the need for rationalisation, and generally to build a consensus on the reform issue. The reform effort countered much potential resistance through the creation of institutions that could effectively lobby potentially recalcitrant groups on behalf of reform. These institutions included the Family Group Practice Association (FGP), Hospital Association, and Licensing and Accreditation Commission.

Some resistance was also expected to the treatment of some social groups with STIs on an anonymous ambulatory basis and to the shift to internationally-recognised standards for treatment of TB, both of which were part of the development of the primary care sector. To address this anticipated resistance, financial incentives were created for case detection and cure of TB patients, including a 60 som payment to a primary health care worker who manages a smear-positive TB patient to a documented cure, and a 30 som payment for the management of a smear-negative patient after treatment completion.

In an effort to pre-empt or appease resistance, various other approaches also were employed. Workshops were held in all regions to inform and discuss with all stakeholders the need for reform and various strategies for reform. Technical Working Groups (TWGs) were established by the MOH for project preparation, drawing key stakeholders from the MOH, MHIF, the associations of FGPs and Hospitals, the Licensing and Accreditation Commission, and other health professionals. Focus groups were conducted with staff members from urban and rural family group practices and family medical centers, with the trainers involved in family medicine education to confirm their continued support for reform. Chairpersons of relevant committees in the Parliament were consulted on a routine basis, as were governors and mayors in the regions. A formal roundtable was held to consult with the head doctors in the Bishkek republican health facilities and city hospitals. Focus groups were held with health professionals in both urban and rural areas.

Despite all of these efforts, at one critical point in mid-2002, it appeared as though opposition to reform would cause some of the key elements of reform to be dramatically altered or abandoned. This opposition emerged from several specific directions: parliamentarians who were physicians and had financial stakes in the "old" system; those who still stressed the superiority of the Soviet system; politically well-connected physicians who were profiting from private practices run out of the tertiary hospitals in Bishkek (this was significant given that these nine national facilities employed 18% of all doctors in practice in the country); and political antagonists whose ultimate interests lay in other issue areas. There was also significant opposition to the family medicine reforms, as many physicians and consumers felt that children and adults should be treated separately, and that the loss of outpatient specialists in pediatrics would result in poorer quality of care and less efficient care. To make matters worse, this opposition to the development of a system based on family medicine was also supported by governments of other Central Asian countries which tried to influence events in the Kyrgyz Republic.

During a peak period of opposition in October 2002, the Kyrgyz Parliament conducted a formal assessment of the Manas health sector reform programme, reaching a conclusion that these reform efforts were "unsatisfactory." It gave no reason for this judgment. The World Bank team successfully mobilised donor response to this opposition, organising a February 2003 Roundtable on health reforms that resulted in a renewed government commitment to reform and a revised action plan, endorsed by Parliament and by the President, for the implementation of reform activities. The personal intervention of the World Bank's Country Director was a key element of the political turnaround. *Outcomes* as a result of the new incentive structures, there was significant capacity reduction in inpatient health care facilities in Issyk-Kul and Chui. Fixed costs were reduced in hospitals from 21.3% of total hospital budgets in 2000 to 12.4% in 2005, allowing expenditures for meals and drugs in hospitals to increase from 18% in 2000 to 20% in 2004. Hospital utility expenditures decreased by 10% from 1999 to 2004.[4] Average length of hospital stay decreased by 12% from 2000 to 2005, with hospitalisation rates for several important chronic diseases declining significantly from 2000 to 2004 (hypertension from 21.5% to 13.9%; peptic ulcer from 45.4% to 37.3%; bronchial asthma from 54.6% to 22%).[5] Between 1999 and 2004, hospital admissions per staff decreased by 50%, and per bed by 25%.[5] The share of unnecessary referrals from primary care facilities to hospitals decreased from 2.5% of total hospital referrals to 0.6%. These outcomes clearly represent a more effective and efficient use of scarce resources.

The vast majority of the population gained access to primary health services through the guaranteed benefits package, and after the introduction of the package, the percentage of the population reporting no access to health care services steadily declined. According to household survey data, the percentage of the population who said that they *needed* health care during the year but did not seek it due to expense or distance to facility fell from 14.7% in 2001, to 5.7% in 2004, and to 3.6% in 2007. Similarly, the percentage of the total population (regardless of whether they said they needed care during the year) who did not seek health care due to expense or distance to facility has fallen from 1.9% in 2001, to 0.9% in 2004, and to 0.6% in 2007.[6] It is reasonable to speculate that the reform programme's interventions prevented access to health care from becoming significantly worse in a context of declining public financing for health care.

The reforms also had an impact on patients' financial burden for hospitalisations, particularly for the poor. Analysis of household surveys conducted both before the benefits package and co-payment reforms were implemented (2001), and then when some regions had experienced reform and some had not (2004), shows that the reforms were successful at limiting the increase in out-of-pocket payments for hospitalisation over that time period by 400 soms for an average household (with the average increase in reform regions at 200 soms, but the average increase in non-reform regions at 600 soms). Furthermore, the reforms had a proportionally greater impact on lower income groups, with the poorest 40% experiencing a significant increase in out-of-pocket payments for hospitalisation in non-reform regions but a slight decline in reform regions. By contrast, out-of-pocket payments increased in all regions for the richest 40%.[7]

The co-payment system, introduced for inpatient care, was intended to substitute formal co-payments for out-of-pocket payments, with exemptions for pregnant women, children under 16, pensioners, and other socially vulnerable groups. The co-payment mechanism aimed to increase the transparency of the system, replacing requirements for unpredictable informal payments with a clear system of benefits and entitlements, and clarifying the responsibility of the state in the provision of health care. As was the case with the single-payer reforms, the co-payments were introduced gradually in four waves: initially in Issyk-Kul and Chui in 2001; in Talas and Naryn in 2002; in Jalal-Abad and Batken in 2003; and finally in Osh and Bishkek in 2003/2004.

Lessons to be Learned

The presence of a clear sector strategy, authored and wholly owned by the MOH, played a key role in achieving donor harmonisation. In the Kyrgyz case, the MOH's role as a leader and coordinator of donor activity, in partnership with the World Bank, was central. Longevity and consistency of donor support, along with clear "division of labour" among donors, has also been essential in an environment where donor presence is strong. These factors have prevented needless duplication of activity, assigned donors to activities best suited to their comparative advantages, and ensured that there is appropriate donor activity across all issue areas.

The political economy of health sector reform inevitably creates both winners and losers. Early and comprehensive anticipation of stakeholder interests, institutional analysis to facilitate understanding of those interests, and the generation of a coherent plan to build support for reform and to persuade and/or co-opt potential opponents has been essential.

One effective mechanism for countering political resistance to reform has been strong and consistent monitoring and evaluation, where analytic results have been generated and disseminated rapidly and effectively, building support for project activities in a politically contentious environment. Positive data and analysis on intermediate project outcomes has generated broad support for further project activities. In the Kyrgyz case, the Issyk-Kul region has become a recognised demonstration site whose successes have prompted other regions to accelerate their participation in the reforms.

Another important tool for overcoming political resistance to reform has been the cultivation and even creation of civil society organisations that have given health professionals and users of the health care system a voice in the decision-making process and a clear sense of affiliation and identity. In other words, supporting potential "winners," and creating pathways to transform "losers" into "winners," has been as important as overcoming or side-stepping recalcitrant "losers." The creation in the Kyrgyz case of the Family Group Practice Association and related organisations has demonstrated the potential long-term impact of institutional development investments that may at first have seemed unsustainable or risky.

The complexity of health care systems dictates that reforms be carefully sequenced. In this case, capacity building in the primary care sector through the family medicine and other primary care reforms was a pre-condition for hospital rationalisation. Revenue gains from financing and service delivery reforms made possible the later benefits package and co-payment schemes, and the changes in revenue collection and pooling were necessary prerequisites to the introduction of new purchasing arrangements.

Conclusion

The Kyrgyz government's success at managing external donors and opposition from domestic groups has enabled consolidation of reform and movement forward. A Manas Taalimi Health Reform Programme was developed in 2005 by the MOH as a successor to the Manas strategy. The name "Manas Taalimi" is significant: Manas is the Kyrgyz national hero, and it was considered desirable to keep that name for the sake of continuity with the prior health care reform programme. "Taalimi" is an ancient Kyrgyz word signifying a vast sense of heritage and legacy. The name Manas Taalimi therefore stresses the extent to which the current reform programme is explicitly based on the lessons learned from the Manas I programme. Manas Taalimi is an extension of the health goals embedded in the 2002 National Poverty Reduction Strategy and Comprehensive Development Framework. The objective of the Manas Taalimi programme is, broadly, to "improve health status through the creation of an effective, comprehensive, and integrated delivery system of individual and public health services, and through increased responsibility of every citizen, family, society, and public administration bodies for the health of each person and for society as a whole."[8] It explicitly aims to institutionalise the reforms initiated under Manas and to strengthen the parts of the health care system that were relatively less emphasised under the earlier strategy. In particular, Manas Taalimi seeks to strengthen the targeting of resources and interventions to groups with worse health outcomes, including Millennium Development Goal outcomes; to implement structural improvements in the public health and health promotion systems; to enhance capacity in the MOH and other relevant institutions in policy formulation, priority setting, policy-based budget planning, and monitoring and evaluation; and to strengthen quality of care with a focus on priority health problems including maternal and child health, cardio-vascular disease, respiratory illnesses, HIV/AIDS, and TB.

Manas Taalimi was developed and refined in an open and transparent manner through extensive stakeholder consultation, including town hall meetings throughout the country, consultations with senior government officials, and numerous formal and informal consultations with health sector donors — although it should be stressed that the core strategy and Programme of Work were developed by the government through a genuinely indigenous process. The government gave extended leave to fifteen key health specialists from the MOH, MOF, MHIF, and other institutions to work on the strategy, providing re-entry guarantees to their original posts once the strategy was completed. The preparation of Manas Taalimi thus overcame any accumulated negative experience and mistrust, evolving as not only a consensus-based technical process, but also a process in which the players knew and understood one another's personalities, institutional constraints, and motivations.

A variety of lessons from the implementation of the Manas programme, as well as the World Bank's two supporting health reform projects, were explicitly applied to the development of follow-on activities. These include: the need to synchronise the financing base and budget formulation and execution systems with health reforms, so that health providers can retain and allocate funds saved through rationalisation of health infrastructure and health budgets can be formed according to output-based formulas; a focus on governance, acknowledging the institutional transformation of the MOH by investing heavily in stewardship functions such as monitoring and evaluation and stressing transparency and accountability in the health sector; a commitment to deepen the rightsizing of the health sector and completing the process of structural reform in Bishkek and Osh cities, where the process remains incomplete; and stress the need for donor coordination, acknowledging that the highly successful informal collaboration supporting Manas should be sustained through an explicit, government-directed Programme of Work and through periodic, formal, structured meetings for sector monitoring and donor coordination. The attention to transparency is particularly important given the acknowledged extent of corruption in the public sector. The follow-on activities put special emphasis on disclosure and transparency and on strengthened complaint handing mechanisms coupled with specific remedial measures.

As in all countries heavily reliant on donor funding and technical expertise, questions have lingered about the sustainability of reform in the eventual absence of donor support. In this case, the Kyrgyz health sector has remained heavily reliant on donor funds, currently amounting to about one-quarter of total public health spending through the SWAp mechanism. It is clear however, that the Kyrgyz health sector is well on its way to being weaned from outside technical assistance. Modern clinical, financial, and administrative practices have been internalised, and it is reasonable to assume that the reform process would be sustained even in the absence of donor persuasion and intervention.

Despite its periods of political turbulence, health sector reform in the Kyrgyz Republic has managed to sustain a steady trajectory of increasing quality and efficiency, maintenance of near-universal access to health care, and improved population health outcomes directly and plausibly attributable to interventions aimed at reforming the system. Overwhelmingly, these remarkable achievements can be traced to the efforts of a small and talented group of Kyrgyz champions of reform, whose skills not only at health policy but also in political negotiations — with both external donors and internal stakeholders — enabled consistent and productive movement forward.

References

1. Meimanaliev A, Ibraimova A, Elebesov B, Rechel B. (2005) *Health Care Systems in Transition: Kyrgyzstan*. European Observatory on Health Systems and Policies, London.
2. World Bank. (2006) Staff Appraisal Report, Kyrgyz Republic, Health Sector Reform Project. Human Resources Division, Country Department III, Europe and Central Asia Region, Report no. 15181-KG, April 22.
3. Jakab M, Manjieva E. (2007) Kyrgyz Republic. In: *Good Practice in Health Financing: Lessons from Reforms in Low and Middle Income Countries*. Health, Nutrition, and Population, Human Development Network, World Bank, Washington.
4. WHO/DfID Manas Health Policy Analysis Project. (2005) Evaluating the Manas health Sector Reform (1996–2005): Focus on Health Financing, Policy Research Paper No. 30.
5. WHO/DfID Manas Health Policy Analysis Project. (Undated) Did Restructuring of Health Facilities Reduce Utility Costs? Policy Brief # 6, http://eng.chsd.med.kg/MyFiles/Policy%20brief6%20Restructuring.E.pdf
6. WHO/DfID Manas Health Policy Analysis Project. (2007) Health, Health-Seeking Behaviour, and Out-of-Pocket Expenditures in Kyrgyzstan, Policy Research Paper No. 46.
7. Jakab M. (2007) Did the Kyrgyz Health Financing Reforms Reduce the Financial Burden of Health Care Seeking for the Poor? In: An Empirical Evaluation of the Kyrgyz Health Reform: Does It Work for the Poor? Ph.D. Dissertation, Department of Health Policy, Faculty of Arts and Sciences, Harvard University, Cambridge, MA.
8. Kyrgyz Republic. (2005) Kyrgyz Republic National Health Care Reform Program "Manas Taalimi" (2006–2010). Bishkek.

18

Yellow Fever and Health Diplomacy: International Efforts to Stop the Urban Yellow Fever Outbreak in Paraguay

Jon Kim Andrus[i], *Alba María Ropero*[ii], *Gladys Ghisays*[iii], *Stacy Romero*[iv], *Barbara Jauregui*[v] *and Cuauhtemoc Ruiz Matus*[vi]

Abstract

A yellow fever outbreak in Paraguay, where there was an insufficient supply of vaccines for the population, led to a unique and diplomatically negotiated global response that rapidly mobilized approximately 3.5 million vaccines from various countries. This case study reviews the efforts behind the process, whereby the Pan-American Health Organization (PAHO) — the World Health Organization's regional arm

[i] Deputy Director, Pan American Health Organization, Washington, DC, USA.
[ii] Regional advisor, Immunization Project, Pan American Health Organization, Washington, DC, USA.
[iii] International advisor, Immunization Project, Pan American Health Organization, Caracas, Venezuela.
[iv] MPH candidate, Global Health Department, George Washington University.
[v] Specialist, Immunization Project, Pan American Health Organization, Washington, DC, USA.
[vi] Senoir Advisor, Immunization Project, Pan American Health Organization, Washington, DC, USA.

for the Americas, together with Paraguay's Ministry of Health and governments from several other countries, managed to deal with the critical and unexpected situation quickly and effectively. The results demonstrate that in health diplomacy good will breeds more good will. Diplomacy and consensus-building skills were required to negotiate an international strategy and convince other countries that they had not only humanitarian, but also vested national interests in helping to control the outbreak in Paraguay.

Introduction

The Yellow Fever (YF) virus causes approximately 200,000 cases of YF and 30,000 case fatalities in both the Latin American and African regions each year where the disease remains endemic.[1] YF is endemic in 13 Latin America and the Caribbean (LAC) countries, with Bolivia, Brazil, Colombia, Ecuador, and Peru considered to be at greatest risk for YF outbreaks.[2] Two modes of YF transmission exist: Jungle YF and Urban YF. Jungle YF is found in tropical rainforest areas where the wild mosquitoes, *Haemagogus*, can infect monkeys with YF virus. Monkeys then serve as the reservoir for other wild *Haemagogus* mosquitoes to become infected with the YF virus. Infected mosquitoes can transmit the virus to humans who enter the rainforest. Because young males are more likely to enter the forest where the monkey reservoir of disease lives, human victims of Jungle YF infection are typically young males who work or hunt in the rainforest. Urban YF occurs when domestic mosquitoes, *Aedes Aegypti,* transmit the virus to humans. Urban transmission does not require monkeys, so outbreaks can be explosive and cause substantial mortality quickly.[1] The epidemiology of urban YF includes: high case fatality rates, both sexes, a wider age-distribution, and more explosive outbreak presentations than the more sporadic jungle YF. Depending upon the quality of surveillance, case fatality rates can be as high as 40%, where nearly four out of every 10 people infected die.

Prior to 2008, the last case of Urban YF in Paraguay was more than 100 years ago in 1904, whilst the last case of Jungle YF in Paraguay was in 1974.[3] The last urban outbreak in the entire hemisphere occurred more than 45 years ago. Despite the elapsed time since the last YF outbreak,

Paraguay started routine vaccination against YF in 2001 along the border areas within close proximity in areas of endemic, or naturally occurring YF in the jungle areas of neighbouring countries, especially Brazil and Bolivia. By 2006, YF vaccine was fully integrated into Paraguay's routine national childhood immunization programme. Additionally, Paraguay had improved YF surveillance efforts across the nation.

The Problem

Between January and May 2008, a total of 28 confirmed YF cases were reported in Paraguay, of which 11 died, for a Case Fatality Ratio (CFR) of 39% (PAHO Epidemiological Bulletin). Four sub-clusters of YF cases were identified. Each cluster was defined as having the same epidemiological link. The first cluster, which started on January 13, 2008, occurred in San Estanislao, San Pedro Department. This cluster consisted of seven YF cases, including five who were hunters with a recent travel history to a nearby jungle. One case resided next to the hunters and the last case worked in their neighbourhood. Because the hunters traveled to an enzootic area within the same region, this cluster was initially classified as Jungle YF transmission.[4]

A second sub-cluster, identified on February 27, 2008, also occurred in the San Pedro Department but in the Santo Domingo and Santa Lucia areas. This sub-cluster consisted of seven cases, of which three died, a CFR of 43%. Most of the cases traveled to attend the funeral of another YF victim and approximately half of the victims were female. Upon collection of mosquitoes in the area, the health authorities found wild mosquitoes, *Haemagogus,* indicative of Jungle YF transmission, as well as the *Aedes Aegypti* mosquito, which characterises Urban YF transmission. Health authorities decided it was not possible to identify with certainty the mode of transmission for this second YF cluster.

The third cluster of nine cases began in early February in the Laurelty neighbourhood of the San Lorenzo District of the Central Department. Of nine cases, five were female and three died. Predominant female gender distribution is consistent with Urban YF transmission. Evidence to support Urban YF transmission came with the identification of *Aedes Aegypti* and no *Haemagogus* wild mosquitoes found.

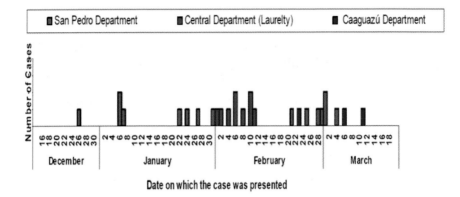

Figure 1.   Epidemic curve of cases of yellow fever in Paraguay, 2008

Source: Pan American Health Organization. Emerging and Reemerging Infectious Diseases, Region of the Americas. Epidemiological Bulletin 2008; 5(5).

The fourth sub-cluster occurred in the Caaguazu Department in late February through early March 2008. The cluster consisted of four cases, three were female and all four died, a CFR of 100%. The YF virus was isolated through polymerase chain reaction from specimens collected from the victims. Both urban and jungle mosquitoes were collected at two of the three sites. Authorities decided it was not possible to conclude with certainty the mode of transmission[4,5] (see Fig. 1).

The number of deaths occurring over a short period of time was alarming to health authorities, as well as to the community at large. A public outcry for immediate vaccination gained momentum. Shortages of vaccine created increasing panic with each passing day. Crowds began daily picketing and protests at the Presidential palace in Asuncion, which is near the epicenter of the outbreak. The government appeared to be on the verge of collapse due to the intense social disruption caused by the outbreaks and the vaccine shortage. The Pan American Health Organization (PAHO), which is the World Health Organization's (WHO) regional arm for the Americas, was requested to mobilise YF vaccine using its Revolving Fund for vaccine purchase. PAHO contacted the global stockpile of YF vaccine in Geneva and found insufficient doses available for use in the Americas. Given the stockpile shortages, PAHO and the Minister of Health (MOH) in Paraguay issued a global alarm for vaccine deployment to Paraguay.

The Local and External Players and Their Roles

The Minister of Health was the key player and is the person ultimately responsible for public health response in Paraguay. The Minister of Health reports directly to the President of Paraguay. The simultaneous occurrence of the sylvatic outbreaks and the urban outbreak caused increasing public alarm and panic. The urban outbreak in Paraguay was the first urban YF outbreak to be reported in the entire hemisphere over the last 45 years. As with all urban outbreaks, the one in Paraguay came with a very high case fatality rate. Moreover, the outbreak occurred right in the back yard of the nation's capital. Public alarm increased when it became apparent that the MOH had only a few thousand doses of yellow fever vaccine available in its supply. The communications officer from the Ministry of Health was challenged to ensure that accurate, transparent information was being provided to the community in a timely manner.

PAHO maintains a local office in Asuncion, Paraguay to provide direct technical cooperation to the MOH on health issues. The Representative of PAHO oversees a staff of public health experts supporting the MOH. The PAHO Representative is the person ultimately responsible for coordinating PAHO's technical cooperation with the Ministry of Health. The Representative is supported by an International Immunization Advisor, an expert in the field of immunization and vaccination. The Advisor also coordinates PAHO's local support from PAHO's Revolving Fund for vaccine purchase (RF).

The RF serves as a mechanism to mobilise and purchase vaccines on behalf of PAHO Member Countrie.[6] Because the RF mechanism is used to purchase vaccines in bulk on behalf of all PAHO Member Countries, the PAHO regional office in Washington, DC manages the day to day operations of the RF. Annually PAHO solicits and collects from each country their most accurate vaccine demand forecasts of country needs. All countries provide PAHO with their vaccine demand forecasts one year in advance of their actual requirements.Then on behalf of Member Countries the RF mechanism uses the leverage of the region-wide vaccine demand to negotiate affordable vaccine prices for countries. Such bulk purchasing greatly supports the numerous smaller countries in the region, especially Paraguay. If these countries had to negotiate prices on their own, vaccine prices would likely be much higher and country programmes would be unlikely to afford the vaccines that they are currently using.

The RF has been in operation serving Member Countries for more than 30 years. Of equal importance to the sustainable supply of effective, safe, and affordable vaccines, the RF has been critical in the region's response to emergency outbreaks of vaccine preventable diseases.[7] Numerous examples include response over the years to jungle YF, seasonal and pandemic influenza, and outbreaks related to importations of polio, measles, and rubella. Without the RF it would have been unlikely for countries of the region to implement plans of action to eradicate polio, measles, and rubella well in advance of other parts of the world.

Limited sources of vaccine were available to help the MOH control the urban YF outbreak in Paraguay. Some possibilities included the global YF vaccine stockpile already mentioned, private industry, or storage supplies in the cold chain of other countries. Two large manufacturers exist for the global supply of YF vaccine. The largest is Sanofi Pasteur of France, followed by Biomanguinhos in Brazil. A third supplier supported by Sanofi Pasteur is located in Senegal to cover national needs.

Sanofi Pasteur of France is a large private multi-national firm with several decades of experience manufacturing vaccines for the global community. Biomanguingos, Brazil, is the other large global supplier of YF vaccine. Biomanguingos has manufactured and provided yellow fever vaccine for use in Latin America and the Caribbean for decades. Biomanguingos is public-private entity whose first responsibility is to maintain YF vaccine supply for the citizens of Brazil. Over the years, the Brazilian MOH has mobilised YF vaccine in response to unexpected shortages of YF vaccine in countries such as Colombia and Venezuela, supporting them in responding to public health emergencies requiring urgent deployment of vaccines.

The YF vaccine global stockpile is a repository of vaccines largely managed in Geneva by a board consisting of representatives of UNICEF, WHO, the Red Cross, and Doctors Without Borders. All these representatives are available on a moments notice to provide technical guidance for the emergency deployment of YF vaccine to countries experiencing outbreaks.

At the time of the outbreak in Paraguay, none of these manufacturers had vaccines available. Only the YF global stockpile had two million

Table 1. Origin of YF vaccine available in Paraguay, 2008

Origin of the Vaccine	Quantity of YF Vaccines
Balance of the Ministry of Health	290,900
Bolivia	50,000
Brazil first delivery	50,000
Brazil second delivery	800,000
Cuba	50,000
Germany	50,000
Global Vaccine Fund of the YF-WHO	2,000,000
Peru	144,430
Venezuela	100,000
Total Vaccines Acquired	3,535,330

doses which were directed to Paraguay. Other players involved in the response to the crisis in Paraguay were high-level Representatives from the MOHs of Venezuela, Cuba, Peru, Brazil, Bolivia, and Germany. Table 1 shows the countries and organisations that finally made YF vaccine available to Paraguay in 2008.

Challenges Faced and the Outcome

Paraguay implemented immediate actions required to control the YF outbreak, including mass vaccination campaigns (starting with the little vaccine they had in their supply), vector control, case investigations, reporting, and follow-up. A PAHO group of experts was convened shortly after the outbreak to evaluate the effectiveness of the outbreak response, to confirm that **urban YF** had indeed occurred, and to mobilise sufficient vaccines and supplies in the face of initial shortages. The PAHO group of experts concluded that the Paraguay response was well coordinated and reduced the likely spread of YF. During the outbreak, the Minister of Health organised daily meetings that included multidisciplinary participation from a team consisting of epidemiologists, vector control experts, and infectious disease experts.[3]

At the onset of the Paraguay urban YF outbreak, there existed a global shortage of YF vaccine. On average, the global stockpile in Geneva contains six million YF vaccine doses. Prior to the outbreak in Paraguay, the recurring outbreaks in Brazil had reduced the available global supply. In January 2008, Brazil prioritised vaccines from Biomanquinhos/Brazil for national use rather than export, and requested an additional four million vaccines from the global stockpile.[8] As a consequence, only two million YF vaccine doses were left in the global stockpile at the time of the beginning of the outbreak in Paraguay.

The routine YF vaccination coverage in Paraguay for the general population was only 24% and along the border areas was around 60% by 2007.[4] For each of the emerging clusters of YF cases, the immediate rapid response included establishing rings of vaccination around the sites of infection. The first ring had an 800 meter diameter and the subsequent concentric rings had 2,400 meter diameters each.[4,5] In addition to these targeted vaccination efforts, Paraguay's Ministry of Health decided to expand the vaccination response to include other susceptible people in the Asunción metropolitan area, in total approximately 1.5 million individuals between the ages of 1 and 59 years.[4] (The total population of Paraguay is approximately 6.350.000 people.) Ultimately, Paraguay expanded its vaccination response to a nationwide campaign targeting all susceptible individuals aged 1 to 59 years who had never received the YF vaccine. In addition to fixed-post vaccination, the campaign also included door-to-door outreach tactics throughout the country. Clearly, the success of this massive initiative was contingent upon readily accessible YF vaccines.

Regarding the availability of YF vaccine as the YF outbreak spread in Paraguay, there were only 300,000 YF vaccine doses available nationally and 50,000 vaccine doses distributed to peripheral vaccination centres. This was far short of the target population of 1.5 million people to be included in the outbreak vaccination response. At the same time, as previously mentioned, the seeming re-emergence of YF in Paraguay induced widespread panic throughout the country. Where vaccines were available, people queued for hours to get their dose. As community tension increased, the demand for vaccines also increased nationwide. Stories appeared on the front pages of newspapers everyday. Television broadcasts also provided daily, rather intense updates of the situation.

In these initial days, PAHO met several times per day with the Minister of Health and his staff. The MOH clearly felt the pressure of media reports, as well as the community response directed at the government. The MOH initially had no clear communication strategy to respond to a national emergency. This situation improved with time, mainly thanks to vaccine availability. PAHO played a key role in activating an accelerated coordination mechanism between partners and countries of the region in order to secure vaccine for Paraguay.

With the reports of additional YF cases in Laurelty, the affected urban area in Paraguay, Brazil shipped 50,000 vaccine doses and Peru shipped 144,430 vaccine doses to Paraguay.[9] The dissemination of information to other countries from technical sources, as well as media and civil society sources of information, enhanced international efforts to mobilise vaccines. But, these shipments, although highly appreciated, fell far short of the large demand being fanned by the flurry of daily media reports.

With PAHO's support, the MOH stayed in almost constant contact with the global stockpile representatives, requesting an immediate release of at least 1.5 million additional YF vaccine doses. Whilst global stockpile discussions progressed, PAHO and the MOH continued their bilateral outreach to other foreign governments. Additional contributions came from Colombia, Cuba, and Germany.[10,11] In total, these efforts resulted in the MOH Paraguay and PAHO mobilising 3,435,330 YF vaccine doses for outbreak response.[9] By May 10, 2008, 2,137,474 individuals had been vaccinated in the country. Paraguay allocated 664,430 doses of vaccine to the central warehouse which is the stockpile for national emergencies.

Lessons to be Learned

The global response to the urban YF outbreak in Paraguay resulted in the rapid mobilisation of approximately 3.5 million YF vaccines. Paraguay was able to implement a timely and rapid vaccination response. These global efforts and contributions constitute a model of health diplomacy, which in all likelihood prevented many more deaths, as well as the potentially disastrous consequences of uncontrolled civil disturbance. The political and technical collaboration led to improved global health because the outbreak was stopped, whilst serving to enhance international relations.[5] Had the outbreak continued, Africa would have faced a serious threat due to insufficient global vaccine supply to respond to potential outbreaks.

With respect to this particular outbreak, there was a delicate balance in the public health response between immediate action with appropriate resources and planning for action without appropriate resources, especially vaccines. Certainly, the planning component progressed whilst tremendous energy went into securing vaccine supply from external sources. Whilst all this was being played out, the public outcry threatened Paraguay's national security. The key players in this process were the Minister of Health and the staff of the Ministry of Health, the PAHO representatives at different levels, as well as representatives from all other countries involved. Control interventions include vaccine and other mitigating measures. Therefore, the collective communication message that evolved focused on mitigating measures, such as vector control around the household, use of repellants and proper protecting clothing. Once sufficient vaccine supply had been secured, mass communication and social mobilisation messages could then be implemented giving instructions to the public regarding where to receive the vaccine. However, until vaccine became readily available the public outcry only got louder and more difficult to manage.

Global health cooperation, derived from health diplomacy, is a national interest and a global good.[5] It was also in the national interest of neighbouring and other countries to donate their available YF vaccine to reduce the risk of imported YF infections. The outbreak in Paraguay transcended its national borders and required global actions to adequately protect the health of the region's population.[12,13] Diplomacy and consensus-building skills were required to convince neighbouring countries that they had not only a humanitarian interest, but also a vested national interest in controlling the outbreak in Paraguay. It is not easy for a country to release limited quantities of a life-saving vaccine intended for its own citizens, for use outside its borders. An importation of infections occurring after the fact could potentially leave national leaders exposed to harsh criticism. Fortunately, this has never been the case. Usually, the voice of reason calls upon immediate action directed at the source of the outbreak to diminish the risk of spread. National leaders change frequently, so these points need to be continually reinforced for each new outbreak or emergency.

By February 27, 2008, after donating the remaining two million YF vaccines to Paraguay, WHO reported that the global stockpile of YF vaccine had been depleted. This reality had severe implications for Paraguay nationally and other nations globally. A highly visible collective response, grounded in solidarity that crossed governments, institutions, and private industry, was essential in making the Paraguayan response possible. Such a response will also be required when responding to future outbreaks, especially given the recent depletion of the global stockpile. PAHO provided technical oversight and also played a coordinating role for all the key stakeholders, including WHO, Paraguay, and neighbouring countries. PAHO and WHO provided the mechanism through which countries could donate and transport their YF vaccines to Paraguay.[12,13] The PAHO Revolving Fund, in particular, aggressively explored all possibilities of vaccine loans or contributions. PAHO and WHO along with the manufacturers have been working on strategies to improve vaccine availability. Nonetheless, it is important to highlight that the current production of YF vaccine is extremely limited, and sufficient vaccine production remains a challenge to maintain both the global stockpile and to reach high vaccination coverage in endemic countries.

At the core of health diplomacy is good health governance which creates a venue whereby compromises and agreements can be reached.[12,13] Compromises were made by each country that donated YF vaccines to Paraguay because they reduced their national capacity to respond to future potential YF outbreaks in their own respective countries. However, the contributing countries acknowledged that by donating vaccines to Paraguay, they were indeed reducing the risk that YF would spread to their own countries. For good health diplomacy to occur effectively, diplomats, public and private sectors, scientists, medical professionals, non-governmental organisations, and civil society must interact to negotiate a clear response strategy.[12,13] Most of these actors were present and all extremely active during the Paraguayan response to YF.

There have been previous experiences of global health diplomacy efforts. Brazil's leading role in YF outbreak response over the years has not gone unnoticed. President Ignacio Lula da Silva has played a role promoting other health initiatives around the world. Most recently Brazil responded to the earthquake crisis in Haiti by sending doctors and nurses from the very onset. Other examples of such humanitarian response are innumerable. In a similar fashion, Thailand in appreciation of the world's generous response to the tsunami, pledged funds to support Haiti's recon-struction. In health diplomacy clearly good will breeds more good will.

Conclusion

Global health diplomacy, global cooperation, and good health governance all occurred during the YF outbreak in Paraguay. Without each of these components, Paraguay would not have had the necessary resources to respond to the outbreak and protect its population from a disease with high case-fatality rates. The Paraguayan government developed an effective and comprehensive response plan to stop transmission of YF nationwide. Given that both jungle and urban YF modes of transmission were present during the outbreaks, the threat of widespread infection was elevated, but was suc-cessfully prevented. The Paraguayan response in conjunction with health diplomacy ought to serve as a model for future health crises worldwide.

References

1. Monath, T. (2005) Yellow Fever Vaccines, *Expert Rev Vaccines* 4 (4): 689–693.
2. World Health Organization. (2001) Yellow Fever Fact Sheet. Retrieved September 3, 2008, Available from: http://www.who.int/mediacentre/fact-sheets/fs100/en/
3. PAHO Group of Experts — Yellow Fever in Paraguay, 22 May 2008. Report to the Minister of Health of Paraguay.
4. Pan American Health Organization. (2008) Emerging and Reemerging Infectious Diseases, Region of the Americas. *Epidemiological Bulletin* 5 (5).
5. Novotny T, Hannah Leslie H, Adams V, and Kickbusch I. (2008) Health Diplomacy: A Literature Review. UCSF/IGCC Project on Health Diplomacy.
6. Andrus JK, Sherris J, Fitzsimmons JW, Kane MA, Aguado T. (2008) Introduction of human papillomavirus vaccines into developing countries–International strategies for funding and procurement, *Vaccine* Suppl 26S: K87–K92.
7. Andrus JK, de Quadros CA, Ruiz Matus C, Luciani S, Hotez P. (2009) New vaccines for developing countries: Will it be feast or famine? *A J Law Med* 35: 311–322.

8. World Health Organization. Epidemic and Pandemic Alert and Response. Yellow fever in Brazil. 5 February 2008. Retrieved March 3, 2009. Available from: http://www.who.int/csr/don/2008_02_07/en/index.html.

9. PAHO Special Report: Yellow Fever in Paraguay, 3 March 2008. Retrieved March 3, 2009. Available from: http://www.reliefweb.int/rw/RWFiles2008. nsf/FilesByRWDocUnidFilename/EDIS-7CGT7P-full_report.pdf/ $File/full_report.pdf.

10. World Health Organization. Transcript of WHO Podcast, 27 February 2008. Retrieved March 3, 2009. Available from: http://www.who.int/mediacentre/ multimedia/podcasts/2008/transcript_28/en/index.html.

11. Center for Disease Control and prevention. (2008) Global Health Diplomacy Summer Workshop, July 21–25.

12. Kickbusch I, Novotny T, Drager N, Silberschmidt G, Alcazar, S. (2007) Global Health Diplomacy: Training across disciplines, Bulletin of the World Health Organization.

13. Kickbusch I, Silberschmidt G, Buss P. (2008) Global Health Diplomacy: The need for new perspectives, strategic approaches and skills in global health, World Health Organization, Retrieved October 15, 2008, Available from: http://www.who.int/bulletin/volumes/85/3/06–039222/en/print.html.

19

Diplomacy and the Polio Immunization Boycott in Northern Nigeria

With scientific evidence and pressure from political allies and religious authority figures, a Nigerian polio vaccine boycott was brought to an end.

Judith R. Kaufmann[i] *and Harley Feldbaum*[ii]

Abstract

The boycott of polio vaccination in three Northern Nigerian states in 2003 created a global health crisis that was political in origin. This paper traces the diplomatic actions that were taken by the Global Polio Eradication Initiative, the United Nations, and the U.S. government, to restart polio vaccination and resolve the crisis. The polio vaccination boycott in Northern Nigeria provides a useful case study of the practice of global health diplomacy. [*Health Affairs* 28, no. 4 (2009): 1091–1101; 10.1377/hlthaff.28.4.1091]

[i] Judith Kaufmann (kaufmannjr2@aol.com) is a visiting scholar at the Global Health and Foreign Policy Initiative, Paul H. Nitze School of Advanced International Studies, in Arlington, Virginia.

[ii] Harley Feldbaum is associate director of this initiative, at its Washington, D.C., office.

IN AUGUST 2003 THE POLITICAL LEADERSHIP of several Northern Nigerian states responded to community pressure and banned federally sponsored polio immunization campaigns. The stoppage was justified by "evidence" that the polio vaccine was contaminated with antifertility drugs intended to sterilize young Muslim girls. The suspension in Northern Nigeria, particularly in Kano State, led to a global outbreak of polio; the disease spread into twenty countries across Africa, the Middle East, and Southeast Asia and caused 80% of the world's cases of paralytic poliomyelitis during the stoppage. The vaccine boycott eventually led to costs of more than US$500 million to control the polio outbreak, and it essentially ended hopes of eradicating polio in this decade (Exhibit 1).[1]

The solution to this global health crisis, caused by internal Nigerian political forces, was not typical: not only was epidemiological information required, but also diplomatic action. Previous literature has examined the political and public health background to the crisis, and the public health response to the vaccination stoppage.[2] What has not been previously reported is how international diplomatic tools were mobilized to end the formal political boycott. There has been much discussion recently of "health diplomacy," but few case studies or little historical examination of how diplomacy and health interact.[3] By examining the diplomatic response to the polio boycott in Nigeria, this paper provides a case study in the use of traditional diplomacy to support global health efforts — an important component of health diplomacy.

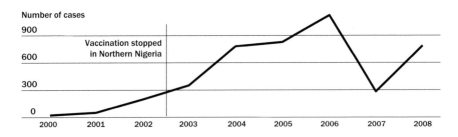

EXHIBIT 1.   Cases of wild poliovirus in Nigeria, 2000–December 2008

Source: World Health Organization/Global Polio Eradication Initiative, "Wild Poliovirus 2000–2009," April 2009, http://polioeradication.org/content/general/casecount.pdf (accessed 10 April 2009).

This case study is based on a literature review, examination of previously unavailable Global Polio Eradication Initiative (GPEI) and U.S. government documents, and thirteen in-depth interviews with people involved in the crisis. Interviews were used to go beyond published accounts of the crisis and to illuminate the experiences, perspectives, and interests of both policymakers and institutions.

Origins of the Vaccine Boycott

Historical political, ethnic, and religious tensions in Nigeria were exacerbated after the April 2003 election, when retired General Olusegun Obasanjo, a born-again Baptist from the southern part of Nigeria, was elected to a second term as president over retired General Muhammadu Buhari, a Muslim northerner. Reflecting and exacerbating these tensions were regional disparities in the provision and use of health services, with poorer health outcomes found in the North.[4]

The *Weekly Trust*, an important northern newspaper, reported that the formal suspension began at a 21 July 2003 meeting of the Jama'atul Nasril Islam (JNI, a northern umbrella group of Muslim organizations):

One of the Emirs presented a memo on the concerns and apprehensions of his people on the allegations that the polio vaccination campaign was being used for the purpose of depopulating developing countries, and especially Muslim countries. ...Although some of the more senior Emirs tried to dismiss the observation as mere rambling by their subjects, the Supreme Council on Sharia implementation in Nigeria led by a respected Kano-based medical doctor, Dr. Datti Ahmed brought the apprehensions into full public glare when . . . he told newsmen that his council had reasons to suspect contamination of the polio vaccines with HIV/AIDS virus, anti-fertility substances and other dangerous elements.[5]

According to then U.S. Ambassador to Nigeria John Campbell, the boycott "was about fear and disaffection at the popular level that fastened on immunization as a precipitant. ...Once the safety of the vaccines became a popular issue, which leaders could not control, they gave in with some reluctance." He continued by saying, "This was not really about technical issues. The issue was Northern Nigeria's thorough disaffection with the Obasanjo government."[6]

A source who has worked closely with the Nigeria polio program said, "This was one of the clearest examples of a public health issue being hijacked for political reasons. ...The bulk of people were sincerely concerned, but clearly the leadership and the encouragement to continue was political." The global polio vaccination campaign had become enmeshed in local Nigerian politics, with northern political leaders ceasing polio immunizations in their states.[7]

Early Response to the Vaccine Boycott

Rumors about safety have plagued many immunization programs, including in the United States, where there are groups and Web sites devoted to theories about the links between immunizations and conditions such as autism.[8] As the United Nations Children's Fund (UNICEF) notes, "Occasionally rumours arise such as a link between immunization and family planning or that vaccination could cause HIV/AIDS. While these rumors are groundless, when they spread, they can severely damage immunization efforts."[9] Generally speaking, local leaders with influence in the community are most effective in countering rumors when they arise.[10]

When rumors about tainted vaccine first began to circulate in Nigeria in 2003, the initial assumption by those involved was that these rumors would be short lived and that tools and lessons learned from other regions would be sufficient to convince those involved to recommit to the campaign.[11] Gianni Murzi, the UNICEF Nigeria director at the time, explained:

> Our own Western-oriented . . . background tells us if vaccine is found to be good, then it's scientifically good, that's it. ...Instead, the population who rejected it was thinking in other terms, and we didn't realize the power of that and how disruptive that could have been. ...We didn't see it coming, and unfortunately that is quite normal.[12]

The United Nations Envoy

Simultaneously, but completely separately, then U.S. Secretary of State Colin Powell and UNICEF headquarters suggested to United Nations (UN) Secretary-General Kofi Annan that he send Ibrahim Gambari, the secretary-general's senior adviser for African affairs, to Nigeria as the secretary-general's special envoy. Normally, the UN Secretariat would not send a national of a country to negotiate in his or her country of origin, for fear of conflict of interest or pressure being put on the individual. However, in this case, most felt that Gambari was uniquely qualified. Gambari's father was a Muslim northerner and Emir of Ilorin, and his mother was a southerner. Gambari has served under virtually all of the surviving former Nigerian presidents, including those with presumed influence in the North, and had managed President Obasanjo's 1991 campaign to be UN secretary-general.

Gambari met with President Obasanjo and the federal minister of health in early 2004. According to Gambari, President Obasanjo approved visits to the Sultan of Sokoto, the Emir of Kano, traditional leaders of the Muslim communities, and former presidents, including General Buhari, saying, "You get to where I find it difficult to get to. They will probably listen to you more than they will listen to me, and you will have access."[13] Gambari presented letters from the secretary-general, appealing for their help and their intervention to resolve the boycott.[14] He spent four hours in heated debate with Datti Ahmed, the doctor who had first called for the suspension of the polio immunization campaign.

Sokoto demonstrated the complexity of the situation. The Sultan of Sokoto is traditionally a spokesman for the region's Muslims on important issues.[15] He is also the head of the JNI. However, the JNI secretary-general was an opponent of polio immunization. Thus, although Gambari felt that the sultan was convinced by the plea that the boycott was hurting children and giving Nigeria a bad name, others within the religious establishment continued to support the boycott.

The sultan did join President Obasanjo at the kick-off of the polio immunization campaign in neighboring Zamfara State in March 2004, and Gambari left Sokoto with assurances from the governor that he would support immunization and would work to convince his colleague, the governor of Kano.

The trip to Kano was, according to Gambari, the most difficult. Gambari describes Kano this way: "Kano has always gone the opposite way politically from the rest of the country. ...Then, of course, they like to give trouble to the central government on an issue where the central government is vulnerable, religion."

Because the governor was of General Buhari's party, it was in his political interest to make things difficult for President Obasanjo. To both the governor and Dr. Ahmed, Gambari's message was simple: "Suppose you are wrong. ...You are going to condemn a whole people to this life of misery. At least consider you may be wrong." Although not immediately successful, Gambari felt that he had created some doubts. Murzi said of Gambari's visit, "With his ability to work in the North, he succeeded in helping us establish a dialogue up North. That visit was instrumental. It opened up the doors for increased conversation."

The GPEI and the Organization of the Islamic Conference

In 2003 the GPEI Secretariat, headquartered at the World Health Organization (WHO) in Geneva, began contact with the Organization of the Islamic Conference (OIC), "an inter-governmental organization grouping fifty-seven States [whose mission is] to safeguard and protect the interests of the Muslim world in the spirit of promoting international peace and harmony among various people of the world."[16] The rationale was that the six remaining polio-endemic countries at the time (Nigeria, Niger, Egypt, India, Pakistan, and Afghanistan) either were majority Muslim or had large Muslim populations, especially in the endemic areas.[17] All but five of the fifty-seven OIC members were polio-free, thanks to advice and support from the GPEI — including advice on choice of vaccines — and could thus counter questions about the efficacy and safety of the polio vaccine and the aims of the eradication initiative.

> *"Ultimately, a number of fatwas, or Islamic religious rulings, were issued on polio vaccination."*

Anand Balachandran, GPEI interagency coordinator and a social scientist, saw that "the OIC, being a political body, was a platform . . . important to defusing the idea that the GPEI and WHO were controlled by Western donors."[18] The secretariat first built a relationship with the OIC ambassador in Geneva, a Senegalese, who played a key role in getting the ambassadors of the OIC countries in Geneva engaged. The

GPEI secretariat then briefed these ambassadors in Geneva, London, and New York. The briefings moved the polio crisis and eradication issues beyond ministers of health to gain broader diplomatic and political support.

The Nigerian boycott, and the continued spread of polio outside Nigeria's borders, made the approach to the OIC more urgent. With the Tenth Islamic Conference scheduled for 16–17 October 2003 in Malaysia, David Heymann, the newly appointed special envoy on polio of the WHO director-general, contacted the Malaysian minister of health, with whom he had worked on severe acute respiratory syndrome (SARS) earlier. The minister and the government of Malaysia put polio on the summit agenda, which was, as Heymann describes it, "quite unusual, particularly in a politically charged atmosphere."[19]

The resolution at the OIC summit urged the remaining polio-endemic OIC countries, including Nigeria, to accelerate their efforts and called on the international community, including OIC members and philanthropic organizations in the Islamic world, to fund the effort.[20] The GPEI continued to share information with the OIC through the ambassadors in Geneva, including evidence on the safety and efficacy of the vaccines.

Quietly, with support from the GPEI, the OIC secretariat and the regional director for WHO's Eastern Mediterranean Regional Organization (EMRO) worked to get religious leaders to speak out on polio. Ultimately, a number of fatwas, or Islamic religious rulings, were issued on polio vaccination.[21] These were important in countering the argument that the vaccine was a Western plot to wipe out Muslims. They also gave, according to Balachandran, "space and options for the political decision makers to move the issue from one of religion concern to the political realm, where they could come up with a deal."[22]

Heymann says of the outreach to the OIC and to other regional organizations, "The most valuable thing was getting the OIC involved and they were helpful in many, many ways as was the African Union. ...Plus getting some Islamic interpretation through the [Islamic] Fiqh [Academy], which was helpful in understanding . . . that the vaccine was safe. We had great help from the Islamic community." Such help took concerted and coordinated outreach by the GPEI.

The U.S. Government

Polio was already on the policy radar screen in the United States in 2003–2004. The U.S. government had decided to make closing the GPEI funding gap a goal of the 2004 G8 Sea Island Summit. One U.S. government official recalls that the U.S. view was that eradicating polio fit perfectly with U.S. interests. The United States was already the largest donor to the GPEI, and the goals of closing the funding gap and eradicating polio by 2005 seemed achievable. Also, the GPEI was a public-private partnership, in line with U.S. government policy preference.

The Centers for Disease Control and Prevention (CDC) had personnel in Nigeria. They reported their concerns about the immunization efforts and the vaccine boycott to the U.S. Department of Health and Human Services (HHS), which suggested to the National Security Council in October 2003 that President George W. Bush send a letter to President Obasanjo, urging him to move forward with the immunization campaign. Others felt that too overt an intervention by the United States could exacerbate the problem in Northern Nigeria, where the war in Iraq had eroded support for the United States and where the polio immunization campaign was seen as a Western plot.[23]

At the same time, the State Department's small office of International Health Affairs (IHA) suggested to the Bureau of African Affairs (AF) an action plan for diplomatic action on polio. Although sympathetic, AF had other priorities. Nigeria was playing an important role in peace-keeping efforts in Sierra Leone and Liberia and had provided safe haven to former Liberian President Charles Taylor, to help end the civil war in that country. The United States had economic interests as well; Nigeria was the fifth-largest supplier of crude oil to the United States, so AF did not focus intently on the polio issue.

However, in January 2004 Secretary of State Powell raised the boycott in a staff meeting and asked for more information. To respond to the request with specific action items, IHA asked for suggestions from the CDC, the U.S. Agency for International Development (USAID), and GPEI. Ellyn Ogden of USAID said that even with all of her experience, including being a part of the team working on the G8 summit, she didn't know what diplomatic tools were available:

> I was having a hard time making that transition from a technical person
> in epidemiology to what tools did State have. ...I didn't know what to

ask for. I didn't know about demarches, I didn't know about briefing notes or cables. I didn't know what State could bring.[24]

William Steiger, the head of the HHS Office of Global Health Affairs, emphasizes the importance of giving policymakers specific actions that can be taken:

> You need to break the situation down into very understandable pieces, preferably with specific outcomes or specific steps to get senior policy-makers to agree or to have their buy-in. If we had just said polio is a disaster but we don't know what to do about it, I don't think we would have gotten anywhere. We were able to say, OK, we have a problem, we think we have a several things that we'd like to have you do. ...It made everybody understand more easily how we could play a role.[25]

Following up on the suggestions, then HHS secretary Tommy Thompson sent a letter to his Nigerian counterpart and made polio a part of his visits to Pakistan, India, and Afghanistan in April 2004. HHS deputy secretary Claude Allen raised the polio issue on a previously scheduled trip to Nigeria, using information from the GPEI to suggest approaches to non-Nigerian Islamic leaders who might be helpful. Secretary Powell met with his Nigerian counterpart in New York and raised the issue of polio, as did senior officials of State when they visited the Middle East and Pakistan. The State Department complemented GPEI efforts with the African Union (AU). In July 2004 Assistant Secretary of State for African Affairs Constance Newman delivered to former president of Mali, Alpha Oumar Konaré, the head of the AU, a letter from Secretary Powell urging action on polio at the 3–6 August Addis Ababa (Ethiopia) summit.

Instructions were sent to the U.S. Embassy in Nigeria, which established a task force to ensure coordination. The chargé d'affaires met with the governor of Kano to urge an end to the boycott. U.S. embassies in the region were asked to discuss polio with their counterparts and to urge host governments to do what they could to turn around the situation in Northern Nigeria.

The End Game?

It is hard to know precisely why the governor of Kano finally ended the boycott. Many of those interviewed for this paper believe that there may have been an internal Nigerian deal. Others say "no," arguing that any deal would have become public knowledge and thus would have threatened the governor's reputation. What is known is that the governor of Kano, by April of 2004 the sole government official opposing immunization, was under increasing pressure. The diplomatic efforts described above ensured that the governor understood the cost to his and Kano State's reputation if the boycott continued. The WHO was able to provide evidence that 80% of global cases of polio paralysis in the world originated in Kano. Or it may simply be that the official boycott had outlived its political usefulness for the Kano government.

Some people feel that another technical action, albeit one with diplomatic ramifications, might have contributed to the resolution. By 2004, countries around the world were asking the WHO and the GPEI, in their technical advisory role, for advice on what steps should be taken "to prevent or limit the international spread of wild poliovirus."[26] While the WHO had been asked by countries for advice, Heymann said that an explicit goal was to make sure that Saudi Arabia understood the potential spread of polio and the role of vaccine in stopping outbreaks, particularly during the January 2005 Hajj (the annual pilgrimage to Mecca, in Saudi Arabia). The WHO sent a *noteverbale* to all WHO members outlining the recommendations that were included in the *Weekly Epidemiological Record* of 6 August 2004.[27] The WHO Representative in Nigeria, among others, made certain that the governor of Kano was aware that travelers from Kano might have to be vaccinated at the airport to travel elsewhere, including to the Hajj. The possibility of Saudi Arabia's instituting WHO recommendations on polio vaccinations undercut the contention that polio immunization was a Western plot to sterilize Muslims.

"Work remains to be done in convincing communities to allow their children to be immunized."

At the same time, the CDC was looking into whether similar restrictions on travels to the United States were advisable. U.S. Ambassador Campbell told the CDC that he was prepared to support such restrictions, if they were scientifically based and necessary for the protection of the U.S. public. He made sure that officials in Nigeria knew of the possibility that the United States would follow the WHO recommendations to require vaccination before travel.

On 30 June 2004, in the same media release in which it announced the consultative process with experts to "evaluate additional measures that might be required to prevent the further international spread of wild poliovirus from Northern Nigeria," the WHO announced that it had been informed by the governor of Kano of "the intention to resume polio immunizations campaigns there in early July."[28]

Other discussions helped achieve a face-saving way to withdraw. Heymann's conversations with the governor of Kano in summer 2004 suggested the use of a panel of pediatricians to recommend restarting vaccination. In addition, UNICEF's ability to quietly divert shipments of polio vaccine produced in Indonesia, a Muslim country, for use in Nigeria allowed the face-saving claim that a safer vaccine was to be used for vaccination (Indonesian-manufactured vaccine had been used for years in Nigeria, even before the boycott began). The idea of supplying vaccine from a Muslim country chosen by the health officials in the North had first surfaced during Gambari's visit.

The boycott began with parents who were disgruntled with the lack of health services. The governor of Kano's decision to allow the resumption of immunization campaigns removed only one barrier to polio eradication in Nigeria. Work remains to be done in convincing communities to allow their children to be immunized.

Global Health Diplomacy Lessons

One person who worked with the GPEI to resolve the boycott said, "The greatest lesson is for the public health community that we are dealing with a political thing."[29] This case study holds a number of lessons for global health and insights into the practice of health diplomacy.

- **Diplomacy as a useful global health tool.** Diplomacy can be a useful tool in pursuing global health efforts. This is particularly true when the challenges to global health efforts are political, rather than scientific, as they were in this case. Resolving problems such as the vaccine boycott, or the sharing of influenza virus samples, will increasingly rely on diplomatic action. However, diplomacy is not a panacea and could not greatly alter the regional health-status disparities in Nigeria that contributed to the boycott.

- **Global, complex undertakings.** Both health and health diplomacy are global and are characterized by great complexity and a highly diverse constellation of actors. This crisis began at the subnational level in Nigeria; affected a global eradication effort supported by other nations, international organizations, and nongovernmental organizations (NGOs); and was only resolved by using diplomacy across these levels to restart vaccinations (Exhibit 2). This global environment makes operationalizing health diplomacy a complex endeavor, because diplomacy may involve numerous and nontraditional actors (such as the OIC) in responding to global health problems.

- **Need to generate action.** The need for actionable suggestions is critical to engaging governments; simply saying that the vaccine boycott was a problem did not generate action. To enact such suggestions, public health professionals need to learn how to approach diplomats and ministries of foreign affairs. Similarly, diplomats require greater training on the role that health can play in foreign policy. Only then will the problems of coordination on global health issues, both within countries and between nations and international institutions, begin to be solved.

- **Science and politics.** Although scientific evidence on the spread of polio was useful in pressuring Kano State to rescind the boycott, the flexibility to address political perceptions of the situation was also critical. Suggesting the use of a panel of pediatricians to give the governor of Kano political cover to retreat from the boycott and diverting vaccine shipments from Indonesia to Nigeria to address Nigerian Muslims' perceptions of the vaccine were unusual but effective actions in restarting vaccination. Notifying the governor of Kano that Saudi Arabia would institute vaccination requirements for the Hajj and enlisting Islamic scholars and fatwas are further examples of well-targeted diplomatic pressure in service of global health.

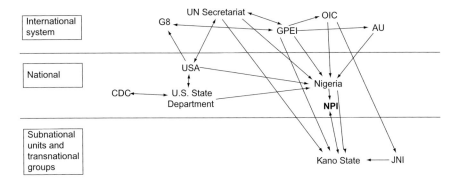

EXHIBIT 2. **Interactions between global actors working to resume polio eradication in Kano State, Nigeria**

Source: Authors' analysis.

Notes: UN is United Nations. G8 is Group of Eight. OIC is Organization of the Islamic Conference. GPEI is Global Polio Eradication Initiative. AU is African Union. CDC is U.S. Centers for Disease Control and Prevention. NPI is National Program on Immunization. JNI is Jama'atul Nasril Islam (Nigeria's umbrella Muslim organization).

Despite the obvious good done by diplomatic efforts, it is important to realize that it was a combination of local and international, technical and diplomatic efforts that eventually led to a resolution of the formal Kano boycott. The end was not quick, and it is hard to ascribe success to any single action. Flexibility; coordination among multiple actors; and a willingness to mix politics, public health, and diplomacy were all a part of the effort. All must be part of the toolbox to address future global health challenges.

The authors gratefully acknowledge the funding provided by the Bill and Melinda Gates Foundation. They thank Scott Barrett and Joshua Michaud of the Global Health and Foreign Policy Initiative, Duza Babafor his help with Exhibit 2, and Anand Balachandranfor help with the timeline (in the online appendix; see Note 7 below).

Notes

1. L. Roberts, "Infectious Disease: Vaccine-Related Polio Outbreak in Nigeria Raises Concerns," *Science* 317, no. 5846 (2007): 1842.

2. See, for example, M. Yahya, "Polio Vaccines — 'No Thank You!' Barriers to Polio Eradication in Northern Nigeria," *African Affairs* 1067, no. 423 (2007): 185–204; A.S. Jegede, "What Led to the Nigerian Boycott of the Polio Vaccination Campaign?" *PloS Medicine* 4, no. 3 (2007): e73; and E. Renne, "Perspectives on Polio and Immunization in Northern Nigeria," *Social Science and Medicine* 63, no. 7 (2006): 1857–1869.

3. I. Kickbusch et al., "Global Health Diplomacy: Training across Disciplines," *Bulletin of the World Health Organization* 85, no. 12 (2007): 971–973; V. Adams, T.E. Novotny, and H. Leslie, "Global Health Diplomacy," *Medical Anthropology* 27, no. 4 (2008): 315–323; and M. Chan, J.G. Store, and B. Kouchner, "Foreign Policy and Global Public Health: Working Together towards Common Goals," *Bulletin of the World Health Organization* 86, no. 7 (2008): 498.

4. Jegede, "What Led to the Nigerian Boycott?"

5. "Nigeria Polio Vaccine: Controversy Over or Renewed?" *Weekly Trust*, 6 March 2004.

6. John Campbell, ambassador to Nigeria, interview, 26 November 2007.

7. A timeline of these events is available in an appendix, online at http://content. healthaffairs.org/cgi/content/full/28/3/1091/DC1.

8. See, for example, the National Vaccine Information Center (NVIC) home page, http://www.nvic.org, and the Global Vaccine Awareness League (GVAL) home page, http://www.gval.com.

9. UNICEF, "Engaging Communities," http://www.unicef.org/immunization/ index_communities.html (accessed 10 April 2009).

10. For example, when rumors about the polio vaccine circulated among Coptic Christians in Alexandria, Egypt, in 2002, vaccinations were done in the churches, to counter the rumors. See B. Hiel, "Egypt Remains Committed as It Closes In on Becoming Polio-Free," *Pittsburgh Tribune-Review,* 3 April 2005.

11. United Nations Children's Fund, Eastern and Southern Africa Regional Office, *Combatting Antivaccination Rumours: Lessons Learned from Case Studies in East Africa,* http://www.path.org/vaccineresources/files/Combatting_Antivac_ Rumors_UNICEF.pdf (accessed 16 January 2009).

12. Gianni Murzi, UNICEF, personal communication, 8 January 2008.

13. Ibrahim Gambari, UN special envoy, interview, 6 December 2007.

14. Press Release, Ibrahim Gambari, 17 March 2004 (received from the GPEI).

15. M. Plaut; "Obituary: The Sultan of Sokoto," 29 October 2006, http://news.bbc. co.uk/2/hi/africa/6096858.stm (accessed 10 April 2009).

16. Organization of the Islamic Conference, "About OIC," http://www.oic-oci. org/page_detail.asp?p_id=52 (accessed 10 April 2009).

17. Since then, two countries, Egypt and Niger, have gone at least a year without a case of indigenous polio.

18. Anand Balachandran, GPEI, interviews, 10 and 12 December 2007, and subsequent e-mail correspondence.

19. David Heymann, World Health Organization, interview, 10 December 2007.

20. UNICEF, "Joint Press Release: Global Polio Eradication Initiative Welcomes OIC Decision to Step Up Effort to Eradicate Polio," http://unicef.org/media/ media_15021.html (accessed 10 April 2009).

21. Fatwas on polio vaccination were issued in late 2003 and early 2004 by Dr. Mohamed Sayed Tantawi, Grand Imam of El Azhar Al Sharif; the Islamic Fiqh Academy (circulated by the OIC); Muhammed Abdul Alim, Grand Mufti of Egypt; and, Abdul Aziz Ibn Abdullah Ibn Baaz, Grand Mufti of Saudi Arabia and president, Committee of Muslim Scholars.

22. Balachandran, personal communication, 21 February 2008.

23. Obasanjo was well known in Washington and appreciated for his commitment to health issues. He stood at President Bush's side when the latter announced the first governmental contribution to the as yet nonexistent Global Fund to Fight AIDS, Tuberculosis, and Malaria, in May 2001.

24. Ellyn Ogden, USAID, interview, 14 November 2007.

25. William Steiger, HHS Office of Global Health Affairs, interview, 17 January 2008.

26. World Health Organization, *Weekly Epidemiological Record,* 32, no. 79 (6 August 2004), pp. 289–290, http://www.who.int/wer/2004/en/wer7932. pdf (accessed 10 April 2009).

27. A *note verbale* is amemorandum, written in the third person and unsigned, used to convey information to a representative of a government.

28. WHO, "Kano, Nigeria, Informs WHO of the Intention to Resume Polio Immunization Campaigns," Press Release, 30 June 2004, http://www.who. int/mediacentre/news/notes/2004/np16/en (accessed 10 April 2009).

29. Anonymous, interview, 12 December 2007.

Contributors

Muhammad Mahmood Afzal, MBBS, DTCD, DHA, MD, worked in the Global Health Workforce Alliance, Geneva in charge of the country team. He started his professional career in the health department of Pakistan where he served in various managerial positions and implemented the Basic Development Needs programme. His book "Model health system in Pakistan" pioneered health systems reforms in the country. He also served in the WHO regional office of the Eastern Mediterranean Region and various WHO country offices including Djibouti, Jordan, Egypt, South Sudan, and the Islamic Republic of Iran. He also developed health systems frameworks for nine districts of Pakistan affected by earthquakes. Dr. Afzal has authored a number of professional publications including strategic documents, technical papers, guidelines and tools, training manuals, frameworks, and evaluation reports.

Jon Kim Andrus, MD, is the Deputy Director of the Pan American Health Organization, Regional Office for the Americas of the World Health Organization (PAHO/WHO). Previously, Dr. Andrus served as lead technical advisor for PAHO's immunization program, with a focus on the poorest communities of the Americas. Formally, he was Professor and Director of George Washington University's Global Health MPH Program. He also holds faculty appointments at the University of California San Francisco (UCSF) and Johns Hopkins Bloomberg School of Public Health. His first overseas assignment began in 1985 as a Peace Corps Volunteer serving as the District Medical Officer of Mchinji District, Malawi. Later, Dr. Andrus worked in key positions on polio eradication in Latin America and

South-East Asia. As Deputy Director of PAHO, he continues to serve as Principle Investigator of the PAHO ProVac Initiative, aimed at enhancing national capacity to make evidence-based decisions for new vaccine introduction. Dr. Andrus has published numerous scientific articles in the fields of vaccines, immunization, and accelerated control of vaccine-preventable diseases. He holds degrees from Stanford University (BS) and the University of California at Davis (MD), and did residencies at the UCSF School of Medicine (family medicine) and at the Centers for Disease Control and Prevention (EIS and preventive medicine).

Rear Admiral Kenneth W. Bernard RADM, MD, USPHS (Ret.) served at the White House from 2002–2005 as Special Assistant to the President for Biodefense and as Assistant Surgeon General. From 2001–2003 he was head of the U.S. Delegation negotiating the Framework Convention on Tobacco Control. From 1998–2001 he was Senior Adviser for Security and Health on President Clinton's National Security Council Staff. His other positions have included Senior Political Adviser to the Director-General of the World Health Organization (2005–2007), International Health Attaché at the U.S. Mission to the UN in Geneva, Associate Director for Medical and Scientific Affairs in the Office of International Health, Department of Health and Human Services, and as International Health Policy Adviser to the Director of the U.S. Peace Corps. Dr. Bernard is a member of the Council on Foreign Relations.

Lai-Ha Chan is Chancellor's Post-Doctoral Research Fellow at the UTS China Research Centre, University of Technology, Sydney, Australia. Dr. Chan's research interests include Chinese international relations, China's participation in global governance as well as non-traditional security issues, particularly infectious diseases. She is the author of "China Engages Global Health Governance: Responsible Stakeholder or System-Transformer?" (New York: Palgrave Macmillan, 2010 forthcoming) and one of the editors of China at 60: Global-Local Interactions (Singapore: World Scientific, 2010 forthcoming). She is currently working on a project with Gerald Chan and Pak K Lee on China and global governance and their joint journal articles appear in Global Public Health, Third World Quarterly, China Security, and Contemporary Politics.

Lucy Chen is the Executive Deputy Director of the Institute for Global Health at Peking University, Beijing, China. She has been supporting the government of China's works in global health especially China's role in the South-South development cooperation since 2008 through evidence building and capacity development.

James N. Class, Ph.D. is former Associate Vice President of International Affairs at Pharmaceutical Research and Manufacturers of America, as well as former Executive Director of the Partnership for Safe Medicines. He was responsible for the creation of the SafeMeds Alert System and weekly SafeMeds News Update and has been involved with the International Medical Products' Anti-Counterfeiting Taskforce and INTERPOL's Intellectual Property Crimes Action Group. He has spoken extensively in the U.S. and elsewhere on policy problems related to counterfeit medicines and strategies to tackle the problem.

Christopher J. Colvin is an anthropologist living and working in Cape Town, South Africa. He has a PhD in socio-cultural anthropology from the University of Virginia and a Masters in Public Health from the University of Cape Town (UCT) in epidemiology. He has lectured in anthropology and public health at Columbia University and several South African universities and was a UCT postdoctoral fellow in health and human rights. He is currently Senior Research Officer in Social Sciences and HIV/AIDS, TB and STIs at UCT's School of Public Health. He also serves as the Program Director for the Health and Community study abroad program at the International Honors Program. His research areas include HIV/AIDS and masculinity, community mobilization and health activism, and community health workers.

Ibadat Dhillon JD, MSPH, LLM serves as the Associate Director, Health Workforce for Realizing Rights: The Ethical Globalization Initiative. Realizing Rights, founded and led by Hon. Mary Robinson, aims to place human rights standards at the heart of global governance. Prior to joining Realizing Rights, Mr. Dhillon spent three years as a Health Scientist at the US Centers for Disease Control and Prevention (CDC). While with the CDC, his work included surveillance projects related to global tobacco control, measles and polio eradication in Lao PDR, and improving maternal and perinatal health care in rural Tanzania. Mr. Dhillon also worked to advance access to ARV drugs through the use of law, globally and in South Africa.

The Honorable Ambassador Mark Dybul, MD, served as the U.S. Global AIDS Coordinator from 2006–2009 heading the President's Emergency Plan for AIDS Relief. Ambassador Dybul is currently Distinguished Scholar and Co-Director of the Global Health Center, The O'Neill Institute for Global and National Health Law, Georgetown University; and inaugural Global Health Fellow, The George W. Bush Institute. In 2008 Ambassador Dybul was a presidentially appointed member of the Board of Trustees of the Woodrow Wilson International Center for Scholars.

Jan Egeland is Director of the Norwegian Institute of International Affairs and Associate Professor at the University of Stavanger. He is co-Chair of the High-level Taskforce on the Global Framework for Climate Services established under the World Climate Conference-3. Until September 2008 Mr. Egeland was Special Adviser to the UN Secretary General for Conflict Prevention and Resolution. In 2003–2006 he was Under Secretary General for Humanitarian Affairs and Emergency Relief Coordinator in the United Nations. Mr. Egeland has been prominent in several peace processes that include the Oslo Agreement between Israel and the PLO (1993) and the Ceasefire Agreement for Guatemala signed in Oslo City Hall in 1996. Mr. Egeland holds a Magister in Political Science from the University of Oslo. He has received a number of awards for his work on humanitarian and conflict resolution issues. In 2008 he published *A Billion Lives — An Eyewitness Report from the Frontlines of Humanity* (Simon & Schuster).

Harley Feldbaum, Ph.D., MPH, is the Director of the Global Health and Foreign Policy Initiative at the Johns Hopkins School of Advanced International Studies. He is an expert on the national security and foreign policy implications of global health issues. He has worked on global health issues for over 10 years, and has consulted for CSIS and the Nuffield Trust on the linkages between health and security. Harley received a degree in Biology with Honors from Wesleyan University, a Masters in Public Health from Johns Hopkins, and a Ph.D. at the London School of Hygiene and Tropical Medicine.

David P. Fidler, J.D., M.Phil., is the James Louis Calamaras Professor of Law and the Director of the Center on American and Global Security at Indiana University. He is one of the world's leading experts on international law and global health. His books include *International Law and Infectious Diseases* (Clarendon Press, 1999), *International Law and Public Health* (Transnational Publishers, 2000), *SARS, Governance, and the Globalization of Disease* (Palgrave, 2004), and *Biosecurity in the Global Age: Biological Weapons, Public Health, and the Rule of Law* (with Lawrence O. Gostin) (Stanford University Press, 2008). Professor Fidler has a J.D. from Harvard Law School, an M.Phil. in International Relations from the University of Oxford, a B.C.L. from the University of Oxford, and a B.A. (University of Kansas).

Gladys Ghisays has a Nursing Degree from the University of the North of Barranquilla, a Postgraduate in Epidemiology of the School of Public Health from the University of Antioquia, and a Masters Degree in Nursing and Health Services Administration from the National University of Colombia. Dr. Ghisays has focused her professional activities in the areas of immunization, epidemiological research, planning, and administration of health programs and implementation of epidemiological surveillance systems. As an advisor in vaccine-preventable diseases, Dr. Ghisays has been in charge of providing technical cooperation to the member countries where she was assigned (Colombia and the Regional Office in the Northern Coast of Colombia, Paraguay, Venezuela, the Netherlands Antilles and Aruba), in order to maintain the orientation of the national processes in accordance with the mandates of PAHO/WHO and to support the development of strategies to increase the effectiveness of the prevention and control measures of preventable diseases through vaccination.

Mark Heywood grew up in Nigeria, Ghana, Botswana and England. He holds a BA (Hons) in English Language and Literature from Balliol College, Oxford University and an MA in African literature from the

University of the Witwatersrand, Johannesburg. Mark joined the AIDS Law Project in 1994, becoming its head in 1997 and executive director in 2006 (now renamed Section 27). In 1998, he was one of the founders of the Treatment Action Campaign (TAC). In 2007, he was elected as deputy chairperson of the South African National AIDS Council. In 2009, Mark was appointed as a member of the Ministerial Advisory Committee on National Health Insurance. Mark has written extensively on HIV, human rights and the law and has been part of the legal teams that have been involved in all the major litigation around HIV and human rights.

Barbara Jauregui is an Argentinian MD, MSc., with eight years of experience in program development/management and applied research, in both governmental and non-profit organisations. Dr. Jauregui is especially skilled at using quantitative tools for analysing and improving systems and processes to promote equity in health. She has been working for PAHO's Immunization Unit since the beginning of 2008. Under direct supervision of the Principal Investigator, Dr. Jon Andrus, she is currently managing the ProVac Initiative in Latin America and the Caribbean (LAC) countries, providing training and technical collaboration in the generation of cost-effectiveness analysis regarding new vaccine introduction. Dr. Jauregui also holds an adjunct associate position at the Global Health Department of the George Washington University.

Rebecca Katz, Ph.D., MPH, is an Assistant Professor of Health Policy and Emergency Medicine at The George Washington University School of Public Health and Health Services. Her research is focused on public health preparedness, and the intersection of infectious diseases and national security. Current research projects are focused on implementation of the International Health Regulations and health diplomacy. She previously worked on Biological Warfare (BW) counterproliferation at the Defense Intelligence Agency, and was an Intelligence Research Fellow at the Center for Strategic Intelligence Research in the Joint Military Intelligence College. She also spent several years as a public health consultant for The Lewin Group working with foundations on community based public health projects, with the federal government on the infectious disease surveillance system, and with local and state health departments on maternal and child health policy. Since September 2004, Dr. Katz has been a consultant to the Department of State, working on issues related to Biological Weapons Convention and disease surveillance. Dr. Katz has a BA from Swarthmore College, an MPH from Yale University, and a Ph.D. from Princeton University.

Judith R. Kaufmann is an independent consultant on using diplomacy to further global health goals. She is also a Visiting Scholar at the Global Health and Foreign Policy Initiative at the Johns Hopkins School of Advanced International Studies. Ms. Kaufmann has previously served as Director of the U.S. Department of State's Office of International Health Affairs, where she was also focal point for the U.S. delegation to the Global Fund to Fight AIDS, TB and Malaria. She has also been advisor on publlic-private partnerships at the Roll Back Malaria Partnership (World Health Organization) and worked on the Partnership on AIDS in Africa at the Joint UN Programme on HIV/AIDS.

Ilona Kickbusch, Ph.D., is Director of the Global Health Programme, Graduate Institute of International and Development Studies, Geneva. Following a distinguished career with the World Health Organization Dr. Kickbusch was Professor and Head of the Division of International Health at Yale University School of Medicine in the Department of Epidemiology and Public Health.

Ambassador John E. Lange (Retired), JD, served as Special Representative on Avian and Pandemic Influenza in the US Department of State from 2006 to 2009. His previous positions included Deputy Inspector General, Deputy Global AIDS Coordinator, and Associate Dean for Leadership and Management at the Foreign Service Institute. From 1999 to 2002, he served as US Ambassador to Botswana. As Chargé d'Affaires, he led the American Embassy in Dar es Salaam at the time of the terrorist bombing on August 7, 1998. Earlier Foreign Service tours included postings in Geneva, Lomé, Paris, and Mexico City. Following his retirement in 2009, Ambassador Lange joined the Global Health Program of the Bill & Melinda Gates Foundation as Senior Program Officer for Developing-Country Policy & Advocacy.

Bryan A. Liang, MD, PhD, JD, is Executive Director and Shapiro Distinguished Professor, Institute of Health Law Studies, California Western School of Law; Co-Director and Professor of Anesthesiology, San Diego Center for Patient Safety, University of California, San Diego School of Medicine. His work includes stints in the EU studying managed care and complementary social health insurance and in Taiwan assisting in health insurance access and reform. He has addressed diverse international bodies including the Asian Pacific Economic Cooperation Community, Organisation of Economic and Community Development, and the World Intellectual Property Organisation on health issues in developed and developing countries.

Tim Mackey, MAS, is a Ph.D. candidate in the Global Health Program, University of California, San Diego-San Diego State University and a Senior Research Associate, Institute of Health Law Studies, California Western School of Law. His work focuses on international global health initiatives and health diplomacy in a range of areas, including patient safety and the drug supply, Orphan Diseases, and conflicts of interest. His thematic assessments involve transforming the concept of international to global using training in Political Science and the perspective of a Japanese national having lived in over half a dozen countries.

Cuauhtémoc Ruiz Matus, MD is a Mexican physician who graduated from the School of Medicine of the National Polytechnic Institute, and specialized in epidemiology at the School of Public Health of Mexico. He is also a graduate of the Public Entity Management Program of the National Public Administration Institute. Dr. Ruiz Matus worked in the Mexican's Ministry of Health for 25 years. During the last 10 years, he served as Chief of Staff to the Undersecretary for Health Prevention and Promotion at the Ministry of Health. He is currently Senior Advisor of the Comprehensive Family Immunization Project, at the Pan American Health Organization/World Health Organization (PAHO/WHO).

Ahmad Mukhtar is the lead negotiator for the government of Pakistan at the Permanent Mission of Pakistan to the WTO in Geneva, Switzerland. Mr. Mukhtar deals with the negotiating areas of Trade in Services (GATS) that includes Health and related Services and the Intellectual Property (TRIPS) among others. He has special interest in public health related issues in the context of liberalization and commercialization of various services including health and related aspects.

Anna Muldoon has worked in medical publishing, HIV/AIDS grant analysis, and most recently at the intersection of public health and national security issues. Her recent research focuses on the history and impact of the International Health Regulations, US biosecurity policies, and the public health impact of emerging technology. She is currently finishing a Master's in Public Health at George Washington University and works for both the Department of Health Policy and the Department of Health and Human Services' Assistant Secretary for Preparedness and Response.

Luvuyo Ndimeni, MA, is the Deputy Permanent Representative (Deputy Ambassador) of the South African Permanent Mission to the UN and Other International Organizations in Geneva and one of the original members of the group of seven countries that conceptualized the Oslo Ministerial Declaration on Global Health and Foreign Policy. Deputy Ambassador Ndimeni was the drafter of the resolution "Global Health and Foreign Policy" and its lead negotiator at the United Nations in 2008 and 2009.

Stacy Romero graduated with her Bachelor of Arts in Molecular, Cellular, and Developmental Biology and Integrative Physiology from the University of Colorado in 2008. She is currently a Master of Public Health candidate at The George Washington University in Global Health Communications and is serving as a Peace Corps health education volunteer in Albania.

Alba María Ropero Alvarez, MPH, is currently serving as a Regional Advisor in the Comprehensive Family Immunization Project of the Pan American Health Organization (PAHO) in Washington DC, a post she has held since 2002. In her role as Regional Advisor, Alba María provides technical and strategic support to strengthen national and regional capacity for the prevention of vaccine-preventable diseases in the Americas.

Alba María is the primary PAHO focal point for influenza yellow fever, and hepatitis B vaccines as well as for Vaccination Week in the Americas, an eight-year-old annual initiative which aims to promote equity and access to vaccination and Pan-Americanism, by targeting hard-to-reach populations in the Region. Alba María worked in Paraguay as an international immunization consultant for PAHO and in the Ministry of Health of Colombia, where she was responsible for communicable disease programs at the national level. Alba Maria received her Master of Public Health degree from the Universidad del Valle in Colombia, and also completed a certificate program in Epidemiology for Public Health Managers at the Bloomberg School of Public Health at Johns Hopkins University.

Ellen Rosskam, Ph.D., MPH, is Senior Advisor and Consultant for the Global Health Programme, Graduate Institute of International and Development Studies, Geneva, Switzerland, and Senior Scholar at the Woodrow Wilson International Center for Scholars, Washington, DC. following a long career as a Senior Social Protection Specialist at the International Labour Organization. Dr. Rosskam is an Associate of the Center for Social Epidemiology, California; Adjunct Professor, University of Massachusetts, Lowell; and Visiting Senior Fellow, University of Surrey, Faculty of Health and Medical Sciences. She is also Vice President and Foreign Advisor for the Center for Institutional Reform, Russian Federation, and International Advisor to the Terve Eesti HIV/AIDS Foundation, Estonia.

Mubashar Sheikh, MBBS, MPH, is Executive Director of the Global Health Workforce Alliance, hosted by the World Health Organization, Geneva. Dr. Sheikh served in the Ministry of Health Pakistan in various key positions, and designed and implemented a nationwide community-based Lady Health Workers' programme. In 1998, Dr. Sheikh joined the Eastern Mediterranean Office of WHO as Regional Adviser and initiated Community Based Initiatives (CBI). In 2004, he was assigned to the WHO office in Iran as Country Representative, where he also served as the UN Resident Coordinator and Representative for the FAO. Dr. Sheikh has contributed in various committees and task forces at the national, regional, and international levels, and is the author of numerous policy documents, training manuals, and guidelines.

Allyn L. Taylor, JD, LLM, JSD is a Visiting Professor of Law at Georgetown University Law Center and an Adjunct Professor of International Relations at the Johns Hopkins Paul H. Nitze School of Advanced International Studies (SAIS). Previous positions include health policy and legal adviser at the World Health Organization where Dr. Taylor was the senior legal advisor for the negotiation of WHO's first treaty, the WHO Framework Convention on Tobacco Control (FCTC), In the early 1990s she initiated the idea of the FCTC with the late Professor Ruth Roemer. Dr. Taylor has also served as a legal consultant to The World Bank, the Organization of American States, the Pan American Health Organization, the Overseas Development Council, the Framework Convention Alliance, the National Campaign for Tobacco Free Kids, Realizing Rights: The Equitable Globalization Initiative and the International Union Against Cancer. She has published extensively on global health law and policy concerns. Most recently, Dr. Taylor worked with WHO as the legal adviser for the negotiation and implementation of the WHO Global Code of Practice on the International Recruitment of Health Personnel. She has published extensively on global health law and policy concerns.

Jonathan B. Tucker, Ph.D., is a Senior Fellow in the Washington, D.C. office of the James Martin Center for Nonproliferation Studies (CNS) of the Monterey Institute of International Studies, where he specializes in biological and chemical weapons issues. Among his many publications, he is the author of the book *Scourge: The Once and Future Threat of Smallpox* (Grove/Atlantic, 2001) and the article "The Smallpox Destruction Debate: Could a Grand Bargain Settle the Issue?" (*Arms Control Today*, March 2009). Before joining the CNS staff in 1996, Dr. Tucker worked at the U.S. Department of State, the congressional Office of Technology Assessment, and the Arms Control & Disarmament Agency. From 1993 to 1995, he served on the U.S. delegation to the Chemical Weapons Convention Preparatory Commission in The Hague, and in 1995 he was a United Nations biological weapons inspector in Iraq.

Judyth L. Twigg, Ph.D., MA, is professor of government and public affairs at Virginia Commonwealth University (VCU). She also currently serves as a senior associate with the Russia and Eurasia Program at the Center for Strategic and International Studies, a senior adviser to the Eurasia Program of the Social Science Research Council, and a consultant to the World Bank and U.S. federal government. In 2009 and 2010, Twigg chaired the Public Health Working Group of the Civil Society Summits that took place in tandem with the Obama-Medvedev meetings in Moscow and Washington. She was a member of the 2005 Council on Foreign Relations Task Force on U.S.-Russia relations and was one of 12 recipients of the 2005 State Council on Higher Education in Virginia's Distinguished Faculty Award. She recently published a book on *HIV/AIDS in Russia and Eurasia*, and she is currently working on a project that compares health systems reform in Russia, the Kyrgyz Republic, and Georgia. Dr. Judyth Twigg holds a B.S. in physics from Carnegie Mellon University, an M.A. in political science and Soviet studies from the University of Pittsburgh, and a Ph.D. in political science and security studies from MIT.

Jin Xu is working at the President's Office, Peking University Health Science Center, Beijing, China. Mr. Xu had worked as a coordinator for the "Healthy China 2020" Strategic Research Project under the leadership of Professor Qide HAN, and was a research assistant to Professor Ling Li from Peking University for a project on China's Health Care System Reform, before assisting Lucy CHEN in organising the WHO-IGH joint research on new initiatives for South-South health collaboration.

Howard A. Zucker, MD, J.D., served as Assistant Director-General of the World Health Organization (2006–2008) and was in charge of the Health Technology & Pharmaceuticals cluster. In addition, he was the Representative of the Director-General for Intellectual Property, Innovation, and Public Health. In this capacity he led the Intergovernmental Working Group (IGWG) for the WHO. He has served as Deputy Assistant Secretary of Health at the US Department of Health and Human Services, as a White House Fellow, and as an Institute of Politics Fellow at Harvard Kennedy School. He is presently a pediatric cardiac anesthesiologist at the Albert Einstein College of Medicine in NYC, Adjunct Professor at Georgetown University Law School, and Senior Advisor in the Division of Global Health & Human Rights at Massachusetts General Hospital.

Index

433